# Management of Fecal Incontinence for the Advanced Practice Nurse

Donna Z. Bliss
Editor

# Management of Fecal Incontinence for the Advanced Practice Nurse

Under the auspices of the International Continence Society

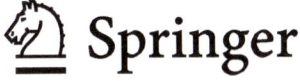 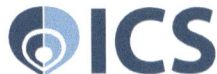

*Editor*
Donna Z. Bliss
School of Nursing
University of Minnesota School of Nursing
Minneapolis
MN, USA

ISBN 978-3-030-08078-5          ISBN 978-3-319-90704-8   (eBook)
https://doi.org/10.1007/978-3-319-90704-8

Printed on acid-free paper

This Springer imprint is published by the registered company Springer International Publishing AG part
of Springer Nature.
The registered company address is: Gewerbestrasse 11, 6330 Cham, Switzerland

# Foreword

In the 45 years since the start of the International Continence Society, continence nursing has come a long way, from virtual invisibility to leadership in services and care for people living with incontinence. Yet even within the continence field, fecal incontinence has remained poorly visible, with considerably less research and development of interventions and services than for urinary incontinence. Nurses who specialize in continence care are not always advanced practitioners in managing fecal incontinence. This book aims to change this.

The size of the problem of fecal incontinence is huge, both in numbers of people affected and in its life-limiting effects, which literally ruins lives. There can be few, if any, more embarrassing and humiliating symptoms, with leaked feces and bowel function a taboo across nearly all cultures. This is true across diverse patient groups and ages. Prevalence is 50% and above among frail older adults in care homes. In people with bowel disorders such as inflammatory bowel disease, fecal incontinence affects at least one quarter. After surgery for colorectal cancer or radiotherapy for pelvic cancers, fecal incontinence often prevents a return to normal life even if the cancer is cured.

All too often the symptom is accepted, even expected, by nurses and patients alike. Medical developments have focused largely on the anal sphincter which we can visualize and measure its quality, function, and sensation. Yet results of surgical approaches, such as anal sphincter repair, have remained often disappointing, especially in the long term. Newer developments, such as sacral nerve stimulation, sphincter bulking, and implanting stem cells, while promising, have yet to pass the test of time and become generalized in use beyond pioneering centers, and it is known that results in generic practice are always less impressive than initial results that enthusiasts suggest.

Tackling fecal incontinence is undoubtedly a task for a multidisciplinary team. Gastroenterologists, colorectal surgeons, radiologists, physiotherapists, dietitians as well as nurses all have important roles on such a team. Devising a referral and care pathway is important to ensure coordination and effective use of resources. But many colleagues have a limited range of options for fecal incontinence. Interventions tend to focus on the anatomy and function rather than the whole person. Both medications and surgery are poorly developed and inappropriate or ineffective for many patients. Specific products are few and have limited uses.

Within a multidisciplinary team, nurses are often best placed to help patients both improve symptoms and to enhance coping skills, thereby improving quality of life. Nurses are often in the closest contact with patients who trust nurses in revealing intimate issues or discussing symptoms they have told nobody else about. Nurses offer the combination of empathetic listening, holistic assessment, and practical techniques that are needed. We are also likely to be in a position to coordinate the team and help the patient navigate the care system.

However, achieving optimal care for fecal incontinence is far more than just using common sense and generic knowledge. We are starting to develop a body of specialist knowledge and skills to enable us to make a real difference to people with fecal incontinence. We also have techniques from related nursing areas of ostomy and bladder management and skin care which can be adapted and applied. This book is a treasure trove of information and techniques to help with this.

Yet we still have a long way to go to find effective strategies and nursing interventions across the full range of patients who experience fecal incontinence. Public awareness is limited, and unlike urinary incontinence, commercial interests have been slow to recognize the opportunity and develop products. The research base for our practice remains woefully inadequate compared with the massive scale of the problem. We are starting to understand the complexity of the physical, psychological, and social underpinnings and consequences of fecal incontinence. But we have yet to find the best ways to improve nursing assessment and management of the many different patients who present to us. And we are a very long way from identifying all those who need our help.

This book is a major contribution to advanced nursing knowledge on fecal incontinence, pulling together in one place the current state of the art for assessing and managing its symptoms. It will help us to progress and speak the same language, fostering our debates and common understanding. I commend all nurses who are, or aspire to be, advanced nurse practitioners in this much neglected field. I wish I had this book when I started to work with these patients.

King's College London, London, UK                                    Christine Norton

# About this Book

The aim of this book is to serve as a resource to advanced practice nurses interested in evidence-based management of fecal incontinence. An international group of nurses and physician colleagues who are expert in the management of fecal incontinence collaborated in offering their expertise for this book. Notably, the International Continence Society (ICS) has provided its endorsement of the book.

The book represents the current evidence and best practices for the management of fecal incontinence across different patient groups. The authors aimed to provide the essential knowledge and practice guidance needed by the advanced practice nurse to diagnose and manage fecal incontinence in various clinical settings and patient groups. They identified and shared exemplars from different countries and developed case studies to highlight the information discussed. Chapter 12 explains common surgeries to treat fecal incontinence for the advanced practice nurse following patients who receive surgical intervention. Chapter 13 summarizes the treatment of incontinence-associated skin damage (i.e., dermatitis and pressure injury), and Chapter 14 addresses the management of fecal incontinence in the presence of urinary incontinence. In addition, the authors determined that clarifying the roles of the generalist, specialist, and advanced practice nurse in continence care would be beneficial in providing a contextual framework for this book. In so doing, they acknowledged the various levels of nurses involved in continence care and the important contributions to care made by each. Chapter 2 proposes a conceptualization of these roles and organizes necessary competencies by role.

I would like to express my sincerest gratitude to all the authors who generously shared their expertise, collaborated on writing teams, and wrote chapters to produce this outstanding book. I would also like to thank the student assistants from the University of Minnesota: Megan Cavanaugh, Elise Gannon, and Haeyeon Lee who assisted in formatting all chapters and references and enabled us to meet our deadlines. We appreciate the review of the ICS members in assisting us to produce the highest quality product. Those reviewers are Veronika Geng, Master in Health Science/Nursing Science, RN, Head of the Advisory Centre for Nutrition and Digestion for spinal cord injured people in the Manfred-Sauer-Foundation, Germany; Joanne Hoyle, Adult Specialist Nurse, Bladder and Bowel UK; ÖZGE ÖZ, Research Assistant and PhD student, Ondokuz Mayis University, Public Health Nursing Dept., Samsun, Turkey; and Debbie Yarde, MA, BSc (Hons), RGN, ONC, Clinical Lead, bowel and bladder care service, Northern Devon NHS Healthcare

Trust, Barnstaple, Devon, UK. Our aim is to assist advanced practice nurses globally to deliver excellent continence care at an advanced level and to improve the lives of patients with fecal incontinence. I thank all who contributed to those efforts.

Minneapolis, MN, USA                                                    Donna Z. Bliss

# Contents

1   **Fecal Incontinence: Definition and Impact on Quality of Life** . . . . . . . . . 1
    Cynthia Peden-McAlpine, Melissa Northwood, and Donna Z. Bliss

2   **Advanced Practice Continence Nursing** . . . . . . . . . . . . . . . . . . . . . . . . . 15
    Joan Ostaszkiewicz, Cynthia Peden-McAlpine, Melissa Northwood,
    Sharon Eustice, Donna Z. Bliss, and Kaoru Nishimura

3   **Epidemiology of Fecal Incontinence** . . . . . . . . . . . . . . . . . . . . . . . . . . . 49
    Maria Helena Baena de Moraes Lopes, Juliana Neves da Costa,
    Vera Lúcia Conceição de Gouveia Santos, and Jaqueline Betteloni
    Junqueira

4   **Normal Defecation and Mechanisms for Continence** . . . . . . . . . . . . . . . 63
    Mônica Milinkovic de la Quintana, Tania das Graças de Souza Lima,
    Vera Lúcia Conceição de Gouveia Santos, and Maria Helena Baena
    de Moraes Lopes

5   **Clinical Assessment and Differential Diagnosis
    of Fecal Incontinence and Its Severity** . . . . . . . . . . . . . . . . . . . . . . . . . . 77
    Kathleen F. Hunter, Tamara Dickinson, and Veronica Haggar

6   **Management of Fecal Incontinence in Community-Living Adults** . . . . 93
    Frankie Bates, Donna Z. Bliss, Alison Bardsely, and
    Winnie Ka Wai Yeung

7   **Management of Fecal Incontinence in Frail Older Adults Living
    in the Community** . . . . . . . . . . . . . . . . . . . . . . . . . . . . . . . . . . . . . . . . . . 127
    Kathleen F. Hunter, Melissa Northwood, Veronica Haggar, and
    Frankie Bates

8   **Management of Fecal Incontinence in Older Adults in
    Long-Term Care** . . . . . . . . . . . . . . . . . . . . . . . . . . . . . . . . . . . . . . . . . . . 149
    Lene Elisabeth Blekken, Anne Guttormsen Vinsnes,
    Kari Hanne Gjeilo, and Donna Z. Bliss

9   **Management of Fecal Incontinence in Adults
    with Neurogenic Bowel Dysfunction** ........................... 171
    Tamara Dickinson, Sharon Eustice, and Nikki Cotterill

10  **Management of Fecal Incontinence in Acutely Ill
    and Critically Ill Hospitalized Adults** ......................... 187
    Marcia Carr and Kathleen F. Hunter

11  **Management of Fecal/Anal Incontinence During Pregnancy
    and Postpartum** ............................................... 211
    Christina Hegan and Marlene Corton

12  **Surgical Management of Fecal Incontinence and Implications
    for Postoperative Nursing Care** ............................... 241
    Sarah Abbott and Ronan O'Connell

13  **Management of Skin Damage Associated with Fecal and  Dual
    Incontinence** .................................................. 257
    Mikel Gray, Donna Z. Bliss, and Sheila Howes Trammel

14  **Management of Urinary Incontinence in the Presence of Fecal
    Incontinence** .................................................. 291
    Sandra Engberg

**Epilogue** ........................................................ 307

# Fecal Incontinence: Definition and Impact on Quality of Life

1

Cynthia Peden-McAlpine, Melissa Northwood, and Donna Z. Bliss

**Abstract**

This chapter defines fecal incontinence and describes the impact of fecal incontinence on quality of life using evidence from qualitative research studies. Quality of life related to the experience of men and women with fecal incontinence is described. Five domains of quality of life when living with fecal incontinence were synthesized from the literature and organized into a model. These domains are living with fecal incontinence related to (i) relationships; (ii) time and planning; (iii) body issues, self-esteem, and body image; (iv) sexuality, and (v) diet issues. Key points from each domain are highlighted in this chapter. Implications for advance practice nurses assisting patients to manage fecal incontinence are explained.

**Keywords**

Fecal incontinence · Quality of life · Lived experience · Qualitative research

## 1.1 Definition of Fecal Incontinence

Fecal incontinence is the involuntary loss of feces [1]. This simple, revised definition was recently adopted by the international, interdisciplinary committee of fecal incontinence clinical and research experts of the 6th International Consultation on

C. Peden-McAlpine · D. Z. Bliss (✉)
University of Minnesota School of Nursing, Minneapolis, MN, USA
e-mail: peden001@umn.edu; bliss@umn.edu

M. Northwood
Saint Elizabeth Health Care, Hamilton, ON, Canada

Aging, Community and Health Research Unit, School of Nursing,
McMaster University, Hamilton, ON, Canada
e-mail: northwm@mcmaster.ca

© Springer International Publishing AG, part of Springer Nature 2018
D. Z. Bliss (ed.), *Management of Fecal Incontinence for the Advanced Practice Nurse*,
https://doi.org/10.1007/978-3-319-90704-8_1

1

Incontinence (ICI-6) and the International Continence Society (ICS) [1]. Other definitions of fecal incontinence have included a criterion for an amount or duration of
leakage or judgment that the loss of feces is a social or hygienic problem. Fecal
incontinence is a unique problem that is one of four types of bowel incontinence; the
other types being anal incontinence, flatus incontinence, and mucus incontinence
(see Box 1.1). Flatus incontinence is the involuntary loss of intestinal gas (or flatus).
Mucus incontinence is the involuntary loss of mucus from the rectum. Anal incontinence, which is the involuntary loss of feces, flatus and/or mucus, has the broadest
definition, possibly encompassing the other types of bowel incontinence. There are
also subtypes of each of the types of bowel incontinence including passive, urge,
and functional incontinence. Passive fecal incontinence is the loss of feces without
sensing or being consciously aware of the loss. Urge fecal incontinence is the loss
of feces associated with defecation urgency. Functional incontinence is the loss of
feces due to associated problems of limited mobility or cognitive impairment [1].

---

**Box 1.1: Types of Bowel Incontinence**
- Anal incontinence
- Fecal incontinence
- Flatus incontinence
- Mucus incontinence
  - Subtypes of each type
  - Passive
  - Urge
  - Functional

Adapted from Bliss et al. 2017 [1].

---

## 1.2 Overview of the Impact of Fecal Incontinence

Fecal incontinence is a distressing problem as it is unpredictable, embarrassing, and
associated with stigma [1, 2]. As the next section of this chapter reveals, fecal incontinence decreases quality of life and can have a considerable negative impact on all
aspects of the concept of self, well-being, and social and public interaction. Fecal
incontinence complicates other health problems such as urinary incontinence,
dementia, critical illness, systemic neuropathic diseases (e.g., diabetes), and
obstetrical injury, to name a few. Fecal incontinence is also a major risk factor for
other problems such as skin damage due to irritation and inflammation or pressure
(see Chap. 13). It requires self-management by the afflicted individual and increases
the burden of care by family members, and its development can be the tipping point
for admission into a nursing home [3–6]. Clinical staff are challenged by the care
and complexity required for managing urinary incontinence, especially for older
adults with multiple chronic health problems, and it seems reasonable to assume
that fecal incontinence presents similar if not greater challenges [7, 8].

Individuals with fecal incontinence desire to have more control over this problem in order to live a more normal life and retain their personal dignity [9]. However, many individuals with fecal incontinence and their caregivers lack health literacy about fecal incontinence [10] limiting their ability to search for resources and communicate with health-care providers [11, 12]. The main components of health literacy are being able to communicate with a health-care provider, understand information and make choices about treatment, access, health information, navigate the health-care system, and seek care, manage chronic health conditions, and engage in symptom self-management [13, 14]. The World Health Organization extends the notion of health literacy to disease prevention and health promotion as well as to health care, an idea which has been adopted by many European countries [15]. The low health literacy about fecal incontinence of patients and caregivers is exemplified in their lack of knowledge of the terms and their meaning by which clinicians and published studies refer to their problem [16]. Informal family or friend caregivers of those with fecal incontinence desire to increase their knowledge and care capacity for managing fecal incontinence and skin problems associated with its occurrence [10, 12]. The need and opportunities for advanced practice nurses to manage fecal incontinence in any health-care setting is great.

### 1.2.1    Impact of Fecal Incontinence on Quality of Life

The experience of fecal incontinence for men and women has been difficult, and it has affected their quality of life in many negative ways. People with fecal incontinence have described how it has affected their relationships. They perceive that it has threatened their social acceptability and privacy in relationships. Women have described feelings of fear and shame before they enter into new relationships. People with fecal incontinence have described anxiety about the potential social isolation they may experience and are very cautious about who they tell about their incontinence. Additionally, people with fecal incontinence talk about the significant amount of time they need to spend planning to prevent public accidents. They have also discussed the troubling physical symptoms they experience because of fecal incontinence along with feelings of distorted body image, poor self-esteem, and sexuality concerns.

Although there are many disadvantages to living with fecal incontinence, many people with these symptoms learn coping and management strategies over time [1]. Many want to try to take control of this problem and live a more normal life. There are important implications for advanced practice nurses that can be drawn from the evidence provided below.

### 1.3    Qualitative Research Perspective

Fecal incontinence and its impact on quality of life issues have been studied from a qualitative perspective. The qualitative research evidence presented in this chapter on fecal incontinence and quality of life is helpful to advance practice nurses in understanding these experiences from international patient perspectives. Qualitative evidence can also be used by the advanced practice nurse to inform care planning and decision-making. This research body can additionally influence policy formation. Patient stories can be helpful in sharing the impact of living with fecal incontinence with health-care decision-makers, such as politicians, but due to the stigma with disclosure, it is a challenge to engage patients in sharing their own stories. Thus, the experiences documented in qualitative reports can lend that personal touch to the advance practice nurse's arguments for policy changes.

Qualitative research studies provide a personal perspective of the lives of people who experience the problematic symptom of fecal incontinence and how it affects the quality of their lives by providing insight into the psychological, physical, and social aspects of living with fecal incontinence. The qualitative research evidence also highlights what is important in treatment for a wide variety of clients with a diversity of other chronic conditions. While the advance practice nurse may have garnered these insights from working with her own patient population, the qualitative research findings can serve to inform and extend this personal clinical experience.

An interpretive qualitative approach to research argues that quality of life is a temporal, context-bound subjective phenomenon where the meaning of life experiences illustrates a personal definition of the phenomenon. Human experience such as living with fecal incontinence can be explained in terms of four overlapping domains of human experience: lived time, lived body, lived relationships, and lived space [17]. Peden-McAlpine and colleagues [8, 9] completed two phenomenological studies on community living women and men and interpreted the findings from these studies through these domains of experience.

In the 2013 and 2017 editions of the International Consultation on Incontinence text, Peden-McAlpine, Bliss, and Northwood refined these four domains to offer a new framework of quality of life for people experiencing fecal incontinence [1, 2]. Five domains of the experience of quality of life were thematically derived from the original domains in light of the findings from 19 qualitative studies on people with fecal incontinence. The new domains are living with fecal incontinence related to relationships; living with fecal incontinence related to time and planning; living with fecal incontinence related to bodily symptoms, self-esteem, and body image; living with fecal incontinence related to sexuality; and living with fecal incontinence related to dietary issues (see Fig. 1.1). Findings of each of the five domains of the model of quality of life for people who experience fecal incontinence are summarized after which key points from each domain are correlated with implications for advanced practice nurses.

## 1.4 Quality of Life in the Five Domains of Living with Fecal Incontinence

Each quality of life domain of living with fecal incontinence will be discussed with attention to men and women's perspectives or the perspectives of only women or those only of men depending on the evidence. Implications for the advanced practice nurse-based are offered as key points, based on the evidence from each domain of living, in tables.

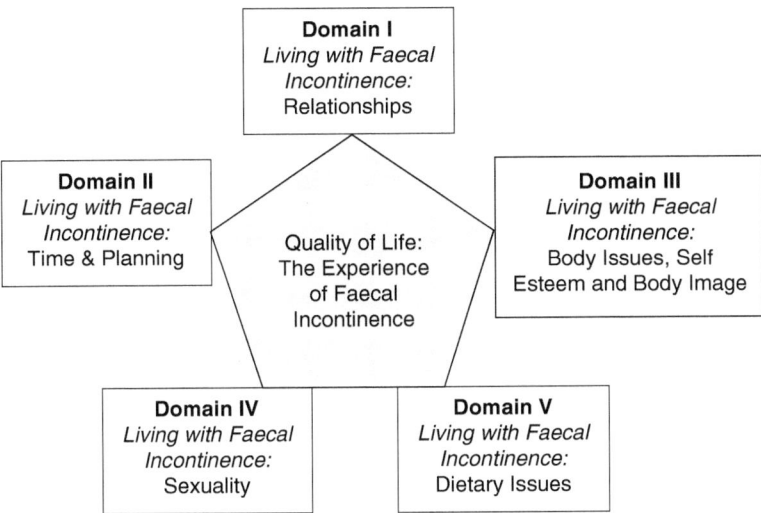

**Fig. 1.1** Model of quality of life: the experience of fecal incontinence

### 1.4.1  Domain I: Living with Fecal Incontinence Related to Relationships

Both men and women perceive that fecal incontinence is a threat to their social acceptability and privacy and that it affects their relationships [9, 18–21] (see Table 1.1). One example given is feeling uncomfortable in "mixed company" (or a group comprised of both men and women) because of the possibility of having a fecal incontinence "accident" (i.e., visible soiling). Individuals report thinking that gender issues are related to the perception of social risk of accidents because of their fecal incontinence [9, 19]. Both men and women suffer from anxiety because of the potential social isolation they may experience because of their symptoms of fecal incontinence [9, 18, 22–26].

Women have concerns about entering into new relationships because of their fear and shame of possibly having to disclose their fecal incontinence [24]. Women feel that fecal incontinence is a very sensitive topic to discuss with others, and it is strongly associated with guilt and shame [21]. Specifically, women may not attend social events and offer excuses not related to their fecal incontinence [21].

Men and women are cautious about who they tell about their problems with fecal incontinence. The selection of these individuals can be a matter of great concern. Family, close trusted friends, and co-workers are often told because they may not be able to completely conceal "their secret" of having fecal incontinence [9, 18, 19]. As part of keeping their secret from others, both men and women describe trying to protect themselves from the unpredictability of having an accident [24].

### 1.4.1.1 Social Support

Social support from spouses is very important for men and women [9, 18, 19, 25]. They attribute their adaptation to fecal incontinence to the loving, empathic, unconditional support they receive from their significant others [27, 28]. Discussing the problems they have experienced because of fecal incontinence with others who also have this problem was described as comforting and allowed conversation about how to manage the problem [9, 19]. The use of humor is a resource to avoid humiliation and embarrassment in dealing with daily symptoms of fecal incontinence even though these feelings of shame and humiliation persist [9, 19, 21, 22, 24].

In general, relationships with health-care professionals are perceived as not helpful in terms of providing advice about symptom management. Men and women report that either no information or misinformation was commonly given by health-care providers [9, 18, 19, 24, 29]. Women specifically describe that they feel embarrassed, humiliated, and marginalized when rude or blaming health-care providers minimize or trivialize their fecal incontinence problems [19, 21, 24, 25]. After years of self-managing their fecal incontinence symptoms, some men and women describe their interactions with the health-care providers as more confident and assertive in regard to decision-making [27], and they now feel comfortable providing support to others with fecal incontinence [27, 28].

**Table 1.1** Recommendations for advanced nursing practice support to quality of life in persons with fecal incontinence related to relationships

| Problems associated with fecal incontinence | Practice implications for the advanced practice nurse |
| --- | --- |
| • Lack of socialization related to fear of public accidents | • Encourage socialization and suggest ways to strengthen coping and prevent accidents in public and support participation in social events (e.g., wear an absorbent product, take an anti-diarrheal medication) |
| • Anxiety related to potential social isolation | • Encourage clients to discuss anxiety concerns about socialization and explore acceptable ways to decrease social isolation |
| • Fear and shame about disclosing fecal incontinence to others | • Acknowledge and address the stigma, embarrassment, fear, and shame related to fecal incontinence both in relationships with family, friends, co-workers, and health-care professionals |
| • Discussing fecal incontinence with others who have the problem was comforting | • Facilitate gender sensitive support groups to promote sharing of practical knowledge of fecal incontinence symptom management |
| • Lack of knowledge by health-care professionals in the treatment of fecal incontinence | • Provide educational materials about fecal incontinence treatment to primary care providers and specialists who may provide care to patients who experience fecal incontinence. For example, the advanced practice nurse could provide rationale for suggested interventions in consultation letters to primary care providers as a strategy to improve knowledge on the topic |

## 1.4.2 Domain II: Living with Fecal Incontinence Related to Time and Planning

Time and planning have significant quality of life implications for men and women with fecal incontinence (see Table 1.2). Hours of time are consumed by people with fecal incontinence, because of the exhaustive planning to prevent public accidents. Time is also a significant issue because of worsening of symptoms with aging and trying to maintain a work life with symptoms of fecal incontinence [1].

### 1.4.2.1 Planning for the Risk of Fecal Incontinence Accidents

Men and women describe spending a significant amount of time planning for and worrying about accidents [9, 19, 21]. They talk about their heightened anxiety about fecal incontinence symptoms and the risk of accidents in public spaces [18, 19, 30, 31]. "Being prepared" is a common theme in discussions related to planning strategies to avoid accidents which include morning bathroom rituals, changing the location of their workstation (relative to the bathroom), altering eating habits (foods and timing), taking a fiber supplement, or using anti-diarrheal products [18, 19, 21, 24, 30]. When going into public places, immediately seeking out the location and availability of a bathroom is a major consideration [9, 18, 19, 21, 24, 29, 30]. Although men and women with fecal incontinence are constantly worried about accidents in public places they do travel. However, travel is limited to familiar places, and significant planning is required prior to travel to prevent potential accidents. Fecal incontinence limits travel for the family [9, 19, 21, 30, 31].

Women are more vigilant with planning to avoid potential accidents in public. They report that the frequency of stool leakage is unpredictable and because of this they need to be vigilant and prepared for the unexpected [19, 24]. Many women discuss packing "kits" of absorbent products, cleansing supplies, and extra clothing as a routine part of planning to leave their home when preparing for an unexpected accident [18, 19].

### 1.4.2.2 Concerns About Aging and Work Life

Many men and women have symptoms for months or years before they seek help for fecal incontinence because of the embarrassment of the symptoms [9, 19]. They discuss their significant worry that their symptoms of fecal incontinence would grow worse with aging in relationship to severity, onset, and duration [9, 19, 30].

Work life presents complicated situations for both men and women and limit some people's abilities to engage in productive work outside the home [9, 19, 26, 29–31]. Women specifically talked about how they postpone business meetings because of their fecal incontinence symptoms [19]. A common reason for early retirement for both men and women is dealing with the symptoms of fecal incontinence [9, 19, 26].

**Table 1.2** Recommendations for advanced nursing practice support to quality of life in persons with fecal incontinence related to time and planning

| Problems associated with fecal incontinence | Practice implications for the advanced practice nurse |
|---|---|
| • Anxiety about fecal incontinence accidents in public places | • Teach practical strategies to manage fecal incontinence symptoms (e.g., morning bowel regimens, altering eating habits (foods and timing), taking fiber supplements, or using anti-diarrheal products, packing absorbent pads, cleansing supplies, and additional clothing) |
| • Limited travel because of fear of accidents | • Discuss potential anxiety about travel with clients and educate about strategies to manage fecal incontinence. Include strategies to cope during travel into care plan |
| • Delayed treatment because of embarrassment of fecal incontinence | • Educate and encourage providers to discuss possible symptoms of fecal incontinence with patients with associated disorders |
| • Work life complications related to fecal incontinence | • Directly ask about anxiety in relation to work situations and encourage planning to accommodate for fecal incontinence (workstation near bathroom and other strategies to effectively manage fecal incontinence discussed above)<br>• Advocate for access to single public toilets in public and work settings<br>• Teach clients about useful phone applications, such as "Go Here," a washroom locator to find toilets when away from home |

## 1.4.3 Domain III: Living with Fecal Incontinence Related to Bodily Symptoms, Self-Esteem, and Body Image

Persons with fecal incontinence experience significant quality of life issues related to the shame and embarrassment of the physical symptoms of fecal incontinence as well as decreased self-esteem and distorted body image [1] (see Table 1.3).

### 1.4.3.1 Stigma

Men and women discuss their perception that poor public knowledge about fecal incontinence causes them to feel stigmatized about their condition [30]. Additionally, they stigmatize themselves because of their inability to control their symptoms [18, 19, 21, 25, 30]. Women in particular feel shame and unworthiness due to fecal incontinence [25, 29]. Some women report the need for psychological consultations because of feeling inadequate and vulnerable [24, 25].

### 1.4.3.2 Body Image

Men and women have negative changes in body image and self-esteem as a result of their inability to control the symptoms of fecal incontinence [9, 19, 21, 24].

They perceive that their emotional life and self-confidence are undermined because of their fecal incontinence and embarrassment [9, 18, 19, 21, 25]. Both men and women have negative feelings associated with living with fecal incontinence such as anger, frustration, injustice, disappointment, hopelessness, despair, and sadness [21]. Men and women avoid talking about the problem or deny fecal incontinence as coping mechanisms to prevent threats to their self-esteem and public embarrassment [25].

Men and women preserve their body image by dressing carefully to conceal a possible fecal incontinence accident. Large diaper-like pads are avoided because of their perceived visibility beneath clothing and small, discreet disposable pads are preferred [9, 19, 24, 31]. Women are particularly attentive to their body image, dress carefully to conceal pads, and wear dark clothing to hide stains if an accident should happen [19, 20, 24, 30].

### 1.4.3.3 Physical Symptoms

Physical symptoms are a major quality of life issue for men and women with fecal incontinence due to the unpredictability of the type, timing, and magnitude of fecal incontinence events [30, 32]. The most troubling bodily symptom for people with both fecal incontinence and irritable bowel syndrome is the sense of urgency to have a bowel movement [30]. Common physical symptoms include skin excoriation at the rectum, sensations in the intestines, itching and burning at the rectum, cramping, feeling of incomplete bowel movements, and odor associated with flatus. Other physical symptoms are leaking stool without defecation sensations and false abrupt, urgent sensations usually indicative of defecation [9, 19, 30, 31].

### 1.4.3.4 Positive Coping

Women who have lived with fecal incontinence for years can establish positive ways of coping. Women maintain hope and optimism by focusing on getting better [21]. For example, women perform self-affirmations, such as "I will not worry what others think of me" or "life has to go on" [21].

Men and women reframe fecal incontinence by asserting control [19, 30]. They focus on controlling all aspects of their life in relationship to the fecal incontinence and avoiding accidents [21, 27]. This involves, early in experience of fecal incontinence, adapting to the presence of obstacles and "making the best of it" [27]. After 10 or more years of living with fecal incontinence, men and women find the addition of multiple chronic conditions poses further challenges to adaptation. However, by using trial and error, adaptation can continue successfully [28]. A sense of mastery and new self-confidence can result from years of successfully self-managing the symptoms of fecal incontinence [27, 28].

**Table 1.3** Recommendations for advanced nursing practice support to quality of life in persons with fecal incontinence related to bodily symptoms, self-esteem, and body image

| Problems associated with fecal incontinence | Practice implications for the advanced practice nurse |
| --- | --- |
| • Stigma of fecal incontinence socially and in health care | • Make a public commitment to speak out against stigmatizing behaviors and language in public and work place<br>• Speak openly about work and challenges of living with fecal incontinence in work as well as social settings |
| • Poor self-esteem related to fecal incontinence | • Ask directly and assess for impact of fecal incontinence on self-esteem<br>• Refer, as necessary, for counseling or psychological support<br>• Encourage use of online support communities, such as Unlocked sponsored by The Simon Foundation for Continence |
| • Negative impact on quality of life from bothersome physical symptoms | • Ask directly about common bodily symptoms in case embarrassment is preventing disclosure by client<br>• Assess for, itemize, and address each bothersome bodily symptom, recognizing variety and range across clients |
| • Poor body image related to fecal incontinence | • Ask directly and assess for impact of fecal incontinence on self-esteem<br>• Model and teach positive self-talk and self-affirmations<br>• Teach practical strategies to maintain positive self-image, such as discreet incontinence products, camouflaging products with darker clothing, etc. |
| • Poor or insufficient coping strategies | • Teach and explain contributing factors to fecal incontinence<br>• Offer range of interventions with client input and choice<br>• Explain what to expect in terms of improvements and the timeline for improvement, emphasizing the positive changes that can come with treatment |
| • Worry the fecal incontinence is not treatable | • Set goals that are meaningful to client and realistic in terms of condition, causes, and available treatment<br>• Assist client to see change and improvements by sharing assessment of progress over time |

### 1.4.3.5 Goal Setting

Positive coping can be enhanced by tailored goal setting. The major goals of people experiencing fecal incontinence are specific and individual, such as, to have fewer dietary restrictions, less fecal leakage especially during exercise, more confidence in controlling fecal incontinence symptoms, and a normal daily routine [33].

### 1.4.4   Domain IV: Living with Fecal Incontinence Related to Sexuality

The negative impact on sexuality affects quality of life for men and women with fecal incontinence (see Table 1.4). In the research context, women share the sexual implications of their fecal incontinence more than men. However, some women are reticent to discuss their sexuality or the effect of their fecal incontinence symptoms on their sexual functioning [19, 24]. Some women experience no changes in their sexual drive [21, 25].

Men and women with fecal incontinence have some strategies to maintain a healthy sexual life. For example, based on patterns of fecal incontinence, the timing of sexual expression can be modified [25]. Cleanliness is a major concern for men and women in regard to sexuality, and they make concerted efforts to wash to avoid smelling [20, 31].

Unfortunately, men and women with fecal incontinence have not find their interactions with health-care professionals about their sexual health helpful. Health-care professionals did not talk about sexual issues concerning fecal incontinence in general and even after surgeries that would affect sexual functioning [20, 26]. This represents a significant knowledge, practice, and research gap for advanced nursing practice.

## 1.4.5   Domain V: Living with Fecal Incontinence Related to Dietary Issues

Eating and diet are significant components of quality of life for people with fecal incontinence (see Table 1.5). The qualitative research participants had numerous strategies for self-management of fecal incontinence related to adding or restricting intake of certain foods, changing ways they prepared food, and modifying the timing of eating [9, 18, 19, 23, 30, 31]. These strategies are discussed in Chap. 6. Box 1.2 provides a clinical exemplar of the care provided by an advanced practice continence nurse for a patient whose body image and self esteem are lowed by their fecal incontinence.

**Table 1.4** Recommendations for advanced nursing practice support to quality of life in persons with fecal incontinence related to sexuality

| Problems associated with fecal incontinence | Practice implications for the advanced practice nurse |
| --- | --- |
| • Avoid sexual intimacy due to fecal incontinence | • Ask directly about impact of fecal incontinence on sexual intimacy<br>• Problem-solve with client strategies to introduce intimacy into their lives, such as discussing fecal incontinence with their partner, establishing pattern of fecal incontinence and timing of sexual activity, and identifying triggering activities and alternative expressions of intimacy |

**Table 1.5** Recommendations for advanced nursing practice support to quality of life in persons with fecal incontinence related to dietary issues

| Problems associated with fecal incontinence | Practice implications for the advanced practice nurse |
| --- | --- |
| • Restrict certain types of foods or eating with others | • Acknowledge and empathize regarding the impact of dietary restrictions and modifications on quality of life<br>• Enquire directly about dietary restrictions<br>• Teach successful diet strategies (refer to interventions in Chap. 6) |

**Box 1.2: Clinical Exemplar: Body Image and Self-Esteem**
Mr. Smith is a 76-year-old man being seen by the home care advance practice continence nurse for assessment and management of his fecal incontinence. Mr. Smith had been experiencing urgent, loose bowel movements for the past 3 or 4 months. He shared with the nurse that he had soiled himself in front of his friends at their weekly euchre tournament. "I have never been so humiliated. How could this stupid, old body let me down like that?" he shared angrily, fighting back tears in his eyes. Mr. Smith had stepped down as euchre team captain and had been avoiding calls from his teammates.

The advance practice continence nurse worked with Mr. Smith to develop a plan to manage his fecal incontinence. She knew, however, that in order for him to feel confident enough to make these changes and return to his previous activities, she had to address Mr. Smith's negative body image and the resultant impact on his self-esteem. The nurse started by acknowledging the huge impact that the public episode of fecal incontinence had on Mr. Smith. She shared with Mr. Smith what she had learned from other clients: it is helpful to develop coping strategies related to both the worry of future incontinence episodes and the actual incontinence.

First of all, the nurse taught Mr. Smith how to engage in progressive relaxation techniques: a simple strategy of counting while deep breathing. Fostering calmness would help Mr. Smith cope proactively with the dread of a future public accident. Also, she suggested he talk to himself positively and not criticize himself or his body as thoughts have real power over feelings. Replace "stupid old body" with "I will figure out ways to work with what my body is doing right now."

Next, the advance practice continence nurse wanted Mr. Smith to feel prepared in the event of future incontinence episodes while working on their treatment plan. She focused on being prepared rather than being fearful of an accident. They discussed strategies such as knowing the closest bathroom when out and traveling with extra clothes and products in a masculine knapsack. The nurse also ensured that Mr. Smith had the right type of incontinence product for his needs, comfort, and physical build. Finally, she suggested that he reach out to his closest friend on his euchre team and confide that "my bowels have not been behaving lately," so he can control the message and enlist help from this friend if needed. None of these discussions or strategies were easy for Mr. Smith, but acknowledging the social impact of his incontinence was critical to fostering hope and engagement with the treatment plan.

# References

1. Bliss DZ, Mimura T, Berghmans B, Bharucha A, Chiarioni G, Emmanuel A, et al. Assessment and conservative management of faecal incontinence and quality of life in adults. In: Abrams P, Cardozo L, Wagg A, Wein A, editors. Incontinence. 6th ed. Bristol: International Continence Society; 2017. p. 1993–2085.

2. Bliss DZ, Mellgren A, Whitehead W, Chiarioni G, Emmanuel A, Santoro G, et al. Assessment and conservative management of faecal incontinence and quality of life in adults. In: Abrams P, Cardozo L, Khoury S, Wein A, editors. Incontinence. 5th ed. The Netherlands: ICUD-EAU; 2013. p. 1444–85.
3. Cassells C, Watt E. The impact of incontinence on older spousal caregivers. J Adv Nurs. 2003;42(6):607–16.
4. Armstrong M. Factors affecting the decision to place a relative with dementia into residential care. Nurs Stand. 2000;14(16):33–7.
5. Tsuji I, Whalen S, Finucane TE. Predictors of nursing home placement in community-based long-term care. J Am Geriatr Soc. 1995;43(7):761–6.
6. Ouslander JG, Zarit SH, Orr NK, Muira SA. Incontinence among elderly community-dwelling dementia patients. Characteristics, management, and impact on caregivers. J Am Geriatr Soc. 1990;38(4):440–5.
7. Jonasson L-L, Josefsson K. Staff experiences of the management of older adults with urinary incontinence. Healthy Aging Res. 2016;5:1–11.
8. Saxer S, de Bie RA, Dassen T, Halfens RJ. Knowledge, beliefs, attitudes, and self-reported practice concerning urinary incontinence in nursing home care. J Wound Ostomy Cont Nurs. 2009;36(5):539–44.
9. Peden-McAlpine C, Bliss DZ, Becker B, Sherman S. The experience of community-living men managing fecal incontinence. Rehabil Nurs. 2012;37(6):298–306.
10. Bliss DZ, Rolnick C, Jackson J, Arntson C, Mullins J, Hepburn K. Health literacy needs related to incontinence and skin damage among family and friend caregivers of individuals with dementia. J Wound Ostomy Cont Nurs. 2013;40(5):515–23.
11. Rolnick SJ, Bliss DZ, Jackson JM. Healthcare providers' perspectives for promoting communication with family caregivers and patients with dementia about incontinence and skin damage. Ostomy Wound Manage. 2013;59(4):62–7.
12. Mullins J, Bliss DZ, Rolnick S, Henre CA, Jackson J. Barriers to communication with a health-care provider and health literacy about incontinence among informal caregivers of individuals with dementia. J Wound Ostomy Cont Nurs. 2016;43(5):539–44.
13. National Institutes of Health. Health literacy 2012. http://www.nih.gov/clearcommunication/healthliteracy.htm.
14. The National Academies of Science, Engineering, Medicine. Health literacy: a prescription to end confusion. What is Health Literacy 2004. https://www.nap.edu/read/10883/chapter/4.
15. Kickbusch I, Pelikan JM, Apfel F, Tsouros A. Health literacy. Copenhagen: WHO Regional Office for Europe; 2013.
16. Patel K, Bliss DZ, Savik K. Health literacy and emotional responses related to fecal incontinence. J Wound Ostomy Cont Nurs. 2010;37(1):73–9.
17. Merleau-Ponty M. Phenomenology of perception (C. Smith, Trans.). London: Routledge Classics; 1962.
18. Collings S, Norton C. Women's experiences of faecal incontinence: a study. Br J Community Nurs. 2004;9(12):520–3.
19. Peden-McAlpine C, Bliss DZ, Hill J. The experience of community-living women managing fecal incontinence. West J Nurs Res. 2008;30(7):817–35.
20. Roe B, May C. Incontinence and sexuality: findings from a qualitative perspective. J Adv Nurs. 1999;30(3):573–9.
21. Olsson F, Bertero C. Living with faecal incontinence: trying to control the daily life that is out of control. J Clin Nurs. 2015;24(1–2):141–50.
22. Cohen DJ, Crabtree BF. Evaluative criteria for qualitative research in health care: controversies and recommendations. Ann Fam Med. 2008;6(4):331–9.
23. Hansen JL, Bliss DZ, Peden-McAlpine C. Diet strategies used by women to manage fecal incontinence. J Wound Ostomy Cont Nurs. 2006;33(1):52–61.
24. Cotterill N, Norton C, Avery KNL, Donovan JL. A patient-centered approach to developing a comprehensive symptom and quality of life assessment of anal incontinence. Dis Colon Rectum. 2008;51(1):82–7.
25. Rasmussen JL, Ringsberg KC. Being involved in an everlasting fight—a life with postnatal faecal incontinence. A qualitative study. Scand J Caring Sci. 2010;24(1):108–15.

26. Rozmovits L, Ziebland S. Expressions of loss of adulthood in the narratives of people with colorectal cancer. Qual Health Res. 2004;14(2):187–203.
27. Wilson M. Living with faecal incontinence: Follow-up to a research project. Br J Nurs. 2013;22(3):147–53. 7p
28. Wilson M. Living with faecal incontinence: a 10-year follow-up study. Br J Nurs. 2015;24(5): 268–74.
29. Norton C, Dibley L. Help-seeking for fecal incontinence in people with inflammatory bowel disease. J Wound Ostomy Cont Nurs. 2013;40(6):631–8.
30. Dibley L, Norton C. Experiences of fecal incontinence in people with inflammatory bowel disease: self-reported experiences among a community sample. Inflamm Bowel Dis. 2013;19(7): 1450–62.
31. Chelvanayagam S, Norton C. Quality of life with faecal continence problems. Nurs Times. 2000;96(31 Suppl):15–7.
32. Norton C, Chelvanayagam S. Bowel problems and coping strategies in people with multiple sclerosis. Br J Nurs. 2010;19(4):220–6.
33. Manthey A, Bliss DZ, Savik K, Lowry A, Whitebird R. Goals of fecal incontinence management identified by community-living incontinent adults. West J Nurs Res. 2010;32(5):644–61.

# Advanced Practice Continence Nursing

2

Joan Ostaszkiewicz, Cynthia Peden-McAlpine,
Melissa Northwood, Sharon Eustice, Donna Z. Bliss,
and Kaoru Nishimura

**Abstract**

This chapter explains the concepts of advanced practice nursing and advanced practice continence nursing. It describes advanced practice nursing and advanced practice continence nursing practice in four countries. It distinguishes between specialist and advanced nursing practice, introduces the reader to the global development of continence nursing as a specialization, describes the role profile of the nurse continence specialist, and proposes a set of competences and education from basic to advanced practice continence nursing care. This chapter includes information about the advanced practice approach to continence care for people with fecal incontinence and concludes with research about the effectiveness of nurses with advanced practice skills in continence care for people with fecal incontinence.

J. Ostaszkiewicz (✉)
School of Nursing and Midwifery, Deakin University, Burwood, VIC, Australia
e-mail: joan.ostaszkiewicz@deakin.edu.au

C. Peden-McAlpine · D. Z. Bliss
University of Minnesota School of Nursing, Minneapolis, MN, USA
e-mail: peden001@umn.edu; bliss@umn.edu

M. Northwood
Saint Elizabeth Health Care, Hamilton, ON, Canada

Aging, Community and Health Research Unit, School of Nursing, McMaster University, Hamilton, ON, USA
e-mail: northwm@mcmaster.ca

S. Eustice
Cornwall Foundation Trust, Cornwall, UK
e-mail: sharoneustice@nhs.net

K. Nishimura
Japan Continence Action Society, Tokyo, Japan

© Springer International Publishing AG, part of Springer Nature 2018
D. Z. Bliss (ed.), *Management of Fecal Incontinence for the Advanced Practice Nurse*,
https://doi.org/10.1007/978-3-319-90704-8_2

**Keywords**
Continence nursing · Advanced practice · Nursing · Specialization · Education
Competence

## 2.1 Introduction

In this book, the term "advanced practice nursing" refers to a specific type of nursing role, whereas the term "advanced nursing practice" refers to the concept of working at an advanced level of practice in nursing. The International Council of Nurses, which is a federation of more than 130 national nurses associations that works to ensure quality nursing care for all, identifies two professional nursing profiles that represent advanced practice nursing: (a) the nurse practitioner and (b) the clinical nurse specialist. Specifically, "a Nurse Practitioner/Advanced Practice Nurse is a registered nurse who has acquired the expert knowledge base, complex decision-making skills and clinical competencies for expanded practice, the characteristics of which are shaped by the context and/or country in which s/he is credentialed to practice" [1]. The International Council of Nurses furthermore identifies five interrelated roles that align with the duties of these two role profiles: (a) clinical practice, (b) consultation, (c) education, (d) leadership, and (e) research [2].

The International Council of Nurses definition of the advanced practice nursing role recognizes that nursing roles and the nature of practice, educational preparation, and regulatory mechanisms vary widely from country to country. At the same time, it is acknowledged that educational preparation for advanced nursing practice is beyond generalist education, i.e., usually a master's degree; is autonomous and independent; and requires advanced clinical competencies and legislation for titling, licensure, credentialing, and specialty certification.

Advanced practice nursing includes specialization but also includes expansion of the scope of practice and educational advancement. It is characterized by role autonomy and health promotion responsibilities along with the diagnosis and management of illness that includes pharmacological and non-pharmacological interventions. The role requires advanced clinical reasoning and organizational leadership [3]. Advanced practice nursing requires a greater depth and breadth of knowledge, a greater degree of synthesis of data, and complexity of skills and interventions than basic nursing practice [4].

Considerable debate centers on the difference between the roles and functions of the nurse practitioner vis-a-vis other nurses with advanced practice skills. According to the findings of a cross-sectional national survey of 5662 Australian nurses, it is possible to distinguish levels of practice within nursing, including the level of advanced practice nursing [5].

Many countries have made significant progress with establishing advanced practice nursing. This chapter describes advanced practice nursing in Australia, Japan, the United Kingdom (UK), and the United States (USA) and discusses the role of the advanced practice nursing in continence care.

## 2.2    Advanced Practice Nursing in Australia

Only one role is regulated in Australia, which is designated as an advanced practice nursing role, i.e., the "nurse practitioner." Nurse practitioners in Australia practice within the regulatory framework established by the Nursing and Midwifery Board of Australia and must adhere to the nurse practitioner standards for practice, the code of ethics, the code of professional conduct, and guidelines regarding professional boundaries, continuing professional development, and recency of practice. In 2016, of the 379,791 nurses and midwives registered with the Nursing and Midwifery Board of Australia, 1477 (0.3%) were nurse practitioners [6].

To be endorsed as a nurse practitioner in Australia, registered nurses must (a) be registered as a registered nurse; (b) have completed 5000 h at the clinical advanced nursing practice level, within the past 6 years; (c) have completed a Nursing and Midwifery Board of Australia-approved program of study leading to endorsement as a nurse practitioner; and (d) demonstrate compliance with the Nursing and Midwifery Board of Australia's nurse practitioner standards for practice [7]. An approved program of study is a postgraduate nursing master's degree that includes Nursing and Midwifery Board of Australia-approved master's level units in advanced health assessment, pharmacology for prescribing, therapeutics, and diagnostics and research (see Table 2.1).

### 2.2.1    Advanced Practice in Continence Nursing in Australia

Australia has approximately 250 registered nurses who specialize in continence nursing and who perform at varying levels of practice, from beginning to advanced. They are professionally represented by the Continence Nurses Society Australia, previously termed Australian Nurses for Continence. Continence Nurses Society Australia is a nonprofit national organization that provides a communication conduit for the activities of the Australian state and territory branches members and provides a single national professional voice that advocates on continence nursing-related issues. In 2000, Australian Nurses for Continence commissioned the development and validation of a suite of competency standards for nurses specializing in continence promotion and the management of incontinence. These standards are currently being updated with reference to the Nursing and Midwifery Board of Australia registered nurse standards for practice [11] and an internationally validated role profile of the nurse continence specialist [12].

A profile of the membership of the Continence Nurses Society Australia reveals titles vary, the most common being "Continence Nurse Advisor." Most continence nurse advisors have completed post-registration accredited education and are employed across a range of practice settings. Some coordinate and manage nurse-led continence services. Very few are nurse practitioners. The following section provides an example of an advanced practice nursing role for the management of fecal incontinence in Australia.

**Table 2.1** Core features of registered nurses working in advanced practice roles in continence care in example countries

| Country | Role titles | Role profile | Registration/certification | Formal education requirements |
|---|---|---|---|---|
| Australia | Nurse practitioner | "Nurse practitioner is an advanced practice nurse endorsed by the Nursing and Midwifery Board of Australia who has direct clinical contact and practices within their scope under the legislatively protected title 'nurse practitioner' under the National Law" [7] (p. 3). The role is qualitatively different from that of the registered nurse because of additional legislative functions and regulatory requirements. The requirements include a prescribed educational level, a specified advanced nursing practice experience, and continuing professional development | The Nursing and Midwifery Board of Australia | Masters of Nursing Practice The equivalent of 3 years' full-time experience (5000 h) at the clinical advanced nursing practice level, within the past 6 years |
| Canada | Clinical nurse specialist | Clinical nurse specialists have expertise in a specialized area and provide expert nursing care for this population [8]. Their role encompasses developing clinical guidelines and policies, promoting evidence-based practice, and providing expert consultation and support to nursing and interdisciplinary teams [8] | Optional certification through the Canadian Nurses Association for specialty areas of practice | Masters of Science in Nursing, Masters of Health Policy or Health Administration, etc. |
| | Nurse practitioner | Nurse practitioners provide direct care focusing on health promotion and treatment and management of health conditions [8]. They can independently diagnose, order, and interpret diagnostic tests and prescribe pharmaceuticals within their legislated scope of practice [8] | Registration class for nurse practitioner through provincial nursing colleges | Masters of Science in Nursing |
| Japan | Certified nurse | Certified nurses "provide high-level nursing practice, and use skilled nursing expertise in specific nursing fields, into society. The roles of Certified Nurses are nursing practice at high level, instruction of nurses, and consultation with nurses" [9] (p. 12) | The Japanese Nurses Association | A credentialing exam |
| | Certified nurse specialist | Certified nurse specialists "contribute to the development of healthcare and welfare as well as to improve nursing science by forwarding Certified Nurse Specialists with specific advanced nursing knowledge and skills into society to provide high-level nursing care efficiently for individuals, families and groups having complex and intractable nursing problems" [9] (p. 11) | The Japanese Nurses Association | A master's program at a graduate school |

| | | | | |
|---|---|---|---|---|
| UK | Advanced nurse practitioner | "The advanced nurse practitioner offers care complementary to that offered by doctors and other healthcare professionals and augments the care that a team can deliver but can also act as a primary care provider" [10] | None | First-degree level recommended |
| | Clinical nurse specialist | Clinical nurse specialists work in a variety of acute and community settings, specializing in particular areas of practice such as general practice, mental health, children's nursing, learning disability nursing, and district nursing; all specialist nurses provide tailored care depending on the patient's level of need. They also provide education and support for patients to manage their symptoms, particularly patients with long-term conditions and multiple morbidities [10] | None | First-degree level recommended |
| | Nurse consultant | "The nurse consultant possesses the full range of integrated expertise necessary to achieve the current government agenda in practice. Through bridging expert nursing practice with learning, evaluation, and measurement in practice and clinical and political leadership, nurse consultants have the skills and expertise to build a culture where quality practice and services are both developed and maintained" [10] | None | Master's degree level recommended |
| USA | Clinical nurse specialist | Clinical nurse specialists integrate care across the continuum through three spheres of influence: patient, nurse, and system. The primary goal of the role is continuous improvement of patient outcomes and nursing care. Responsible and accountable for diagnosis and treatment of health/illness states, disease management, health promotion, and prevention of illness and risk behaviors among individuals, families, groups, and communities [3] | American Nurses Credentialing Center Wound, Ostomy, and Continence Nurses Certification Board Advanced Practice Registered Nurse (APRN CCCN-AP) | Masters of Nursing or Doctor of Nursing Practice |
| | Nurse practitioner | Nurse practitioners practice autonomously in areas as diverse as family practice, pediatrics, internal medicine, geriatrics, and women's health. They provide initial, ongoing, and comprehensive care, including taking comprehensive histories, providing physical examinations and other health assessment and screening activities, and diagnosing, treating, and managing patients with acute and chronic illnesses. This includes ordering, performing, supervising, and interpreting laboratory and imaging studies; prescribing medication and durable medical equipment; and making appropriate referrals for patients and families [3] | American Nurses Credentialing Center Adult Gerontological, or Primary Care, or Family, or Women's Health Gender-Related Nurse Practitioner AGPCNP CCCN-AP Wound, Ostomy, and Continence Nurses Certification Board | Masters of Nursing or Doctor of Nursing Practice |

## 2.2.2  Exemplar of Practice

Donna is a registered nurse with specialized advanced qualifications and experience in continence care for women with bladder, bowel, and pelvic floor dysfunction or injury. She was the first nurse continence specialist to gain the protected title of "Continence Nurse Practitioner" in Australia. This was achieved through the process of portfolio, demonstrated advanced practice, 5000 specialty clinical hours, and completion of master's degree. Donna also has postgraduate qualifications in continence nursing, sexual and reproductive health, gynecology nursing, and midwifery. In 2006, Donna was awarded two scholarships which enabled her to complete a master's certificate in biofeedback and visit continence services in England.

Donna's expertise is firmly grounded in clinical and multidisciplinary practice. She helped establish a continence nurse services at a large tertiary hospital in South Australia and was a trailblazer in the care of women with postpartum or post-gynecological bladder, bowel, or pelvic floor dysfunction or injury. In addition to her clinical leadership role, Donna initiated audits of practice, identified and addressed gaps, developed multidisciplinary policies and protocols, and educated and mentored midwives and nurses. In 2012, Donna completed her Masters of Nurse Practitioner, which complemented her nurse practitioner authorization and clinical work. Her thesis examined the classification of obstetric anal sphincter injuries using endo-anal ultrasound and found many women with obstetric anal sphincter injuries were underdiagnosed, increasing their long-term risk of developing fecal incontinence. Among other resources, Donna developed (a) a digital assessment tool to evaluate anorectal dysfunction and a separate tool for urogenital assessment, (b) clinical practice guidelines for pessary prescription and fitting, (c) and perinatal practice guidelines for the management of obstetric third- and fourth-degree anal sphincter injuries and the assessment and management of voiding dysfunction after childbirth.

## 2.3  Advanced Practice Nursing in Canada

Advanced practice nursing in Canada is an "umbrella term describing an advanced level of clinical nursing practice that maximizes graduate educational preparation, in-depth nursing knowledge and expertise in meeting the health needs of individuals, families, groups, communities, and populations" [11] (p. ii). A national framework defines advanced practice nursing and outlines the competencies and necessary education [8].

Canada has two recognized advanced practice nursing roles: "Clinical Nurse Specialist" and "Nurse Practitioner." Although these roles are critical in advancing nursing knowledge and contributing to the improvement of the healthcare system, they account for less than one percent of the registered nursing workforce in Canada [8, 13]. Although not required, some clinical nurse specialists and "nurse practitioners" pursue certification in their specialty area of nursing practice through the Canadian Nurses Association, for example, enterostomal therapy and gerontological nursing practice. Both roles incorporate clinical, research, leadership, and consultation and collaboration competencies but are distinctly different [8] (see Table 2.1). Moreover, while the title of "nurse practitioner" has additional regulation and title protection in Canada, the title "clinical nurse specialist" does not.

### 2.3.1  Advanced Practice in Continence Nursing in Canada

Canada has approximately 100 registered nurses who are members of the Canadian Nurse Continence Advisors Association. Collectively, they are referred to as "Nurse Continence Advisors." In addition, there are approximately 129 enterostomal therapists who are certified by the Canadian Nurses Association [14, 15]. These nurses perform at different levels of practice. A minority are clinical nurse specialists or nurse practitioners. Clinical nurse specialists or nurse practitioners who specialize in continence care in Canada work across all healthcare sectors, including home and community and acute, chronic, and long-term care. The specialty populations these nurses serve are most commonly urology, gynecology, gerontology, and community [15]. The following section provides a Canadian example of a clinical nurse specialist role for the management of fecal incontinence.

### 2.3.2  Exemplar of Practice

Laura is a clinical nurse specialist at a large tertiary hospital. She is a masters-prepared advanced practice nurse, an enterostomal therapist, and a nurse continence advisor. Laura became interested in continence promotion while working with clients with advanced multiple sclerosis and complicated clinical presentations. She first completed an enterostomal therapy course, and as her interest in continence care developed, she decided to take the nurse continence advisor program. With this credential, Laura established the first nurse-led continence clinic in her setting. Laura then pursued her Master's Degree in Nursing and attributes this education in preparing and enabling her to assume a leadership role in her hospital and at the regional healthcare planning level.

The acute care hospital where Laura is employed requires an advanced practice approach to continence in order to meet the needs of outpatients, inpatients, and older adults living in the community. Laura provides direct clinical care to adult outpatients in her nurse-led continence clinic. As well, she conducts clinical consultation to inpatients in the acute care setting for complex clinical issues related to fecal incontinence. Laura is also the clinical coordinator of satellite community-based continence clinics and home visiting program for community-dwelling adults and, in this capacity, leads and mentors her nursing colleagues. Laura conducted a program evaluation of the community clinics, demonstrating post-clinic involvement improved clients' self-efficacy and reduced costs from emergency room diversion.

Laura has also led research initiatives to evaluate linen and incontinence product use with acute care inpatients and worked with multiple hospital departments to improve client outcomes related to pressure injuries complicated by incontinence. Laura also planned, implemented, and evaluated public education delivered at retirement homes, community groups, and hospitals. In her multifaceted practice, Laura integrates her clinical experience, expert nursing knowledge and theory, and leadership skills to promote continence and enhance quality of life for persons experiencing fecal incontinence in her community.

## 2.4    Advanced Practice Nursing in Japan

Currently, there is no regulation for advanced practice nursing in Japan. The roles that most closely resemble an advanced practice nursing role are the "Certified Nurse" and the "Certified Nurse Specialist." The Japanese Nurses Association [9] states the certified nurse "provides high-level nursing practice, and uses skilled nursing expertise in specific nursing fields, into society. The roles of Certified Nurses are nursing practice at high level, instruction of nurses, and consultation with nurses" (p. 12).

In order to attain national certification as a certified nurse by the Japanese Nurses Association, nurses must have "a certain amount of experience, after obtaining a national license for nurses, and then pass a credentialing examination given by the Japanese Nurses Association after completing the required education program for certification" [9] (p. 12). Nurses can be certified in a range of areas of practice, including oncology nursing, psychiatric mental health, community health nursing, gerontological nursing, pediatric nursing, women's health nursing, chronic care nursing, infection control, and family health and home care nursing. As of July 2015, there were 15,935 nurses registered as certified nurses in Japan. Of these, 2166 were certified in wound, ostomy, and continence nursing.

According to the Japanese Nurses Association [9], the role of the certified nurse specialist is to "contribute to the development of healthcare and welfare as well as to improve nursing science by forwarding Certified Nurse Specialists with specific advanced nursing knowledge and skills into society to provide high-level nursing care efficiently for individuals, families and groups having complex and intractable nursing problems" (p. 11). The Japanese Nurses Association furthermore states the role reflects the following: (a) "excellent nursing practice; (b) consultation with care providers including nurses; (c) coordination among the concerned parties; (d) ethical coordination to protect the rights of individuals, etc., and (e) education of nursing personnel, and research activities at clinical settings" [9] (p. 12).

In order to be certified as a certified nurse specialist in Japan, nurses complete a master's program at a graduate school after obtaining a national license for nurses and then pass the credentialing examination given by Japanese Nurses Association after accumulating a certain amount of experience [9] (p. 12). The system for certifying certified nurse specialists was initiated in 1996. As of 2015, 1466 (0.1% of nurses) were certified as certified nurse specialists; however, none were certified in wound, ostomy, and continence nursing [9] (see Table 2.1).

### 2.4.1  Advanced Practice in Continence Nursing in Japan

The first nurse in Japan to specialize in wound, ostomy, and continence nursing was in the 1980s, and in 1990, the Japan Continence Action Society was established. In 1996, the Japanese Nurses Association developed the first course on wound, ostomy, and continence nursing, which has been completed by over 4000 individuals. In 2016, there were 2303 nurses in Japan who identified as wound, ostomy, and continence nurses. Most specialize in wound and ostomy care, and there are very few with specialist knowledge and skills in the management of incontinence. Those who do specialize in continence care, primarily focus on bladder rather than bowel dysfunction.

Currently, Japan has three advanced practice nurses who specialize in the management of fecal incontinence. They perform comprehensive assessments and provide advice that includes, but is not limited to, dietary information; advice about supplements, laxatives, etc.; instruction about bowel movement posture and bowel habit; advice about skin care and pelvic floor muscle training, including biofeedback; and advice about continence products and psychosocial support. A key barrier to nurse-led specialized services for the management of fecal incontinence in Japan is the lack of national health reimbursement insurance.

### 2.4.2  Exemplar of Practice

Mihoko is a registered nurse and a wound, ostomy, and continence nurse who specializes in the treatment of bowel disease in an acute care setting in Japan. Mihoko's interest in bowel management began when she observed a gap in care for people with a stoma. She found the majority of these patients experienced irritable bowel disease and fecal incontinence. However, at that time, only one nurse was employed to address this area. Mihoko decided to become a wound, ostomy, and continence nurse. She completed a 6-month course in 1998 and commenced work as a wound, ostomy, and continence nurse in 2000 at a large tertiary hospital. Mihoko established a fecal incontinence outpatient clinic. She states three factors led to her desire to provide a specialized service for people with fecal incontinence. Firstly, there was a lack of nursing support for this group of patients; secondly, Mihoko wanted to improve the overall approach to the use of laxatives; and thirdly, the nurse-led clinic was medially supported.

In 2015, Mihoko conducted an audit of her practice revealing 65% of patients received medical advice, 43% were counseled about diet, 24% received advice about skin care, and 4% ($n = 32$) received biofeedback. Biofeedback training resulted in a complete recovery for 56% ($n = 18$), a decrease in symptoms for 10% ($n = 3$), and "no change" for 22% ($n = 7$).

## 2.5    Advanced Practice Nursing in the UK

Advanced nursing practice in the UK has been in development for many years. The UK Royal College of Nursing [10] refers to nurses who work at an advanced practice level as "Advanced Nurse Practitioners" and recommends that "nurses aspiring to this level of practice should undertake a Royal College of Nursing accredited advanced nursing practice program" (p. 4). There is general agreement from the UK health departments that master's level educational preparation is required for advanced nursing practice but is not a registrable qualification as yet. In an effort to strengthen regulation and standardization at advanced levels of nursing practice for patient safety and public protection, in 2017, the Royal College of Nursing launched a credentialing program for UK nurses with a relevant master's qualification who work at an advanced level of practice. While voluntary, the program aims to provide a means to assess the background and legitimacy of nurses to practice at an advanced level through assessing their qualifications, experience, and competence.

Sheer and Wong [16] claim the first advanced practice nursing role was introduced in the UK in 1991 by the Royal College of Nursing with the establishment of a nurse practitioner program focusing on primary healthcare. The impetus for the development of the role was the need to address gaps in the availability of primary care physicians in primary care [17]. Indeed, the establishment of advanced practice nursing roles has been particularly popular in primary care [18]. While the role of an advanced nurse practitioner has gained popularity, the title is unprotected and national regulation isn't in place [19].

Currently, the advanced nurse practitioner in the UK has both prescriptive authority and work autonomy, two role characteristics that are congruent with the International Council of Nurses definition [10]. There is no centralized information on the numbers or distribution of nurses who are employed in advanced practice roles in the UK, and although all such nurses will have been trained to degree level and undertaken postgraduate training in their specialist area, there is a lack of information about their qualifications. At the same time, the Royal College of Nursing states "there is a UK-wide agreed standard for advanced nursing practice which links to a set of competences and transferable skills that can be used across generalist and specialist health care contexts. These competences are about: (a) providing safe, effective person-centred care directly to patients/clients at an advanced level; (b) developing the care context (systems of care) to enable safe, effective person-centered care to be sustained by others; and (c) providing terminology which is understood across all the health professions" [20].

Although advanced nursing practice roles in the UK are not regulated, many nurses nevertheless practice in an area of specialization at varying levels of practice. Role titles vary and educational preparation is inconsistent; however, specialist nurse posts have a distinctive position within the infrastructure of the healthcare delivery system [21]. The Royal College of Nursing [22] states "there is a general consensus in the UK that nurses practicing at specialist level complete a 1-year full-time degree level program concentrating on: clinical nursing practice; care and program management; clinical practice development and clinical practice leadership. The course should cover 50% theory and 50% practice" (p. 2) (see Table 2.1).

## 2.5.1  Advanced Practice in Continence Nursing in the UK

Nurses who specialize in the management of incontinence in the UK are registered nurses and regulated by the Nursing and Midwifery Council. However, supporting nurses in specialist roles has been lacking. In the UK, nurses can choose to become a member of the Association for Continence Advice, which is a professional membership organization providing a mechanism for professional development, networking, and educational opportunities. There is a lack of information about the scope and number of nurses who specialize in continence care across the UK. The National Health Service has a major influence on the overall performance of continence services in the UK and on nurses' abilities to extend the scope of their practice [23].

Although there is limited information about current continence nursing practice in the UK, several documents inform the delivery of continence care broadly. These include the Department of Health "Good Practice in Continence Services" [24], the UK Continence Society "Minimum Standards for Continence Care" [25], and the National Health Service "Excellence in Continence Care Framework" [26]. Collectively, they describe the features of a high-quality integrated continence service as dynamic and involving all practice professionals in prevention, recognition, assessment, and treatment. Access to specialist continence nurses is one of many characteristics of a high-quality integrated continence service.

The "Excellence in Continence Care Framework" [26] differentiates the responsibilities of nursing broadly from the responsibilities of "specialist continence staff." Broad nursing responsibilities are to (a) assess need, (b) prescribe and treat within the sphere of competence, and (c) refer for specialist advice and treatment. The responsibilities of "specialist continence staff" are to:

• Provide clinical leadership of continence services.
• Provide advanced clinical assessment and treatment.
• Advise about the design and delivery of services.
• Develop clinical guidelines and pathways.
• Endorse best practice by teaching.
• Guide and correct practice where necessary.
• Assess and review policies and practices: make recommendations for change.
• Evaluate clinical outcomes [26].

## 2.5.2  Exemplar of Practice

Sharon has been a nurse consultant since 2002, providing clinical care and leadership for a diverse population of people with bladder and bowel problems in an English county. Her role in a primary care setting requires her to have advanced assessment and clinical decision-making skills to meet the needs of children, young people, and adults with varying health problems. She has a Bachelor of Philosophy in Healthcare, a Diploma in Nurse Practitioner, and a Masters of Science in Professional Issues. Completion of the latter and her status as an independent/supplementary nurse prescriber allowed her to expand the scope of her practice.

Sharon's role encompasses clinical expertise and advocacy for research, education, and innovation. She is also passionate about influencing policy and practice related to incontinence. To this end, she has previously chaired the UK Association for Continence Advice and, more recently, was a member of a parliamentary committee that developed a guide setting out how to commission and deliver a quality integrated service which meets patient's needs and is cost-effective to the National Health Service. Sharon is an active and elected member of the International Continence Society Nursing Committee and takes a leading role in activities to promote continence nursing worldwide.

Sharon is currently completing a PhD that focuses on women's experiences of using a new patient-centered device that she designed for women with vaginal prolapse. In 2015, she was named the UK Continence Nurse of the Year for this innovation and has received numerous national awards, including an award for a project that improved the diagnosis and management of urinary tract infections using remote monitoring technology.

## 2.6    Advanced Practice Nursing in the USA

The USA has two recognized advanced practice nursing roles that address continence care: (a) nurse practitioners and (b) clinical nurse specialists. As in Australia and Canada, a national framework (the APRN Consensus Regulatory Model) defines advanced practice nursing and outlines the competencies and necessary education [3]. The key characteristics of advanced practice nursing in the USA are expertise in assessing, diagnosing, and treating complex conditions and the attainment of a master's or doctoral education concentrating in a specific area of advanced nursing practice coupled with practice supervision and ongoing clinical experience [4]. It requires three qualifications:

- Graduate education
- National certification
- Practice focused on the patient and family [27]

Firstly, advanced practice registered nurses (APRNs) must possess a graduate degree (Masters or Doctor of Nursing Practice) with a specialty in an APRN role. Students acquire specialized knowledge about theories and research findings relevant to the core of the chosen specialty. Nationally all APRN curricula have a common educational requirement of three graduate courses: Advanced health/physical assessment, advanced pathophysiology, and advanced pharmacology Practice skills are acquired by faculty supervised clinical practice hours in the specialty area [3]. Most master's programs require a minimum of 500 h, and Doctor of Nursing Practice programs require 1000 h of supervised practice.

The second qualification for recognition of advanced nursing practice is a national certification. National certification exams have been developed by specialty nursing organizations and also by a national nursing certifying body the

American Nurses Credentialing Center. These certification exams are used to determine knowledge of beginning standards of practice for a particular specialty. Certification exams test both knowledge of the specialty content and the APRN role [27]. The third criterion for advanced practice nursing is that the central focus of the role is on the care of patient/family. The intentional focus on the care of the patient/family is one factor that differentiates the APRN role from other nursing roles [27].

In addition to the qualifications for advanced practice, there are core competencies across the four APRN roles. The central competency of advanced practice is direct clinical practice that is distinguished by the following six competencies:

- The use of a holistic perspective
- Formation of therapeutic partnerships with patients
- The use of expert clinical reasoning and skillful performance
- The use of reflective practice
- Reliance of research evidence as a guide to practice
- The use of diverse health and illness management approaches [27] (see Table 2.1)

### 2.6.1   A Consensus Model for APRN Regulation

In 2008, the APRN Joint Dialogue Group and the APRN Consensus Group published a national regulatory and credentialing model for APRN's titled "The Consensus Model for APRN Regulation: Licensure, Certification and Education" (see Fig. 2.1). The model includes role definitions, specifies titles to be used, defines the term "specialty" and population foci, describes future roles, and presents

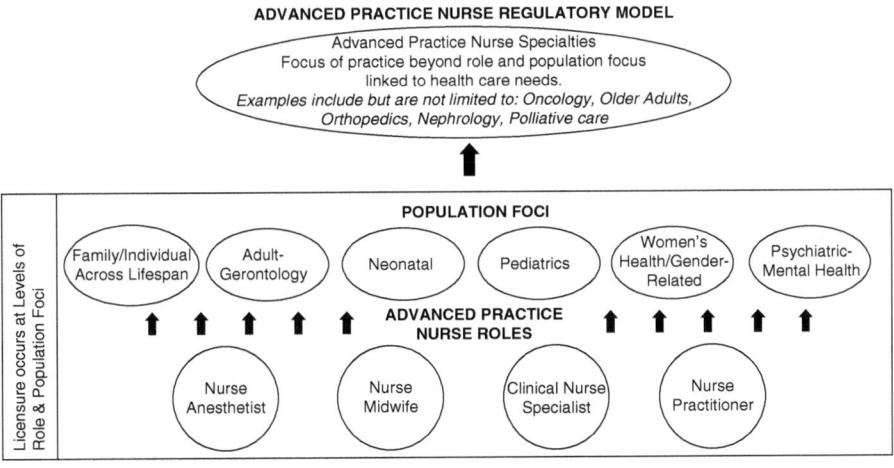

**Fig. 2.1** Consensus Model for advanced practice registered nurses regulation: Licensure, accreditation, certification, and education, National Council of State Boards of Nursing Joint Dialogue Group Report, 2008 (publically available image available from: https://www.ncsbn.org/aprn-consensus.htm [3])

strategies for implementation. The consensus model is supported by 41 nursing organizations. The goal is for all 50 states to adopt the model.

Based on work completed by the APRN Consensus Workgroup and the National Council of State Boards of Nursing, a mechanism that enhances the communication and transparency among APRN licensure, accreditation, certification, and education bodies (LACE) has been developed. LACE signifies the following essential elements:

- Licensure is the granting of authority to practice.
- Accreditation is the formal review and approval by a recognized agency of educational degree or certification programs in nursing or nursing-related programs.
- Certification is the formal recognition of the knowledge, skills, and experience demonstrated by the achievement of standards identified by the profession.
- Education is the formal preparation of APRNs in graduate degree-granting or postgraduate certificate programs.

## 2.6.2 Advanced Practice in Continence Nursing in the USA

There are two roles in which an APRN can apply for advanced practice certification in the specialty area of incontinence care in the USA: (a) the clinical nurse specialist and (b) the certified nurse practitioner. The Wound, Ostomy, and Continence Nurses Certification Board offers an examination for certification as an advanced practice continence nurse (CCNP-AP). Nurses who are already certified as an advanced practice nurse are eligible to take this examination. Other eligibility criteria are certification as a nurse practitioner or a clinical nurse specialist through the American Nurses Credentialing Center. Other certification examinations offered by the Wound, Ostomy, and Continence Nurses Certification Board are in wound and ostomy; the trispecialty of wound, ostomy, and continence; and foot care.

The Wound, Ostomy, and Continence Nurses Certification Board is the certifying body that also offers certification and recertification as a continence specialty nurse at the entry level for registered nurses with a baccalaureate degree who have graduated from one of their accredited continuing education programs. Currently there are six continuing education programs in the USA accredited by the Wound Ostomy and Continence Nurses Certification Board. Nurses may recertify for continence certification or advanced practice certification every 5 years by reexamination or through a professional growth program [28]. The following exemplar of practice illustrates the role of an advanced practice nurse in the USA who specializes in the management of incontinence.

## 2.6.3 Exemplar of Practice

Susan is a family nurse practitioner certified in advanced practice continence care by the Wound, Ostomy, and Continence Nurses Certification Board. She has a Master's Degree in Nursing with a focus on education and oncology. In addition to her clinical practice as a continence nurse practitioner, Susan is a clinical scholar with an academic affiliation. She has presented at national conferences on incontinence in adults and cancer patients. She has several peer-reviewed publications about urinary and fecal incontinence and chapters in undergraduate-level nursing textbooks.

Susan's philosophy of continence care is holistic; she cares for patients by looking at the impact incontinence has on all aspects of their life. Her approach to incontinence care is that it is both an art in caring for the whole person and a science related to utilizing research evidence. As an APRN, Susan is able to be reimbursed by insurers for her care, collaborate directly with medical colleagues, and promote patient education and self-management. She is nationally recognized as a leader in continence care. She has held national leadership positions in several professional organizations and has served as a board member and president on her specialty certification board.

## 2.7 Differentiating Between Specialist and Advanced Nursing Practice

Many nurses specialize in an area of practice, such as incontinence, and function at an advanced level of practice. As nursing has advanced and responded to changes in the healthcare delivery system, specialization has become commonplace. Specialization includes preparation for nursing at an entry level with concentration and experience in a particular area of nursing practice (such as urology or urogynecology). Considerable debate centers on the difference between the role of a nurse with specialist knowledge and skill and the role of the advanced practice nurse.

Nursing specialists develop specialty skills through practice experiences and continuing education. By contrast, advanced practice nursing includes specialization but also includes expansion of the scope of practice and educational advancement. It is characterized by role autonomy, health promotion responsibilities, and the diagnosis and management of illness that includes pharmacological and non-pharmacological interventions. The clinical exemplars in Boxes 2.1 and 2.2 illustrate the differences in practice between the role of a nurse continence specialist and an advanced practice nurse continence specialist.

---

**Box 2.1: Clinical Exemplar: Nurse Continence Specialist**
Mrs. Smith is an 82-year-old woman who referred herself to a continence outpatient program. She had been advised by her primary care provider that "nothing could be done" for fecal incontinence as it is a normal consequence of aging. Mrs. Smith had stopped participating in social activities outside of her home such as a darts league. She was so distressed by the negative impact her incontinence was having on her social life she reached out to her local seniors' community center and learned about the continence program.

The nurse continence specialist from the program conducted an advanced assessment during which Mrs. Smith divulged she had been constipated for most of her adult life and had developed fecal incontinence in her 80s. Her bowel movements were unpredictable, and her stool consistency varied between a hard and formed. The assessment revealed Mrs. Smith had a low fluid intake and a low-fiber diet.

The nurse continence specialist conducted a physical examination and identified factors associated with Mrs. Smith's fecal incontinence. She then developed a conservative management plan in collaboration with Mrs. Smith which included drinking four to five 8-ounce glasses of water over the course of the day gradually increasing her dietary fiber intake up to 25 mg per day limiting her caffeine intake to two cups per day and allowing time after her breakfast to sit comfortably to have a bowel movement.

The nurse continence specialist documented the plan and framed each strategy as a means to achieve Mrs. Smith's goal of resuming her social activities. Gradually with follow-up appointments over the course of 3 months and the support and coaching from the nurse continence specialist, Mrs. Smith's fecal incontinence and constipation were resolved. She monitored her bowel movements and episodes of fecal incontinence on a stool diary reviewed her progress with the nurse at the follow-up visits. She was able to return to her darts league.

**Box 2.2: Clinical Exemplar 2: Advance Practice Nurse Continence Specialist**
John is a 42-year-old man who was referred by his home care coordinator to an advance practice nurse continence specialist for an assessment of fecal incontinence. John has spina bifida and had been managing his bowels with a combination of stimulant and osmotic laxatives, digital stimulation from his home care nurse, and a planned toileting and defecation schedule. Over the past 6 months, John started having multiple episodes of fecal incontinence in between these scheduled visits. John uses a wheelchair and needs support to transfer, so these episodes were undermining his ability to remain in his home and contribute to his community by volunteering at the local children's hospital.

The advance practice nurse continence specialist conducted a health history and physical assessment, which suggested that John may have a fecal impaction. She also ordered an X-ray of his abdomen that revealed multiple pockets of stool and gas but not a complete obstruction. She prescribed an oral laxative preparation. After a few days of evacuation of both hard and watery stool, John's bowel function returned to normal and he was continent. The period of continence did not last long, however.

The advance practice nurse continence specialist and John discussed an alternative treatment: a trans-anal irrigation system. John was concerned that the equipment cost would not be covered by his government disability program. The advance practice nurse continence specialist wrote the order and completed the necessary paperwork requesting coverage for John's trans-anal irrigation supplies from his government disability program. The application was rejected. She then liaised with the case worker to approve a trial period of the new product arguing it was cost-neutral and had potential to improve John's quality of life.

Next, the advance practice nurse continence specialist provided education to the home care nurses working with John. She arranged joint home visits with each of the three nurses to support them in learning to use the equipment. Each nurse had their own unique worries (e.g., could the anchoring rectal catheter balloon break and harm John) that had to be addressed to meet John's goal to be continent and out in the community.

After using the equipment for a month, John was having bowel movements on a regular schedule and was continent in between. The government continued funding the product and, consequently due to the advance practice nurse continence specialist's advocacy, funded other clients for this equipment. The advance practice nurse continence specialist developed a protocol for the home care agency to share with its nurses that outline the procedures for trans-anal irrigation, including consultation with the advance practice nurse continence specialist, for clients requiring this approach to their fecal incontinence.

## 2.8   The Global Development of Continence Nursing as a Specialization

Continence nursing has been considered a specialization within nursing for many years. The first continence nursing specialist role was established in the UK, under the title "continence advisor" in the early 1970s in response to lengthy urological waiting lists. In 1990, Roe [29] reported there were more than 214 nurses who specialized in continence care working throughout the UK. One of the first publications to describe the role was based on a mixed methods study undertaken by Rhodes and Parker [30]. Using the UK Royal College of Nursing framework to articulate the core functions of the clinical nurse specialist in 1991–1992, Rhodes and Parker [30] reported the nurses who specialized in continence care worked to varying degrees in clinical, educational, consultative, managerial, and research roles. Specifically, over 90% performed clinical, consultative, and educational roles and 73% carried a personal caseload, and of these, caseload size ranged from less than 10 clients to over a hundred, with an average of 96 and a mode of 50. The majority (73%) fulfilled a research function at some level.

Fader et al. [31] identified two types of continence nursing specialist roles in the UK which varied according to the key focus and role autonomy. While some nurses who specialized in continence care visited clients in the community or residential care homes and focused on product management, other roles focused on continence promotion and offered nurse-led services.

The specialist continence nursing role also emerged and developed in Australia, Canada, and many other countries, including the USA. According to Brink et al. [32], the first continence clinic established in the USA was in 1983 at the University of Michigan, and an early survey conducted in that country found nurses who specialized in bladder, bowel, and pelvic floor dysfunction had very diverse educational backgrounds and worked under a wide range of different service models, such as ambulatory care settings (47%), acute care hospitals (34%), home care settings (21%), and consultation to nursing homes (16%) [32]. The nurses cited a lack of recognition for the role, lack of reimbursement for nursing services, and insufficient resources to establish continence practices as key barriers to effective service provision.

In contrast to the UK and US models, continence nursing specialization in Canada was linked to the development of a formal academic qualification and postgraduate nursing program [33]. Skelly and Kenny [33] reported on the education of 37 nurses titled "Nurse Continence Advisors" which was funded by the Ontario Ministry of Health in 1995.

A more recent evaluation of continence services provides further insights into the specialist role of the nurse in the management of incontinence. In 2003 Milne and Moore [34] explored and described continence services in Canada and several other countries. The researchers identified the following types of continence service models: physiotherapy delivered continence services, multidisciplinary continence services, and nurse-led continence services. The latter differed in terms of providing outreach care. While nurse-led continence services were generally located in community centers and acute care centers, some also provided home-based care.

## 2.9    The Role Profile of the Nurse Continence Specialist

A more recent understanding of the role of nurses who specialize in the management of incontinence and other bladder, bowel, and pelvic floor disorders was developed by Paterson et al. [12]. Using a mixed methods approach characterized by consensus and consultation, Paterson et al. [12] developed and validated a role profile, titling these nurses as "Nurse Continence Specialists." The findings revealed that continence nursing is a specialty that is a distinct and defined area of nursing practice, that it requires an application of specially focused knowledge and skill sets, and that it is based on a core body of nursing and/or midwifery knowledge, which is being continually expanded and refined. Nurse continence specialists have a broad base of nursing experience combined with a specialized theoretical and experiential knowledge of bladder, bowel, and pelvic floor dysfunction with a focus on incontinence. It is this combination of theoretical and experiential knowledge that enables the nurse continence specialist to make complex decisions across all of the determinants of health and well-being to promote bladder, bowel, and pelvic floor health and manage dysfunction [12]. The project represents an important first step in the process of international recognition for nurses with specialized knowledge and skill in research, education, and practice in the care of people with urinary and fecal incontinence and other bladder, bowel, and pelvic floor dysfunction.

## 2.10   Competencies for Basic to Specialist Continence Nursing Care

Arguably, many individuals have a role to play in addressing the nursing care needs of individuals with bladder, bowel, and pelvic floor dysfunction. This includes nurses working at varying levels of practice, across varying healthcare settings, as well as non-nurses who care for patients. We identify four broad levels of continence nursing practice:

1. Basic continence nursing care (i.e., nursing aides or technicians, licensed practical or vocational nurses)
2. Skilled continence nursing care (i.e., registered nurses)
3. Specialist continence nursing care (i.e., registered nurses who are certified as continence nurse advisors/specialists/nurse continence specialists)
4. Advanced practice continence nursing care (i.e., advance practice nurse continence specialist, i.e., registered nurses who are certified as clinical nurse specialists/nurse practitioners/continence nurse practitioners)

Further work is needed to assess interest in and feasibility of reaching international agreement about the core knowledge and skill (i.e., competencies) required at these different levels of practice. In the interim, we propose the following set of continence nursing care competencies (see Table 2.2). The competencies for basic continence nursing care practice were sourced from the Nevada State Board of Nursing [35]. Competencies for skilled nursing care are derived from an Australian national consultation that resulted in guidelines for the inclusion of core continence content in undergraduate nursing and midwifery curriculum [36]. These guidelines consist of five recommended core elements and multiple criteria. Competencies for registered nurses who specialize in continence care are drawn from a role description of the wound, ostomy, continence nurse or continence care nurse published by the Wound, Ostomy, and Continence Nurses Society [37].

**Table 2.2** Competencies for basic to specialist continence nursing care

| Basic continence nursing care competencies | Skilled continence nursing care competencies | Specialist continence nursing care competencies |
|---|---|---|
| • Knowledge of key anatomy and physiology of the urinary and digestive systems<br>• Knowledge of normal and abnormal symptoms and when to report<br>• Uses continence products appropriately<br>• Identifies urinary incontinence and common reasons why people become incontinence<br>• Describes nursing care for incontinence<br>• Performs perineal care/peri-care<br>• Explains the relevance of fluid intake<br>• Describes types of catheters and drainage bags<br>• Understands risk of CAUTI<br>• Empties catheter drainage bag/cleans tube<br>• Performs catheter care for males and females<br>• Identifies factors affecting bowel elimination<br>• Explains bladder retraining and the role and responsibility of the CNA<br>• Demonstrates ability to record urinary output<br>• Discusses straining urine<br>• Describes the purpose and performs a bladder scan<br>• Describes measures to help a client regain normal bowel function<br>• Explains why the various types of enemas are given and describes the administration of each<br>• Knowledge of colostomy and ileostomy and associated conditions as an ostomy is a treatment for fecal incontinence<br>• Describes care of an established colostomy | • Knowledge and awareness about incontinence<br>• Knowledge about how to prevent incontinence and promote continence<br>• Knowledge and assessment skills<br>• Clinical reasoning skills<br>• A plan of care that is based upon the best evidence available | • Performs a focused assessment<br>• Obtains a relevant history<br>• Performs bedside testing of bladder filling and sensation<br>• Measures post-void residual urine by catheterization or bladder scan<br>• Synthesizes data related to incontinence to identify individuals at risk, reversible causes, types of urinary incontinence, and common bowel dysfunctions that contribute to fecal and/or urinary incontinence<br>• Diagnoses urge, stress, mixed, and/or functional urinary incontinence<br>• Uses/recommends appropriate management strategies<br>• Educates and counsels patients, families, and staff regarding management techniques<br>• Monitors therapeutic effects of medication<br>• Provides pelvic floor rehabilitation and reeducation via electrical muscle stimulation and biofeedback, in some settings<br>• Evaluates outcomes of interventions and reports to the primary care provider<br>• Refers for recurrent urinary tract infections, hematuria, pelvic organ prolapse, urinary retention, and pelvic pain syndromes<br>• Monitors overall quality of care |

## 2.11    Competencies for Advanced Practice Continence Nursing Care

According to a role description of the Wound, Ostomy, and Continence Nurses Society [37], nurses, who specialize in continence care and who work in advanced practice roles, possess the competencies of nurses who specialize in continence management; however, they have additional advanced competencies in accordance with an advanced level of education at the master's level and with state practice regulations. These competencies are described in Box 2.3.

## 2.12    An Advanced Practice Approach to Continence Care for People with Fecal Incontinence

A review of literature reveals an absence of a holistic framework for an advanced nursing practice approach to fecal incontinence [38]. Drawing on the International Council of Nurses' description of advanced nursing practice [2], we propose that this approach requires competencies in the categories of clinical practice, research,

---

**Box 2.3: Competencies for Advanced Practice Continence Nursing Care**
- Performs a comprehensive physical assessment that may include a pelvic examination for masses, prolapse, and urethral hypermobility, a digital rectal exam of the prostate, and a neurologic assessment
- Synthesizes data
- Uses/recommends appropriate management strategies including the following interventions:
  - Interprets diagnostic studies such as urodynamic studies and studies of bowel motility and elimination
  - Prescribes pharmacologic treatment for common conditions of the urinary tract and bowel such as urinary tract infection, overactive bladder, constipation, and diarrhea
  - Provides care for common gynecological conditions such as vaginitis and pelvic organ prolapse (i.e., fitting and management of pessaries)
  - Performs complex, multichannel urodynamic studies with or without fluoroscopic imaging
  - Performs anorectal manometry studies
  - Provides initial conservative interventions regarding lifestyle modifications
  - Provides secondary conservative interventions such as pelvic floor rehabilitation and reeducation via electrical muscle stimulation and biofeedback [37] (p. 4)
- Participates as a member of multidisciplinary specialty teams offering tertiary treatments

leadership, and consultation. Moreover, advanced continence nursing care for people with fecal incontinence is likely to differ by geographic location, practice setting, individual skill expertise, and client needs. We developed a set of competencies for advanced nursing practice for the management of fecal incontinence using existing resources: the International Council of Nurses categories for advanced practice nursing [2], the Canadian Nurses Association framework [8], guidelines from the International Consultation on Incontinence [39], guidelines for assessment and management of fecal incontinence and quality of life in adults [40], guidelines for the management of constipation from the Registered Nurses Association of Ontario [41], and recommendations from a nursing consultation about research on incontinence [42] (see Table 2.3).

**Table 2.3** Advanced nursing practice competencies for the management of fecal incontinence

| Competency category | Illustration of enactment of competencies |
| --- | --- |
| Clinical practice | • Perform an advanced assessment of fecal incontinence including health history and physical examination<br>• Diagnose and manage the type of fecal incontinence in a wide range of patient presentations and complex situations while considering sociological, psychological, and physiological processes<br>• Assess and manage skin damage associated with fecal incontinence<br>• Identify and implement research-based interventions to improve client care related to fecal incontinence |
| Research | • Contribute to the identification of priority areas for continence nursing research<br>• Conduct research on priority areas in order to generate new knowledge to support nursing practice<br>• Disseminate research findings and promote their translation into practice<br>• Evaluate current practice at system level in relation to inclusion of emerging research findings related to fecal incontinence |
| Leadership | • Advocate for individuals with fecal incontinence in the public policy domain (such as importance of accessible bathrooms in public and employment spaces)<br>• Identify the learning needs of nurses and other members of the healthcare team related to fecal incontinence and develop programs and resources to meet those needs (such as best practice guidelines)<br>• Evaluate programs in practice settings related to fecal incontinence (such as toileting support for older adult inpatients with mobility impairments) and develop solutions with the interdisciplinary team |
| Consultation | • Collaborate with other disciplines to synthesize qualitative and quantitative research on fecal incontinence (e.g., by participating in international consultations)<br>• Provide consultation to other healthcare providers in practice setting related to complex clients with fecal incontinence<br>• Collaborate with interdisciplinary teams to develop quality improvement strategies related to fecal incontinence |

## 2.13   Education for Advanced Nursing Practice in Continence Care for People with Fecal Incontinence

Educational preparation is foundational to advanced nursing practice and is what differentiates advanced from specialist and generalist nursing practice. The knowledge and skills required to practice at an advanced level to care for people with fecal incontinence are related to the key competencies of advanced nursing practice and a defined scope of practice [2]. Direct clinical care is the core competency, and research, leadership, and consultation competencies support the delivery of this care to persons with fecal incontinence [2].

As previously indicated, the minimum educational requirement for advanced nursing practice has historically been a master's degree [2]. However, nursing scholars in the USA have recently called for a "doctor of nursing practice degree" as the entry degree for advanced nursing practice, and this concept has been explored in wound, ostomy, and continence nursing communities of practice [43].

While many nurses and advanced practice nurses have a clinical focus in continence care, education about incontinence (including fecal incontinence) in graduate and undergraduate programs is scant [36, 44]. A national review of educational content about incontinence in undergraduate nursing curriculum in Australia found the majority of nursing academics were unlikely to possess foundational knowledge in incontinence and would require external support from advanced practice nurses in incontinence in order to integrate continence promotion concepts into their courses [36].

There are a limited number of nursing faculties that offer postgraduate programs that prepare RNs to practice at an advanced level in continence nursing. Few focus on the management of incontinence alone, and even less focus on fecal incontinence. In Australia, La Trobe University School of Nursing and Midwifery offers a Masters of Nursing course that has a special focus on urology and continence nursing. It is a 1.5-year, full-time or 2–3-year, part-time award with exit options available at either the graduate certificate, postgraduate diploma, or Masters of Nursing level. The course is delivered online, and students need to be working with people who have bowel and/or bladder health problems.

Similar to other countries profiled in this text, at this point in time, Canada does not have graduate-level programs that prepare nurses for advanced practice nursing roles in continence. To address this curricular gap, Canadian clinical nurse specialists and nurse practitioners working with specialized populations such as older adults, women, or wound care typically pursue post-basic education programs to develop their expertise in continence promotion either as nurse continence advisors or enterostomal therapists. The Nurse Continence Advisor Continuing Education Certificate Program offered by distance education at McMaster University in Hamilton, Ontario, is a 1-year program that combines academic study with preceptored and independent clinical practice. This program is the only university-based program for educating nurse continence advisors in Canada. The Canadian Association for Enterostomal Therapy Academy is an online continuing educational resource that prepares registered nurses to practice in wound, ostomy, and continence nursing. This 1-year program includes both online and practical components.

Key barriers to the establishment and sustainability of highly specialized courses for advanced nursing practice such as postgraduate nursing programs on incontinence are competing fiscal priorities and the limited availability of nursing academics to champion and teach these programs. For example, the Faculty of Medicine, Nursing, and Health Sciences at Flinders University in Australia previously offered a highly acclaimed, articulated, continuing, and postgraduate education program on incontinence. The Graduate Certificate in Nursing (continence nurse advisor) was an 18-unit program that provided the opportunity for individuals from any professional background who were working in health-related areas to deepen the knowledge base on which their practice was grounded. The Graduate Diploma in Nursing (continence nurse advisor) distance education course articulated with the Graduate Certificate in Nursing and the Masters of Nursing. The graduate diploma equipped nurses with the knowledge and skills in the area of continence nursing and extended their general theoretical preparation in nursing knowledge and research. The continence nurse advisor specialization was identified on the student's transcript of academic record and on the parchment presented to the student on completion of the course. The articulated nature of the program was particularly important as many students were hospital trained.

Despite evidence from the National Institute for Clinical Effectiveness [45] about the importance of incontinence, there is a paucity of educational preparation for both generalist and specialist nurses in the UK about incontinence. The education that is available about fecal incontinence is woven into curricula that tends to focus mainly on bladder dysfunction and is usually offered to nurses and other healthcare professionals as a 1-day study event, with or without accreditation. This gap in education could lead to variations in care [46]. Indeed, recent national audits of practice in UK hospitals, community, and care homes reveal considerable variation in the quality of continence care, particularly for older people [47]. The findings exposed gaps in best practice and suggested that continence care was poorly organized, with inadequate training. Although change is yet to be strengthened for post-registration training and indeed advanced nursing practice, the UK Nursing and Midwifery Council [48] is committed to improving preregistration standards of education, which has an opportunity to steer a fit-for-purpose workforce.

According to Schober [2], the curriculum to support the preparation of nurses for advanced nursing practice should include core theory courses, clinical core courses, and specialty courses. Arguably, courses should reflect the context of the country, the academy, and the local requirements of specialty practice (such as aging, chronic illness, dementia care, oncology, etc.) [2, 49]. Core theory courses could be more broad-based components of graduate nursing programs and include education about a theoretical approach to nursing, research methodology, health education, and health policy [49]. The specific curriculum required to advance clinical skills in the management of fecal incontinence should include an overview of fecal incontinence and the gastrointestinal system, information about advanced physical assessment, and management of fecal incontinence, including advanced pharmacology. It should also offer a mentored clinical practicum experience that is purposefully designed to develop advanced nursing practice skills related to fecal incontinence [49].

Table 2.4 lists a set of clinical topics for inclusion in a curriculum for an advanced nursing practice approach to fecal incontinence. Consistent with the approach used to

**Table 2.4** Clinical topics for inclusion in a curriculum to support the preparation of nurses for advanced nursing practice in the management of fecal incontinence

| Unit | Content |
|------|---------|
| Overview of fecal incontinence | • Prevalence<br>• Incidence<br>• Risk factors<br>• Associated chronic conditions<br>• Social impact<br>• Healthcare system approach<br>• Clinical practice guidelines |
| Gastrointestinal system | • Anatomy and physiology<br>• Normal evacuation<br>• Pathophysiology<br>• Internationally standardized terminology |
| Advanced physical assessment | • History<br>• Physical<br>• Standardized questionnaires<br>• Secondary assessments (i.e., manometry)<br>• Anal inspection<br>• Abdominal palpation<br>• Neurological examination<br>• Digital rectal examination |
| Management | • Patient goals<br>• Diet and fluid<br>• Bowel habit<br>• Advanced pharmacology<br>• Incontinence products<br>• Practical coping strategies |

develop advanced nursing practice competencies described in Table 2.4, the topic list was developed with reference to the International Council of Nurses categories for advanced practice nursing [2]; the Canadian Nurses Association framework [8]; guidelines from the International Consultation on Incontinence [39] including guidelines for the assessment and management of fecal incontinence and quality of life in adults [40], as well as guidelines about the management of constipation from the Registered Nurses Association of Ontario [41]; recommendations from a nursing consultation about research on incontinence [42]; and a key publication by Rogalski [49].

## 2.14   The Effectiveness of Nurses with Advanced Practice Skills in Continence Care for People with Fecal Incontinence

Nurses play a pivotal role in generating foundational knowledge about incontinence; in implementing and evaluating conservative interventions to prevent, improve, and treat incontinence; and in disseminating evidence-based interventions, as well as translational methods to embed these interventions into everyday practice. The effects of nursing interventions on the frequency and severity of urinary incontinence and pelvic floor symptoms are established [50]; however, there is limited evidence about outcomes for people with fecal incontinence. Table 2.5

**Table 2.5** Experimental studies that describe the outcomes of nursing interventions for the management of fecal or anal incontinence

| Study | Aim | Design | Sample/setting | Intervention | Findings | Nurses title, qualification, and role |
|---|---|---|---|---|---|---|
| Bartlett et al. (2015) [51] | To assess the effect of supplementary home-based biofeedback for fecal incontinence | Randomized controlled trial | 75 community-residing adults from an outpatient clinic in Australia | Standard biofeedback + perineometer at home compared to standard biofeedback | Supplementary home biofeedback did not result in greater clinical improvement for the intervention group as a whole. A subanalysis revealed younger age was associated with better outcomes | Not reported |
| Bliss et al. (2013) [52] | To assess outcomes of care by certified WOC nurses for home healthcare (HHC) patients | Descriptive and comparative | 449,170 episodes of care from a national convenience sample of 785 HHC agencies in the USA with 447,309 adult non-maternity patients between Oct. 1, 2008, and Dec. 31, 2009 | Usual care by WOC nurses | Significant improvements for patients cared for by a WOC nurse, despite having more frequent and severe problems than other patients. HHC patients not cared for by WOC nurses, with less-severe wound and incontinence problems, also improved | Certified WOC nurses |

| | | | | | | |
|---|---|---|---|---|---|---|
| Goodman et al. (2013) [53] | To test if a clinical benchmarking tool (Essence of Care) improves bowel-related care | Quasi-experimental | Older people living in six care homes in the UK | A clinical tool compared to advice about continence services contact details | No significant reduction in bowel-related problems, although one care home had fewer avoidable episodes of fecal incontinence | District nurses and care home staff |
| Harari et al. (2004) [54] | To evaluate treatment of constipation and fecal incontinence in persons who have survived a stroke | Randomized controlled trial | 122 community-dwelling and 24 in-patient rehabilitation persons in UK who had had stroke within 4 years and bowel dysfunction | One-time assessment by nurse followed by targeted patient and caregiver education, provision of booklet, summary of diagnosis, and treatment to physician | Percentage of normal bowel movements as graded by patients was higher in intervention group; no significant reduction in fecal incontinence. At 12 months, intervention patients more likely to have made diet and fluid modifications and sought physician care for bowel concerns | "Nonspecialist study nurse" with education in bowel management |

(continued)

**Table 2.5** (continued)

| Study | Aim | Design | Sample/setting | Intervention | Findings | Nurses title, qualification, and role |
|---|---|---|---|---|---|---|
| Northwood et al. (2014) [55] | To evaluate a program of five NCA-led continence clinics | Program evaluation (pre-post design) | Five NCA-led continence clinics in Southern Ontario, Canada, and the older adult clients who attended these clinics during the evaluation period | NCAs performed a comprehensive, standardized assessment, identified contributing factors of urinary and fecal incontinence, and taught conservative, behavioral methods | Improved self-efficacy (measured by the Geriatric Self-Efficacy for Urinary Incontinence), goal achievement (measured by goal attainment scaling), 50% reduction in incontinence product costs and 78% reduction in laundry | NCAs |
| Norton et al. (2003) [56] | (a) To assess the effects of biofeedback compared to attention control, (b) identify important elements of biofeedback and, (c) determine if patients with anal sphincter disruption are less likely to respond to biofeedback than patients with an intact sphincter | Randomized controlled trial | 71 people with fecal incontinence attending an outpatient clinic in the UK | (a) Standard care (advice), (b) advice plus instruction about sphincter exercises, (c) hospital-based computer-assisted sphincter pressure biofeedback, (d) hospital biofeedback plus electromyelogram biofeedback at home | No differences in outcomes between the groups at the end of treatment or at 12 months | Nurse-led management by a specialist nurse |

| | Aim | Design | Sample | Intervention | Results | Provider |
|---|---|---|---|---|---|---|
| Ostaszkiewicz et al. (2010) [57] | To assess the effects of an individualized, multimodal, conservative intervention on symptom severity and quality of life in community-dwelling adults with constipation and lower urinary tract symptoms | Within-subject, pretest-posttest design and purposeful recruitment | 27 community-dwelling adults aged 35–83 years (mean age, 63.85 years) with lower urinary tract symptoms and constipation who presented to a community-based nurse-led continence service in Australia | Individualized conservative treatment of constipation that comprised advice on dietary supplementation, fluid intake, exercise, position to defecate, the gastrocolic reflex, and over-the-counter laxatives | Significant reductions in the severity of overall constipation symptoms measured by the PAC-SYM ($T = 75.5$, $P < 0.01$.) and in overall quality of life as measured by the PAC-QOL ($T = 48.5$, $P < 0.01$) | Nurse-led management by specialist nurse |
| Tappin et al. (2013) [58] | To assess routine consultant pediatrician-led care against minimum standards and develop and evaluate a nurse-led intervention | Audit followed by service development and evaluation | Case notes of 30 children (aged 1–13 years) referred to secondary care in Scotland | A nurse-led intervention focused on self-help using NICE guideline support compared to routine consultant pediatrician care | No statistically significant differences between intervention and comparison groups for constipation, passing a stool that would block the toilet, having retentive withholding behavior or painful defecation in last week, being better than prior to first clinic visit, still taking medication or Movicol | An experienced pediatric nurse who had been a generic health visitor for years, with experience using a prescriptive psychological intervention |

identifies full-text English language randomized controlled trials, quasi-experimental studies, or cohort studies that describe the outcomes of nursing interventions for the management of fecal or anal incontinence. As information about the nurse's qualifications and role is limited, it is unclear if the nurse's role is consistent with the International Council of Nurse's definition of advanced nursing practice.

The best available evidence about the effectiveness of nursing intervention for the management of fecal incontinence is based on two randomized controlled trials. The most recent of these was a trial of home-based biofeedback in a sample of 75 community residing adults in Australia [51]. Thirty-nine adults were randomized to standard biofeedback combined with the use of a perineometer, and 36 were randomized to standard biofeedback protocol (control). The nurse conducted an assessment, i.e., a medical, surgical, and medication history including bowel problems and habits, as well as diet, fiber, and fluid intake. Anorectal function and proctometrographic evaluation were assessed using clinic manometric equipment, and relaxation (diaphragmatic) breathing was taught. Patients were advised to practice relaxation breathing for 7–10 min at least twice/day and complete a bowel chart/food diary for the following week. Intervention participants were also instructed in the use of the perineometer and in how to perform rapid and sustained anal sphincter and pelvic floor muscle exercises. The researchers reported supplementary home biofeedback did not result in greater clinical improvement for the intervention group as a whole; however, continence and the quality of life of younger people in the intervention group were significantly better than those of their control counterparts.

Norton et al. [52] compared nurse-led biofeedback with standard care in a randomized controlled trial of 171 patients with fecal incontinence. The participants were randomized to one of four groups: (a) standard care (advice), (b) advice plus instruction on sphincter exercises, (c) hospital-based computer-assisted sphincter pressure biofeedback, and (d) hospital biofeedback plus the use of a home electromyelogram biofeedback device. There were no differences in outcomes between the groups at the end of treatment or at 12 months. Neither pelvic floor exercises nor biofeedback was superior to standard care supplemented by advice and education. Box 2.4 summarizes the main points discussed in this chapter for the attention of the advanced practice nurse caring for the patient with fecal incontinence.

**Box 2.4: Summary Points**
- Advanced practice nursing includes specialization but also includes expansion of the scope of nursing practice and educational advancement. It is characterized by an advanced level of education and responsibilities, role autonomy, and the diagnosis and management of illness as well as health promotion, which include pharmacological and non-pharmacological interventions.
- Continence nursing is a specialty that is a distinct and defined area of nursing practice that requires the application of specialty-focused knowledge and skill sets. It is based on a core body of nursing and/or nurse midwifery knowledge that is being continually expanded and refined.

- Many registered nurses specialize in the management of incontinence and other bladder, bowel, and pelvic floor disorders and work in clinical, educational, consultative, managerial, or research roles.
- Registered nurses who specialize in continence care who work in advanced practice roles possess the competencies both of nurses who specialize in continence management and those in an advanced practice role. They have an advanced level of education at the master's or DNP level and in accordance with professional and legal regulations.
- There is a need to develop educational programs that prepare registered nurses to practice at an advanced level in continence nursing. In some countries, there is also a need to develop formal educational programs for the continence nurse specialist.
- This chapter proposes a set of competencies for advanced nursing practice for the management of fecal incontinence as well as a list of topics for inclusion in an associated curriculum.
- The effects of nursing interventions on the frequency and severity of urinary incontinence and pelvic floor symptoms are well established; however, further research is required to establish the efficacy of nursing interventions for people with fecal incontinence.

## References

1. International Council of Nursing Nurse Practitioner/Advanced Practice Nursing Network. Definition and characteristics of the role. http://international.aanp.org/Practice/APNRoles.
2. Schober M. Introduction to advanced nursing practice: an international focus. Cham: Springer International; 2016.
3. National Council of State Boards of Nursing. Advanced practice registered nurses: consensus model for APRN regulation: licensure, accreditation, certification and education. 2008. https://www.ncsbn.org/aprn-consensus.htm.
4. The American Nurses' Association. Scope and standards of advanced practice registered nursing. 2nd ed. Silver Spring, MD: American Nurses Association; 2010.
5. Gardner G, Duffield C, Doubrovsky A, Adams M. Identifying advanced practice: a national survey of a nursing workforce. Int J Nurs Stud. 2016;55(Suppl C):60–70.
6. Nursing and Midwifery Board of Australia. Registrant data. 2016. http://www.nursingmidwiferyboard.gov.au/About/Statistics.aspx.
7. Nursing and Midwifery Board of Australia. Registration standard: endorsement as a nurse practitioner. 2016. http://www.nursingmidwiferyboard.gov.au/Registration-Standards/Endorsement-as-a-nurse-practitioner.aspx.
8. Canadian Nurses Association. Advancing nursing practice: a national framework. 2008. https://cna-aiic.ca/~/media/cna/page-content/pdf-en/anp_national_framework_e.pdf.
9. Department of International Affairs of the Japanese Nursing Association. Nursing in Japan. Tokyo: Japanese Nursing Association; 2016. p. 1–17.
10. Royal College of Nursing. Advanced nurse practitioners: An RCN guide to advanced nursing practice, advanced nurse practitioners, and program accreditation. https://www.rcn.org.uk/professional-development/publications/pub-003207.
11. Nursing and Midwifery Board of Australia. Registered nurse standards for practice. 2016. http://www.nursingmidwiferyboard.gov.au/Codes-Guidelines-Statements/Professional-standards/registered-nurse-standards-for-practice.aspx.

12. Paterson J, Ostaszkiewicz J, Suyasa IGPD, Skelly J, Bellefeuille L. Development and validation of the role profile of the nurse continence specialist: a project of the International Continence Society. J Wound Ostomy Cont Nurs. 2016;43(6):641–7.
13. Martin-Misener R, Bryant-Lukosius D. Guest editors' reflections on progress in the development of advanced practice nursing in Canada. Nurs Leadersh. 2016;29(3):6–13.
14. Canadian Nurses Association. Number of valid CNA certifications by specialty/area of nursing practice and province or territory. 2017. https://www.cna-aiic.ca/-/media/cna/page-content/pdf-en/cert_by_specialty_and_area_2010_e.pdf.
15. Eggertson L. Inspiring confidence to overcome incontinence. Nurse continence advisors help their patients regain control. Can Nurse. 2014;110(7):18.
16. Sheer B, Wong FKY. The development of advanced nursing practice globally. J Nurs Scholarsh. 2008;40(3):204–11.
17. Pulcini J, Jelic M, Gul R, Loke AY. An international survey on advanced practice nursing education, practice, and regulation. J Nurs Scholarsh. 2010;42(1):31–9.
18. Sibbald B, Laurant M, Reeves D. Advanced nurse roles in UK primary care. Med J Aust. 2006;185(1):10–2.
19. King R, Tod A, Sanders T. Regulation of advanced nurse practitioners: understanding the current processes in the UK. Nurs Stand. 2017;32(14):43–50.
20. Royal College of Nursing. RCN's position on advanced nursing practice. https://my.rcn.org.uk/data/assets/pdf_file/0017/290231/RCN_position_on_advanced_nursing_pratice.pdf. 2009.
21. Wickham S. What history can teach us today, looking at the development of advanced nursing practice and clinical nurse specialism. Int J Nurs Clin Pract. 2017;4(222):2.
22. Royal College of Nursing (RCN). RCN factsheet: Specialist nursing in the UK. 2013. http://www.rcn.org.uk/__data/assets/pdf_file/0018/501921/4.13_RCN_Factsheet_on_Specialist_nursing_in_UK_-_2013.pdf.
23. All Party Parliamentary Group for Continence Care. Continence care services England 2013: survey report. 2013.
24. Department of Health, editor. Good practice in continence services. Department of Health: London; 2000. https://www.nhs.uk/chq/Documents/2015%20uploads/DH%20-%20Good%20practice%20in%20continence%20services.pdf.
25. The United Kingdom Continence Society (UKCS). Minimum standards for continence care in the UK. 2015. http://www.ukcs.uk.net/wp-content/uploads/2016/04/15091716_Revised_Min_Standards_for_CC_in_UK.pdf.
26. The National Health Service England. Excellence in continence care framework. 2015.
27. Hamric AB, Hanson CM, Tracy MF, O'Grady ET. Advanced practice nursing: an integrative approach. 3rd ed. Philadelphia, PA: Saunders/Elsevier; 2013.
28. Wound Ostomy and Continence Nursing Certification Board. https://www.wocncb.org/.
29. Roe BH. Development of continence advisory services in the United Kingdom. Scand J Caring Sci. 1990;4(2):51–4.
30. Rhodes P, Parker G. The role of the continence adviser in England and Wales. Int J Nurs Stud. 1995;32(5):423–33.
31. Fader M. Practice in England. In: College U, editor. Unpublished manuscript presented at the 31st Annual Conference of Wound, Ostomy, and Continence Nurses ed. London; 1999.
32. Brink C, Wells T, Diokno A. A continence clinic for the aged. J Gerontol Nurs. 1983;9(12):651–5.
33. Skelly J, Kenny K. The impact of the nurse continence advisor on continence care. Clin Eff Nurs. 1998;2(1):4–10.
34. Milne JL, Moore KN. An exploratory study of continence care services worldwide. Int J Nurs Stud. 2003;40(3):235–47.
35. Nevada State Board of Nursing. Nursing assistant training program. 2006. p 1–34.
36. Paterson J. Consultation, consensus and commitment to guidelines for inclusion of continence into undergraduate nursing and midwifery curricula. The Commonwealth Department of Health and Ageing: Adelaide; 2006.
37. Wound Ostomy and Continence Nurses Society Position Statement. Role of the wound ostomy continence nurse or continence nurse in continence care. J Wound Ostomy Cont Nurs. 2009;36(5):529–31.

38. Norton C. Nurses, bowel continence, stigma, and taboos. J Wound Ostomy Cont Nurs. 2004;31(2):85–94.
39. Abrams P, Cardozo L, Wagg A, Wein A, editors. Incontinence. 6th ed. Bristol: International Continence Society; 2017.
40. Bliss DZ, Mimura T, Berghmans B, Bharucha A, Chiarioni G, Emmanuel A, et al. Assessment and conservative management of fecal incontinence and quality of life in adults. In: Abrams P, Cardozo L, Wagg A, Wein A, editors. Incontinence. 6th ed. Bristol: International Continence Society; 2017. p. 1993–2085.
41. Registered Nurses Association of Ontario (RNAO). Prevention of constipation in the older adult population. Toronto, ON: Registered Nurses Association of Ontario; 2011. www.rnao.org/bestpractices/
42. Bliss DZ, Norton CA, Miller J, Krissovich M. Directions for future nursing research on fecal incontinence. Nurs Res. 2004;53(6S):S15–21.
43. Pieper B, Colwell J. Doctoral education for WOC nurses considering advanced practice nursing. J Wound Ostomy Cont Nurs. 2012;39(3):249–55.
44. McClurg D, Cheater F, Eustice S, Burke J, Jamieson K, Hagen S. A multi-professional UK wide survey of undergraduate continence education. Neurourol Urodyn. 2012;32(3):224–9.
45. National Institute of Health and Care Excellence (NICE). Fecal incontinence: the management of fecal incontinence in adults. 2007. https://www.nice.org.uk/guidance/cg49.
46. Harari D, Norton C, Lockwood L, Swift C. Treatment of constipation and fecal incontinence in stroke patients. Stroke. 2004;35(11):2549–55.
47. Royal College of Physicians (RCP). National audit of continence care (NACC): pilot audit evaluation report. London: Royal College of Physicians; 2012.
48. Nursing and Midwifery Council (NMC). Consultation on education framework: standards for education and training. 2017. https://www.nmc.org.uk/education/education-consultation/framework/.
49. Rogalski NM. A graduate nursing curriculum for the evaluation and management of urinary incontinence. Educ Gerontol. 2005;31(2):139–59.
50. Du Moulin M, Hamers J, Paulus A, Berendsen C, Halfens R. The role of the nurse in community continence care: a systematic review. Int J Nurs Stud. 2005;42(4):479–92.
51. Bartlett L, Sloots K, Nowak M, Ho Y-H. Supplementary home biofeedback improves quality of life in younger patients with fecal incontinence. J Clin Gastroenterol. 2015;49(5):419–28.
52. Bliss DZ, Westra BL, Savik K, Hou Y. Effectiveness of wound, ostomy and continence-certified nurses on individual patient outcomes in home health care. J Wound Ostomy Cont Nurs. 2013;40(2):135–42.
53. Goodman C, Davies SL, Norton C, Fader M, Morris J, Wells M, et al. Can district nurses and care home staff improve bowel care for older people using a clinical benchmarking tool? Br J Community Nurs. 2013;18(12):580–7.
54. Harari D, Husk J, Lowe D, Wagg A. National audit of continence care: adherence to National Institute for Health and Clinical Excellence (NICE) guidance in older versus younger adults with faecal incontinence. Age Ageing. 2014;43(6):785–93.
55. Northwood M, Skelly J. Improving continence care for older adults in the community: chronic care model mobilized. Perspectives. 2014;37(1):15–8.
56. Norton C, Chelvanayagam S, Wilson-Barnett J, Redfern S, Kamm MA. Randomized controlled trial of biofeedback for fecal incontinence. Gastroenterology. 2003;125(5):1320–9.
57. Ostaszkiewicz J, Hornby L, Millar L, Ockerby C. The effects of conservative treatment for constipation on symptom severity and quality of life in community-dwelling adults. J Wound Ostomy Cont Nurs. 2010;37(2):193–8.
58. Tappin D, Nawaz S, McKay C, MacLaren L, Griffiths P, Mohammed TA. Development of an early nurse led intervention to treat children referred to secondary paediatric care with constipation with or without soiling. BMC Pediatr. 2013;13:193.

# Epidemiology of Fecal Incontinence

**3**

Maria Helena Baena de Moraes Lopes, Juliana Neves da
Costa, Vera Lúcia Conceição de Gouveia Santos,
and Jaqueline Betteloni Junqueira

**Abstract**
This chapter will present an overview of the epidemiology of fecal incontinence in different populations and countries of the world. Findings are limited to studies published in the last 5 years (2012–2017). The majority of the studies were carried out with women and adults and in outpatient settings. Only one article was found that reported the prevalence of fecal incontinence in children, and the sample was a very specific subgroup, i.e., children with attention deficit hyperactivity disorder. The prevalence data vary widely depending on the population studied and the setting. The variation in rates also reflects the different methodologies adopted for investigating the phenomenon, such as the theoretical and operational definition of the type of incontinence and data collection procedures, among other aspects.

**Keywords**
Anal incontinence · Fecal incontinence · Epidemiology · Incidence · Prevalence

## 3.1 Prevalence and Incidence of Fecal Incontinence

According to the 6th International Consultation on Incontinence and International Continence Society, fecal incontinence is the involuntary loss of feces, and anal incontinence is the involuntary loss of feces, flatus, and/or mucus [1] (see Chap. 1). In addition, the Rome III Diagnostic Criteria for Functional Gastrointestinal

M. H. B. de Moraes Lopes (✉) · J. N. da Costa
Faculty of Nursing, University of Campinas, Campinas, SP, Brazil

V. L. C. de Gouveia Santos · J. B. Junqueira
School of Nursing of the University of São Paulo, São Paulo, SP, Brazil
e-mail: veras@usp.br

Disorders includes the diagnosis "functional fecal incontinence," defined as "recurrent and uncontrolled elimination of fecal material in an individual with development corresponding to at least four years of age, associated with one or more of the following: abnormal functioning of normally enervated and structurally intact sphincter muscles; discrete structural abnormality and/or innervation of the sphincter muscles; normal or altered bowel habit (for example, fecal retention or diarrhea) and psychological causes." For this classification, it is necessary to exclude structural or neurogenic abnormalities as causes of incontinence [2].

Frequency rates of fecal incontinence—prevalence and incidence—reflect the different methodologies adopted for investigating the phenomenon, such as the theoretical definition of the condition, the population studied, and the means of data collection, among other aspects, besides the real variations of occurrence. The systematic review by Sharma et al., 2016, confirms this assertion, showing that the prevalence of fecal incontinence varied widely depending on the methods used for data collection and the definition of incontinence adopted (type and frequency of episodes of fecal incontinence) [3]. When calculating the combined prevalence rate of functional fecal incontinence studies, defined according to ROMA II criteria, the authors obtained 5.9% (95% CI 5.6–6.3) in adults residing in the community [4].

Another systematic review investigated the relationship between obstetric trauma of the anal sphincter (episiotomy and third and fourth degree perineal laceration) and 25 anal incontinence after vaginal delivery and showed a significant relationship between perineal trauma (episiotomy [OR, 1.74; 95% CI, 1.28–2.38; $Q = 8.9$; $p < 0.26$; $I(2) = 21.4$] and third- or fourth-degree perineal laceration [OR, 2.66; 95% CI, 1.77–3.98; $Q = 27.9$; $p = 0.002$; $I2 = 64.1$]) and anal incontinence [5].

The present chapter will present an overview of the epidemiology of fecal and/or anal incontinence in different populations and countries of the world established through a review conducted in the databases Embase, CINAHL, Web of Science, Lilacs, and PubMed, in the last 5 years (2012–2017). Search terms used were *fecal incontinence* OR *epidemiology* AND *prevalence* OR *incidence* and the uncontrolled term *anal incontinence*. Studies with cross-sectional, cohort, or case control designs, clinical trials, or systematic reviews that described the prevalence and/or incidence of fecal incontinence were included. Editorials or case studies were excluded. Results were supplemented with published studies known or referred to the authors who were not identified by the search. The literature search identified 44 studies, and two additional ones were referred for a total of 46 studies. Of the total number of studies found, 20 investigated fecal incontinence, 25 anal incontinence, and one examined anal and fecal incontinence. Studies are organized by clinical setting, i.e., community, hospital, and nursing home.

## 3.2    Community-Living People

The prevalence of fecal incontinence in the general adult population has been reported to be approximately 10% [6]. Prevalence of fecal incontinence in various groups of adults in the community in different countries in recent studies ranged from 14.7% to 19.5% [7–12]. In studies only of women, the rates were 4.7 % [8] and

**Table 3.1** Prevalence of fecal and anal incontinence in the community by year, country, and population

| Country | Author, year of publication | Population | Type of incontinence | Prevalence |
|---|---|---|---|---|
| USA | Brown et al., 2012 [16] | Women aged 45 years or over (community) | Anal | 18.8% |
| USA | McKeown et al., 2013 [13] | Children with ADHD (military database) | Fecal | 0.9% |
| USA | Matthews et al., 2013 [7] | Women (community) | Fecal | 4.7% |
| USA | Townsend et al., 2013 [17] | Adults (community) | Anal | 20% |
| Australia | Halland et al., 2013 [8] | Older women (82–87 years) (community) | Fecal | 9.7% |
| Singapore | Lim et al., 2014 [14] | Adults (community) | Anal | 4.7% |
| Brazil | Santos et al., 2014 [9] | Adults (community) | Fecal | 3.6% (4% for women and 3% for men) |
| Finland | Lehto et al., 2014 [15] | Adults (community) | Anal | 58% |
| USA | Ditah et al., 2014 [18] | Adults (community) | Anal | 8.39% (9.4% for women, 7.3% for men) |
| USA | Wu et al., 2015 [19] | Adults (community) | Anal | 8.2% (women) and 8.4% (men) |
| Australia | Ng et al., 2015 [10] | Adults (community) (review) | Fecal | 7.7% (2–20.7%) 8.9% (women) 8.1% (men) |
| USA | Noelting et al., 2016 [11] | Adults (community) | Fecal | 10% |
| USA | Andy et al., 2016 [20] | Adults (community) | Anal | 11.2% (women) and 8.6% (men) |
| New Zealand | Sharma et al., 2016 [3] | Adults (community) (review) | Fecal | 1.4–19.5% |
| Netherlands | Meinds et al., 2017 [12] | Adults (national database) | Fecal | 7.9% |

*ADHD* attention deficit hyperactivity disorder

9.7% [9]. In the only study found of children, the prevalence of fecal incontinence was 0.9% [13]. Prevalence of anal incontinence in the community in different countries was 4.7% to 58% [14–20]. In studies conducted only with women, the rate of anal incontinence was 18.8% [16] (see Table 3.1).

## 3.3   Hospitals and ICUs

The prevalence of preexisting fecal incontinence or the incidence of new onset fecal incontinence in acute care is difficult to determine due to the dearth of research in this area. Nair et al., 2000, reported a point prevalence for fecal incontinence of 12%

on an audit of older adult patients on medical units in an Australian hospital [21], while Bayón García et al., 2012, found a prevalence of 9–37% in a large multisite study of European critical care units [22]. In a prospective study of 152 patients on acute and critical care units in a US hospital, Bliss and colleagues, 2000, reported a cumulative incidence of fecal incontinence of 33% [23].

Risk factors for fecal incontinence in hospitalized patients included loose or liquid stool, severity of illness, and older age [23]. Akpan et al., 2007, reported loose stools as more prevalent in a sample of UK hospitalized older adults with fecal incontinence than those in rehabilitation, nursing home, or home settings [24]. These authors also reported functional disability as more prevalent in the hospitalized group. Factors that are barriers to assessment and management of fecal incontinence in the acute care setting include poor understanding and recognition of geriatric syndromes [21], lack of assessment of fecal incontinence by generalist nurses and physicians [21, 25], lack of adoption of standardized assessment and protocols on admission and throughout the patients' stay in hospital in the acute care setting [22], and practitioner omission or patient declining a focused physical examination including digital rectal exam [24, 25]. Patients in critical care are at a high risk for fecal incontinence with most experiencing at least one episode [26, 27].

The prevalence of fecal incontinence in different groups of outpatients was 6.4% to 12.1% [10, 28] while in hospitalized patients it ranged from 2.2% to 37% [22, 28, 29]. The prevalence of anal incontinence ranged from 8.3% to 8 7% in various outpatient groups [30–39] and from 6.1% to 50% in inpatients [40–42] (see Table 3.2). The population of patients (ambulatory or hospitalized) with anal incontinence was eminently female. Prevalence was high in postpartum women (16.5% and 50%) [31, 42] and those with irritable bowel syndrome (69%) [37] (see Table 3.2).

**Table 3.2** Prevalence of fecal and anal incontinence in outpatients or hospitalized patients by year and country

| Country | Author, year of publication | Population | Type of incontinence | Prevalence |
|---|---|---|---|---|
| Germany (n = 94), Italy (n = 165), Spain (n = 144), UK (n = 127) | Bayón García et al., 2012 [22] | Adults (intensive care unit) | Fecal | General = 9–37% Germany = 36.9% Italy = 11.7% Spain = 8.7% UK = 13.6% |
| South Africa | Naidoo et al., 2012 [41] | Pregnant women (hospitalized) | Anal | 6.1% |
| South Korea | Kang et al., 2012 [28] | Adults (outpatient) | Fecal | 6.4% (6.8% of women; 6.2% of men) |
| Spain | Parés et al., 2012 [30] | Patients with obesity (outpatient) | Anal | 32.7% |
| USA | Alsheik et al., 2012 [39] | Adults (outpatient) | Anal | 12% |

**Table 3.2** (continued)

| Country | Author, year of publication | Population | Type of incontinence | Prevalence |
|---|---|---|---|---|
| Sri Lanka | Rajeshkannan et al., 2013 [31] | Women postpartum (outpatient) | Anal | 16.5% |
| Malaysian | Roslani et al., 2014 [32] | Adults (outpatient) | Anal | 8.3 (women and men) |
| Australia | Ng et al., 2014 [10] | Adults (outpatient) | Fecal | 12.1% |
| Norway | Johannessen et al., 2014 [40] | Pregnant women (hospitalized) | Anal | 24% |
| UK | Harari et al., 2014 [25] | Adults (audited in hospital inpatient and outpatient, primary care, and care home) | Fecal | 56% (patients incontinent every day/night at hospital or primary care) |
| Brazil | Murad-Regadas et al., 2014 [33] | Women (outpatient) | Anal | 79% |
| Chile | Guzman et al., 2015 [34] | Women (outpatient) | Anal | 14% |
| Denmark | Bogeskov et al., 2015 [42] | Postpartum women (hospital database) | Anal | 50% |
| USA | Meyer et al., 2015 [35] | Women (outpatient) | Fecal/Anal | 10% fecal, 87% anal, 2.3% flatus |
| Austrian | Shahin and Lohrmann, 2015 [28] | Adults (hospitalized) | Fecal | 6.5% |
| Chile | Sanguineti et al., 2016 [36] | Adults (outpatient) | Anal | 31% |
| Czech Republic | Huser et al., 2017 [29] | Postpartum women (hospitalized) | Fecal | 3.7% after vaginal delivery; 2.2% after cesarean delivery |
| USA | Markland et al., 2017 [37] | Women with irritable bowel syndrome (outpatient) | Anal | 69% |
| Lebanon | Ghandour et al., 2017 [38] | Women (outpatient) | Anal | 39.8% |

## 3.4    Nursing Home, Long-Term Acute Care, and Other Long-Term Care Institutions

Since the review by Wagg et al., 2013 [43], some new studies were identified reporting the prevalence of fecal incontinence in nursing homes or long-term care facilities (see Table 3.3). The studies confirm the high prevalence rate already known and varied around 42% [44–46]. Saga et al., 2013, reviewed studies from 1980 up to 2011 on prevalence and associations of fecal incontinence in nursing home patients [44]. Prevalence rates in nursing homes varied from 10% to 67%, concentrated between 40% and 55%. However, the reported data were limited by lack of a coherent definition of fecal incontinence, including different frequency labeling, poor definition of the institutional units (the nursing homes), and poor descriptions of patient characteristics [44]. Little is known about the fecal incontinence incidence rates in the nursing home population, with one past study reporting a rate of 20% during a 10-month period [47].

In the population living in long-term care institutions, the prevalence of fecal incontinence is higher (up to 42%) [44–46] compared to other settings (see Table 3.3). The prevalence of anal incontinence has even higher rates (54–57%) [48, 49]. This may be explained in part by the fact that both fecal incontinence and anal incontinence are associated with functional impairment and dementia, which are more common reasons for the institutionalization of the elderly [50, 51].

In summary, the prevalence data for fecal and anal incontinence presented varied widely depending on the population studied and the place; the majority of

**Table 3.3** Prevalence of fecal and anal incontinence in long-term care facilities by year and country

| Country | Author, year of publication | Population | Type of incontinence | Prevalence |
|---|---|---|---|---|
| Norway | Saga et al., 2013 [44] | Adults (institutionalized) (review) | Fecal | 42.3% |
| Australia | Halland et al., 2013 [8] | Older women (82–87 years) (institutionalized) | Fecal | 14.1% |
| USA | Bliss et al., 2013 [46] | Adults (65 years and older) (at admission to an institution) | Fecal | Any fecal incontinence[a] = 35–38%, Only fecal incontinence[b] = 8–9% |
| Brazil | Jerez-Roig et al., 2015 [45] | Adults (institutionalized) | Fecal | 42.68% |
| Czech Republic | Ihnát et al., 2016 [48] | Adults (institutionalized) | Anal | 57.1% |
| Norway | Blekken et al., 2016 [49] | Adults (institutionalized) | Anal | 42.1–54% |

[a]Any fecal incontinence (fecal incontinence with or without urinary incontinence)
[b]Only fecal incontinence (without urinary incontinence)

the studies were carried out with women and adults, in outpatient follow-up. There was only one article that evaluated the prevalence of fecal incontinence in children in a very specific subgroup (attention deficit hyperactivity disorder).

## 3.5    Incidence of Anal and Fecal Incontinence

Only a few studies about the incidence of fecal or anal incontinence were found in the literature in the last 5 years [15, 39–41, 52, 53]. Events such as postpartum are a focus of the incidence studies [40, 41, 52]. The rates of incidence are presented in Table 3.4.

## 3.6    Factors Associated with the Presence of Anal or Fecal Incontinence

There are a large number of factors associated with the presence or occurrence of fecal incontinence or anal incontinence, which include acquired abnormalities or congenital malformations, degenerative or functional conditions, and neurological diseases [53–56]. Table 3.5 summarizes these factors.

**Table 3.4** Incidence of fecal and anal incontinence in different settings by year, country, and population

| Country | Author, year of publication | Population | Type of incontinence | Incidence |
|---|---|---|---|---|
| South Africa | Naidoo et al., 2012 [41] | Women 6 weeks postpartum (hospital) | Anal | 61.1%; persistence of symptoms after 6 months = 6.4% |
| USA | Alsheik et al., 2012 [39] | Adults (outpatient) | Anal | 3% |
| Finland | Lehto et al., 2014 [15] | Adults (outpatient) | Fecal | 1% per year (all women) |
| Norway | Johannessen et al., 2014 [40] | Women 1 year after childbirth | Anal | 2.2% with three or more symptoms 1 year postpartum |
| USA | Richter et al., 2015 [52] | Primiparous women with obstetric anal sphincter injury 6, 12, and 24 weeks postpartum | Anal | 7% (6 weeks) 4% (12 weeks) 9% (24 weeks) General incidence = 24% (24 weeks) |
| USA | Bliss et al., 2017 [53] | Adults (nursing home residents with urinary incontinence) | Fecal | 8.7% |

**Table 3.5** Factors associated with the occurrence of anal or fecal incontinence

| | |
|---|---|
| • Advanced age [10, 14, 19, 28, 32, 54, 57] | • Malnutrition [57] |
| • Anal sphincter injury during labor [41] | • Menopause [55] |
| • Anal sphincter trauma (obstetrical or perineal injury, prior surgery) [56] | • Mobility impairment [55] |
| • Anorectal surgery [9] | • Multiparity [19, 55, 57] |
| • Cognitive impairment and dementia [48, 54, 55] | • Multiple comorbidity [17, 49] |
| • Constipation [9, 56] | • Neurological disorders [17, 54, 55] |
| • Chronic illness [54, 55] | • Obesity [54, 55] |
| • Decreased physical activity [54] | • Pelvic floor anatomical disturbances (rectal prolapse) [54] |
| • Depression [19, 39] | • Pelvic or abdominal radiation therapy [56] |
| • Diabetes mellitus type 2 [7, 17, 18, 54, 55] | • Poor general health [55] |
| • Diarrhea or loose/liquid stool consistency [9, 10, 19, 23, 28, 54, 57] | • Pressure injury stage 1 [57] |
| • Functional limitation [16, 57] | • Prostate surgery [55] |
| • Gynecological surgery (hysterectomy) [9, 19] | • Race/ethnicity (varies by setting) [7, 17, 53] |
| • Gestation [16] | • Smoking [17, 54] |
| • Inappropriate cholecystectomy [54] | • Spinal cord injury [57] |
| • Inflammatory bowel disease [40, 54] | • Stroke [9] |
| • Limitations in daily activities [55] | • Symptom of rectal urgency [54] |
| • Lower urinary tract symptoms and infections in women [55] | • Urinary incontinence [10, 17, 18, 48, 54] |

## 3.6.1 Age

Age above 50 years was considered as an independent factor associated with fecal incontinence in the studies of Kang et al., 2012, and Lim et al., 2014 [14, 28]. In a study conducted by Townsend et al., 2013, with elderly women, the prevalence of anal incontinence increased significantly with age, from 9% in women aged 62–64 years to 17% in women aged 85–87 years [17].

In a cross-sectional study conducted by Ditah et al., 2014, the prevalence of anal incontinence in community-living individuals increased with age from 2.91% among 20- to 29-year-old participants to 16.16% (14.15–18.39%) among participants 70 years and older [18]. In study of Wu et al., 2015, in both sexes, the prevalence of all incontinence types increased with age [19].

Roslani et al., 2014, found that anal incontinence was present in 18.7% of subjects older than 65 years, compared to 9.7% in those aged 45–64 years, 6.0% in those 24–44 years old, and 5.1% in subjects aged 18–24 years [32].

## 3.6.2 Sex

In relation to differences in prevalence of anal or fecal incontinence by sex, results are mixed, with most studies showing no difference by sex while others show a difference (see Tables 3.1 and 3.2). Differences in the sample studied, incontinence definition, or other methodological factors may explain variation. Townsend et al., 2016, found some differences in the pathophysiological mechanisms of fecal incontinence between sexes [58]. These authors observed that anal structural sphincter abnormalities were uncommon among men (M, 37%, vs. W, 77%; $p < 0.001$), but impaired rectal sensation (M, 24%, vs. W, 7%; $p = 0.001$) and functional disturbances of evacuation (M, 36%, vs. W, 13%; $p = 0.001$) were more frequent in men than in women [58].

### 3.6.3   Race

The prevalence of anal incontinence was 50% less in Black community-living women than in White women (6% and 12%, respectively), and there are other variables that increased their chances of occurrence, such as pregnancy, high body mass index, reduced physical activity, functional limitations, current smoking, type 2 diabetes mellitus, systemic arterial hypertension, neurological diseases, and urinary incontinence [17].

Bliss et al., 2013, examined the prevalence of fecal incontinence at nursing home admission by race and ethnicity using various definitions related to fecal incontinence that have been commonly reported in the literature: "only fecal incontinence, dual incontinence (both urinary incontinence and fecal incontinence), any fecal incontinence (fecal incontinence with or without urinary incontinence), and any incontinence (urinary incontinence and/or fecal incontinence and/or dual incontinence) [53]." Bliss et al., 2013, found differences among racial/ethnic groups despite different definitions. For example, the prevalence of any fecal incontinence in White nursing home admissions (36%) was similar to that of American Indian admissions (37%), whereas Asian, Black, and Hispanic admissions had higher rates (54%, 58%, and 49%, respectively) [53]. The rate of having only fecal incontinence was 9–10% in White, Asian, and American Indian nursing home admissions but was 13–14% in Black and Hispanic admissions [53].

### 3.6.4   Structural and Neurological Impairments

The most common structural causes of fecal or anal incontinence are obstetric injuries, especially associated with vaginal delivery, anorectal surgeries, hemorrhoids, fistulas, and fissures, among others [9, 54, 59]. A systematic review showed significant associations between perineal trauma (episiotomy [OR, 1.74; 95% CI, 1.28–2.38; $Q = 8.9$; $p = 0.26$; $I^2 = 21.4$] and third- and fourth-degree perineal laceration (OR, 2.66; 95% CI, 1.77–3.98; $Q = 27.9$; $p = 0.002$; $I^2 = 64.1$) and anal incontinence [5].

Among the neurological alterations, pudendal neuropathy (arising from radiation, diabetes, and chemotherapy), spinal column surgeries, dementia, and central nervous system injuries such as stroke, trauma, tumors, infections, and congenital lesions are described [9, 59].

Diabetes mellitus is one of the chronic diseases that affects the peripheral nervous system and was pointed out as a risk factor for fecal or anal incontinence [7, 17, 18, 32, 55]. In a study conducted with patients seeking treatment at the general surgical, obstetrics and gynecology, and antenatal specialist outpatient clinics, the authors found anal incontinence was more prevalent among diabetics than nondiabetic patients (13.9% vs. 7.6%, $p = 0.026$) [32].

### 3.6.5   Functionality

In 588 long-term institutions in the Czech Republic, the prevalence of fecal incontinence was 57.1% ($n = 336$), and there were important associated factors such as reduction of physical mobility, mental/cognitive alterations (especially dementias), general state of health decline (presence of four or more comorbidities), urinary incontinence, and long stay in these institutions [48].

In another study by Blekken et al., most of the variation in anal incontinence rates was explained by differences in patient characteristics such as deficiencies in daily living activities, cognitive impairment, diarrhea, and not participating in activities, being the most important [49].

### 3.6.6   Consistency of Feces

Some conditions are considered as independent factors associated with the occurrence of fecal or anal incontinence, such as diarrhea [10] and/or loose or liquid stool consistency [23], altered bowel habits of irritable bowel syndrome [28, 54], inflammatory bowel disease, constipation with paradoxical diarrhea (fecal impaction), and overflow incontinence [28].

### 3.6.7   Urinary Incontinence

The frequent association between anal or fecal incontinence and urinary incontinence probably reflects a common etiologic pathway (common innervations, support structures) and many common factors such as advancing age, function, and neurodegenerative diseases [18]. In a study conducted by Ditah et al. 2014, community-living participants who were incontinent of urine were over three times more likely to report anal incontinence (OR 3.24, 95% CI 1.73–6.08) [18]. Similarly, in nursing home residents, Bliss et al., 2017, showed that having urinary incontinence was the strongest predictor of developing subsequent fecal incontinence (i.e., dual incontinence) [53]. The hazard of developing dual incontinence for residents with urinary incontinence was 1.3 times greater than the hazard for those who were continent.

## 3.6.8 Hospitalization

The factors associated with fecal incontinence in the hospital setting were female sex, advanced age, low body mass index (BMI), hospitalization diagnoses such as dementia and spinal cord injury, stage 1 pressure injury, and functional limitation [57].

Pressure injury can be defined as "localized damage to the skin and underlying soft tissue usually over a bony prominence or related to a medical or other device. The injury occurs as a result of intense and/or prolonged pressure or pressure in combination with shear. The tolerance of soft tissue for pressure and shear may also be affected by microclimate, nutrition, perfusion, co-morbidities and condition of the soft tissue" [60]. So, pressure injury would be a consequence of the damage caused by leaked urine and/or feces to the skin. In fact, results of Lachenbruch et al., 2016, who analyzed data of 176,689 hospital patients from a cross-sectional cohort database, showed that the prevalence of pressure injuries was 4.1% for continent and 16.3% for incontinent patients [61]. As wound severity increased, the odds ratios for pressure injury also increased, mainly in patients with fecal incontinence.

## 3.6.9 Other Factors

Smoking, obesity, and cholecystectomy emerged as potentially modifiable factors associated with anal incontinence which also included comorbidities such as diabetes [30, 54, 55].

## References

1. Bliss DZ, Mimura T, Berghmans B, Bharucha A, Chiarioni G, Emmanuel A, et al. Assessment and conservative management of faecal incontinence and quality of life in adults. In: Abrams P, Cardozo L, Wagg A, Wein A, editors. Incontinence. 6th ed. Bristol: International Continence Society; 2017. p. 1993–2085.
2. Apêndice B. Os critérios diagnósticos de Roma III para os distúrbios gastrointestinais funcionais. Arq Gastroenterol. 2012;49(Suppl 1):64–8.
3. Sharma A, Yuan L, Marshall RJ, Merrie AEH, Bissett IP. Systematic review of the prevalence of faecal incontinence. Br J Surg. 2016;103(12):1589–97.
4. Bharucha AE, Wald AM. Transtornos anorretais. Arq Gastroenterol. 2012;49:51–60.
5. LaCross A, Groff M, Smaldone A. Obstetric anal sphincter injury and anal incontinence following vaginal birth: a systematic review and meta-analysis. J Midwifery Womens Health. 2015;60(1):37–47.
6. National Institute for Health and Care Excellence (NICE). Faecal incontinence: management of faecal incontinence in adults. 2007. https://www.nice.org.uk/guidance/cg49
7. Matthews CA, Whitehead WE, Townsend MK, Grodstein F. Risk factors for urinary, fecal, or dual incontinence in the Nurses' Health Study. Obstet Gynecol. 2013;122(3):539–45.
8. Halland M, Koloski NA, Jones M, Byles J, Chiarelli P, Forder P, et al. Prevalence correlates and impact of fecal incontinence among older women. Dis Colon Rectum. 2013;56(9):1080–6.

9. Santos VL, Domansky RC, Hanate C, Matos DS, Benvenuto CV, Jorge JM. Self-reported fecal incontinence in a community-dwelling, urban population in southern Brazil. J Wound Ostomy Cont Nurs. 2014;41(1):77–83.

10. Ng K-S, Sivakumaran Y, Nassar N, Gladman MA. Fecal incontinence: community prevalence and associated factors—a systematic review. Dis Colon Rectum. 2015;58(12):1194–209.

11. Noelting J, Eaton JE, Choung RS, Zinsmeister AR, Locke G, Bharucha AE. The incidence rate and characteristics of clinically diagnosed defecatory disorders in the community. Neurogastroenterol Motil. 2016;28(11):1690–7.

12. Meinds RJ, van Meegdenburg MM, Trzpis M, Broens PM. On the prevalence of constipation and fecal incontinence, and their co-occurrence, in the Netherlands. Int J Colorectal Dis. 2017;32(4):475–83.

13. McKeown C, Hisle-Gorman E, Eide M, Gorman GH, Nylund CM. Association of constipation and fecal incontinence with attention-deficit/hyperactivity disorder. Pediatrics. 2013;132(5):e1210–5.

14. Lim JW-M, Heng C, Wong MT-C, Tang C-L. Prevalence of faecal incontinence in the community: a cross-sectional study in Singapore. Singapore Med J. 2014;55(12):640–3.

15. Lehto K, Ylönen K, Hyöty M, Collin P, Huhtala H, Aitola P. Anal incontinence: long-term alterations in the incidence and healthcare usage. Scand J Gastroenterol. 2014;49(7):790–3.

16. Brown HW, Wexner SD, Segall MM, Brezoczky KL, Lukacz ES. Accidental bowel leakage in the mature women's health study: prevalence and predictors. Int J Clin Pract. 2012;66(11):1101–8.

17. Townsend MK, Matthews CA, Whitehead WE, Grodstein F. Risk factors for fecal incontinence in older women. Am J Gastroenterol. 2013;108(1):113–9.

18. Ditah I, Devaki P, Luma HN, Ditah C, Njei B, Jaiyeoba C, et al. Prevalence, trends, and risk factors for fecal incontinence in United States adults, 2005–2010. Clin Gastroenterol Hepatol. 2014;12(4):636–43.e2.

19. Wu JM, Matthews CA, Vaughan CP, Markland AD. Urinary, fecal, and dual incontinence in older U.S. adults. J Am Geriatr Soc. 2015;63(5):947–53.

20. Andy UU, Vaughan CP, Burgio KL, Alli FM, Goode PS, Markland AD. Shared risk factors for constipation, fecal incontinence, and combined symptoms in older US adults. J Am Geriatr Soc. 2016;64(11):e183–8.

21. Nair B, O'Dea J, Lim L, Thakkinstian A. Prevalence of geriatric 'syndromes' in a tertiary hospital. Australas J Ageing. 2000;19(2):81–4.

22. Bayón García C, Binks R, De Luca E, Dierkes C, Franci A, Gallart E, et al. Prevalence, management and clinical challenges associated with acute faecal incontinence in the ICU and critical care settings: the FIRST™ cross-sectional descriptive survey. Intensive Crit Care Nurs. 2012;28(4):242–50.

23. Bliss DZ, Johnson S, Savik K, Clabots CR, Gerding DN. Fecal incontinence in hospitalized patients who are acutely ill. Nurs Res. 2000;49(2):101–8.

24. Akpan A, Gosney MA, Barrett J. Factors contributing to fecal incontinence in older people and outcome of routine management in home, hospital and nursing home settings. Clin Interv Aging. 2007;2(1):139–45.

25. Harari D, Husk J, Lowe D, Wagg A. National audit of continence care: adherence to National Institute for Health and Clinical Excellence (NICE) guidance in older versus younger adults with faecal incontinence. Age Ageing. 2014;43(6):785–93.

26. Dobb GJ. Diarrhoea in the critically ill. Intensive Care Med. 1986;12(3):113–5.

27. Beitz JM. Fecal incontinence in acutely and critically ill patients: options in management. Ostomy Wound Manage. 2006;52(12):56–8, 60, 62–6.

28. Kang H-W, Jung H-K, Kwon K-J, Song E-M, Choi J-Y, Kim S-E, et al. Prevalence and predictive factors of fecal incontinence. J Neurogastroenterol Motil. 2012;18(1):86–93.

29. Huser M, Janku P, Hudecek R, Zbozinkova Z, Bursa M, Unzeitig V, et al. Pelvic floor dysfunction after vaginal and cesarean delivery among singleton primiparas. Int J Gynaecol Obstet. 2017;137(2):170.

30. Parés D, Vallverdu H, Monroy G, Amigo P, Romagosa C, Toral M, et al. Bowel habits and fecal incontinence in patients with obesity undergoing evaluation for weight loss: the importance of stool consistency. Dis Colon Rectum. 2012;55(5):599–604.
31. Rajeshkannan N, Pathmeswaran A. Prevalence of postpartum anal incontinence: a cross sectional study in Northern Sri Lanka. Ceylon Med J. 2013;58(2):76–9.
32. Roslani AC, Ramakrishnan R, Azmi S, Arapoc DJ, Goh A. Prevalence of faecal incontinence and its related factors among patients in a Malaysian academic setting. BMC Gastroenterol. 2014;14(1):95.
33. Murad-Regadas S, Dealcanfreitas I, Regadas F, Rodrigues L, Fernandes G, Pereira JJ. Do changes in anal sphincter anatomy correlate with anal function in women with a history of vaginal delivery? Arq Gastroenterol. 2014;51(3):198.
34. Guzmán RRA, Kamisan Atan I, Shek KL, Dietz HP. Anal sphincter trauma and anal incontinence in urogynecological patients. Ultrasound Obstet Gynecol. 2015;46(3):363–6.
35. Meyer I, Richter HE. Impact of fecal incontinence and its treatment on quality of life in women. Womens Health. 2015;11(2):225–38.
36. Sanguineti MA, Bocic AG, Domínguez CC, Abedrapo MM, Azolas MR, Llanos BJL, et al. Prevalencia de incontinencia fecal en personas que acuden a policlinicosde un hospital universitario. Rev Chil Cir. 2016;68:51–7.
37. Markland AD, Jelovsek JE, Rahn DD, Wang L, Merrin L, Tuteja A, et al. Irritable bowel syndrome and quality of life in women with fecal incontinence. Female Pelvic Med Reconstr Surg. 2017;23(3):179–83.
38. Ghandour L, Minassian V, Al-Badr A, Ghaida RA, Geagea S, Bazi T. Prevalence and degree of bother of pelvic floor disorder symptoms among women from primary care and specialty clinics in Lebanon: an exploratory study. Int Urogynecol J. 2017;28(1):105–18.
39. Alsheik EH, Coyne T, Hawes SK, Merikhi L, Naples SP, Kanagarajan N, et al. Fecal incontinence: prevalence, severity, and quality of life data from an outpatient gastroenterology practice. Gastroenterol Res Pract. 2012;2012:947694.
40. Johannessen HH, Wibe A, Stordahl A, Sandvik L, Backe B, Morkved S. Prevalence and predictors of anal incontinence during pregnancy and 1 year after delivery: a prospective cohort study. BJOG. 2014;121(3):269–79.
41. Naidoo TD, Moodley J, Esterhuizen TE. Incidence of postpartum anal incontinence among Indians and black Africans in a resource-constrained country. Int J Gynecol Obstet. 2012;118(2):156–60.
42. Bøgeskov RA, Nickelsen CN, Secher NJ. Anal incontinence in women with recurrent obstetric anal sphincter rupture: a case control study. J Matern Fetal Neonatal Med. 2015;28(3):288–92.
43. Wagg AS, Chen LK, Kirschner-Hermanns R, Kuchel GA, Johnson Y, Ostaszkiewicz J, et al. Incontinence in the frail elderly. In: Abrams P, Cardozo L, Khoury S, Wein A, editors. Incontinence. 5th ed. Arnhem: ICUD-EAU; 2013. p. 1001–100.
44. Saga S, Vinsnes AG, Morkved S, Norton C, Seim A. Prevalence and correlates of fecal incontinence among nursing home residents: a population-based cross-sectional study. BMC Geriatr. 2013;13:87.
45. Jerez-Roig J, Souza DLB, Amaral FLJS, Lima KC. Prevalence of fecal incontinence (FI) and associated factors in institutionalized older adults. Arch Gerontol Geriatr. 2015;60(3):425–30.
46. Bliss DZ, Harms S, Garrard JM, Cunanan K, Savik K, Gurvich O, et al. Prevalence of incontinence by race and ethnicity of older people admitted to nursing homes. J Am Med Dir Assoc. 2013;14(6):451.e1–7.
47. Chassagne P, Landrin I, Neveu C, Czernichow P, Bouaniche M, Doucet J, et al. Fecal incontinence in the institutionalized elderly: incidence, risk factors, and prognosis. Am J Med. 1999;106(2):185–90.
48. Ihnát P, Kozáková R, Rudinská LI, Peteja M, Vávra P, Zonča P. Fecal incontinence among nursing home residents: is it still a problem? Arch Gerontol Geriatr. 2016;65.(Suppl C:79–84.
49. Blekken LE, Vinsnes AG, Gjeilo KH, Norton C, Mørkved S, Salvesen Ø, et al. Exploring faecal incontinence in nursing home patients: a cross-sectional study of prevalence and associations

derived from the Residents Assessment Instrument for Long-Term Care Facilities. J Adv Nurs. 2016;72(7):1579–91.

50. Whitehead WE, Borrud L, Goode PS, Meikle S, Mueller ER, Tuteja A, et al. Fecal incontinence in U.S. adults: epidemiology and risk factors. Gastroenterology. 2009;137(2):512–7. e2

51. Rey E, Choung RS, Schleck CD, Zinsmeister AR, Locke GR 3rd, Talley NJ. Onset and risk factors for fecal incontinence in a US community. Am J Gastroenterol. 2010;105(2):412–9.

52. Richter HE, Nager CW, Burgio KL, Whitworth R, Weidner AC, Schaffer J, et al. Incidence and predictors of anal incontinence after obstetric anal sphincter injury in primiparous women. Female Pelvic Med Reconstr Surg. 2015;21(4):182.

53. Bliss DZ, Gurvich OV, Eberly LE, Harms S. Time to and predictors of dual incontinence in older nursing home admissions. Neurourol Urodyn. 2018;37:229–36.

54. Bharucha AE, Dunivan G, Goode PS, Lukacz ES, Markland AD, Matthews CA, et al. Epidemiology, pathophysiology, and classification of fecal incontinence: state of the science summary for the National Institute of Diabetes and Digestive and Kidney Diseases (NIDDK) workshop. Am J Gastroenterol. 2015;110(1):127–36.

55. Australian Institute of Health and Welfare. Incontinence in Australia: prevalence, experience, and cost 2009. Bulletin No. 112. Cat. No. AUS 167. Canberra: AIHW; 2012.

56. Muñoz-Yagüe T, Solís-Muñoz P, Ciriza de los Ríos C, Muñoz-Garrido F, Vara J, Solís-Herruzo JA. Fecal incontinence in men: causes and clinical and manometric features. World J Gastroenterol. 2014;20(24):7933–40.

57. Shahin ES, Lohrmann C. Prevalence of fecal and double fecal and urinary incontinence in hospitalized patients. J Wound Ostomy Cont Nurs. 2015;42(1):89–93.

58. Townsend DC, Carrington EV, Grossi U, Burgell RE, Wong JYJ, Knowles CH, et al. Pathophysiology of fecal incontinence differs between men and women: a case-matched study in 200 patients. Neurogastroenterol Motil. 2016;28(10):1580–8.

59. Ruiz NS, Kaiser AM. Fecal incontinence-challenges and solutions. World J Gastroenterol. 2017;23(1):11.

60. The National Pressure Ulcer Advisory Panel (NPUAP). NPUAP Pressure Injury Stages. 2016. http://www.npuap.org/resources/educational-and-clinical-resources/npuap-pressure-injury-stages/.

61. Lachenbruch C, Ribble D, Emmons K, VanGilder C. Pressure ulcer risk in the incontinent patient: analysis of incontinence and hospital-acquired pressure ulcers from the International Pressure Ulcer Prevalence™ Survey. J Wound Ostomy Cont Nurs. 2016;43(3):235–41.

# Normal Defecation and Mechanisms for Continence

**4**

Mônica Milinkovic de la Quintana, Tania das Graças de Souza Lima, Vera Lúcia Conceição de Gouveia Santos, and Maria Helena Baena de Moraes Lopes

**Abstract**

The mechanism of fecal continence is a complex process, composed of a series of events, which are influenced by the consistency, volume, and speed with which the fecal material reaches the rectum; the sensitivity and distensibility of the rectum vault; and factors related to the sphincter muscles, which involve sensorial and mechanical components that require muscular and nervous integrity. The defecatory mechanism is complex and involves a sequence of events, which integrates smooth and striated muscle and the central, somatic, autonomic, and enteric nervous systems. Normal defecation involves the rapid, semivoluntary emptying of the rectum and a variable part of the colon, and it requires a high degree of coordination to achieve the evacuation of solid or semisolid feces. In this chapter, anatomical and physiological components of the anorectal portion of the gastrointestinal tract will be explained, according to their relevance to maintain continence.

**Keywords**

Fecal incontinence · Defecation · Constipation · Diarrhea

M. M. de la Quintana (✉)
Nipo Brasileiro Hospital, São Paulo, SP, Brazil

T. das Graças de Souza Lima
University of Rio de Janeiro, Rio de Janeiro, Brazil

V. L. C. de Gouveia Santos
School of Nursing, University of São Paulo, São Paulo, SP, Brazil
e-mail: veras@usp.br

M. H. B. de Moraes Lopes
Faculty of Nursing, University of Campinas, Campinas, SP, Brazil

© Springer International Publishing AG, part of Springer Nature 2018
D. Z. Bliss (ed.), *Management of Fecal Incontinence for the Advanced Practice Nurse*,
https://doi.org/10.1007/978-3-319-90704-8_4

## 4.1    Introduction

Fecal continence is an extremely important function of the digestive system, which involves the transport of fecal material, the ability to delay defecation to a socially appropriate location and moment, and finally the defecation of the body's wastes.

There are anatomical structures and physiological conditions that allow continence to be achieved. These functions transform intestinal contents into soft or pasty stools and transport fecal matter through the colon to the rectum, where it is stored until the desire for defecation is triggered through sensory and reflex mechanisms. Defecation is voluntarily delayed until the socio-environmental situation allows for that. All this activity with involuntary and conscious components is extremely complex and can lead to multiple forms of fecal incontinence when one or more of these components fail.

Fecal continence is maintained by the structural and functional integrity of the anorectal and pelvic floor neuromuscular components. Although they represent a short segment of the gastrointestinal tract, the anus and rectum have complex anatomy and physiology and are extremely important for continence; therefore, any change in their anatomy or physiology can lead to incontinence. For many patients suffering from anorectal diseases, fecal continence represents a "challenge" rather than a daily physiological act in their lives.

## 4.2    Anatomical Structures

### 4.2.1    Rectum

The rectum is a muscular tube measuring 12–15 cm and serves to store the feces that arrive from the sigmoid colon. Its muscle arrangement allows it to function both as a reservoir, being able to accommodate passive distension, and as a stool propellant.

Rectal capacity is a parameter reflecting the overall size of the reservoir whereby a more spacious reservoir allows for storage of more stool [1]. Rectal compliance is a parameter reflecting the distensibility of the rectal wall, i.e., the ratio of a change in volume to a change in pressure ($\Delta$volume/$\Delta$pressure) [1]. The compliance and hence the capacity of the rectum are related to produce defecation. As rectal distension increases, rectal compliance falls. The rectum tolerates volumes up to about 300 ml without showing any marked change in intraluminal pressure [2].

During stretching, there is a decrease in anal resting pressure in a process called the anal-rectal inhibitory reflex, whose amplitude and duration increase with rectal distension. The ability of the rectum to passively accommodate distension during transient sudden increases in intrarectal pressure contributes to the maintenance of pressure levels relatively lower than those of the anal canal. A compliant rectum, therefore, is essential for maintaining continence [3], and changes in rectal compliance may contribute to incontinence [4]. Rectal perception and adaptation to distension are widely heterogeneous in people suffering from fecal incontinence [3, 5]. Some studies show that rectal compliance is lower in incontinent patients [3, 6, 7], but this finding was not confirmed by other studies [8, 9].

The contractile response involves the contraction of the external anal sphincter. When rectal complacency is compromised, a small volume of feces can generate a high intrarectal pressure, which causes incontinence by overcoming anal resistance [10]. In addition, a decrease in rectal capacity and the maximum tolerable volume is directly related to the increase in defecation frequency and decrease in continence, due to an increase in rectal pressure at lower volumes.

## 4.2.2  Anal Canal

The study of the anatomy of the anorectal region can be defined as the analysis of the elements involved in the morphology of the segment described as the anal canal.

The anal canal is understood to be the final segment of the digestive system where its physiological occlusion occurs due to the tonus of two concentric muscular cylinders, namely, the external anal sphincter and internal anal sphincter. At its upper end, the muscular structure of the anal canal includes the innermost bundle of the levator muscle of the anus, called the puborectal bundle, which relates directly to the upper portion of the external anal sphincter muscle [11].

The anal mucosa is configured into folds with vascular cushions (expansions of vascular tissue within the mucosa) that can expand to form a seal that aids in maintaining resting anal tone and promoting continence [12, 13]. The anal vascular cushions contribute to approximately 15% of the resting anal tone [12].

The extension of the anal canal varies as a function of the individual tonicity as it is influenced by the action of the musculature. Its function emphasizes the importance of the participation of the puborectal bundle of the levator ani muscle. This bundle is a main factor in maintaining continence through its anterior traction of the limit of the anal canal. The length of 4 cm for the extension of the anal canal, from its lower end in the anal orifice to its upper opening in the rectal ampulla, can be described as "normal". Its length varies according to the individual's age and sex [11].

## 4.3  The Pelvic Floor and the Sphincter Apparatus

The set of muscular structures that act in the anorectal region are composed of four muscles related to each other [11]:

- Levator ani muscle
- Internal anal sphincter
- External anal sphincter
- Longitudinal anal muscle

### 4.3.1 Levator Ani Muscle

The pelvic diaphragm is comprised of two muscles that occlude the inferior opening of the bony pelvis, the levator ani muscle and the coccygeus muscle, the latter with no relevant function in fecal continence. The levator ani muscle is the main muscle responsible for the support of the rectum and for assisting in fecal continence [14].

The levator ani muscle is funnel shaped, with an anterior funnel. On its posterior inner surface rests the rectum, extending from the coccyx to its inferior opening in the anal canal. The levator ani muscle is composed of three distinct bundles: two acting on the rectum support, like a net, anchored in an anteroposterior insertion on the fascia of the internal obturator muscle, by means of a structure described as the tendinous arch [15].

These bundles are described as the iliococcygeus muscle posteriorly and pubococcygeus muscle anteriorly. The third bundle, called the puborectalis muscle, is located inferiorly to the two bundles described. It has a muscular handle shape with bilateral anterior insertions on the posterior surface of the pubis. Its posterior arch faces the anal canal, where it fuses with the upper extremity of the external anal sphincter. Its contraction in conjunction with the external anal sphincter exerts anterosuperior traction, causing angulation between the rectum and the anal canal (anorectal angle) [15, 16] (see Fig. 4.1).

The anorectal angle is formed by the longitudinal axis of the anal canal and the posterior wall of the rectum. It presents around 90°, under normal resting conditions, whereas with voluntary squeeze of the external anal sphincter and puborectalis muscle, the angle becomes more acute (70°) in order to close off the anal canal and maintain continence. The angle becomes more obtuse during defecation, through the relaxation of puborectal and pelvic floor muscles, resulting in alignment of the rectum with respect to the anal canal [4] (see Fig. 4.2).

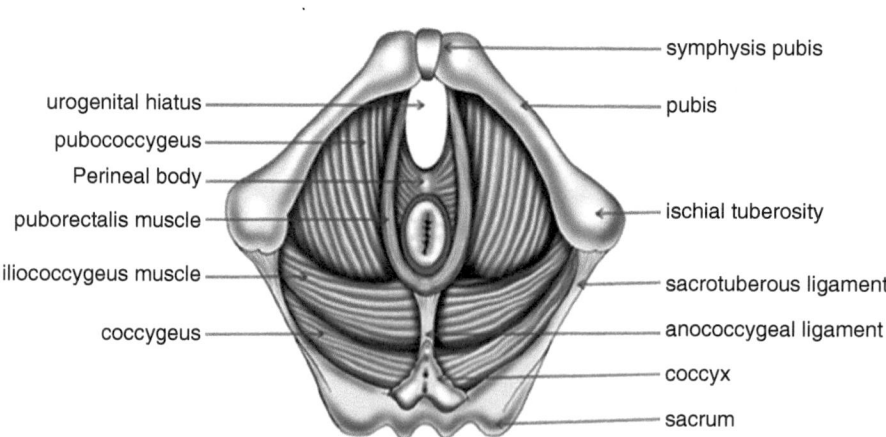

**Fig. 4.1** Pelvic floor, containing the muscles and ligaments

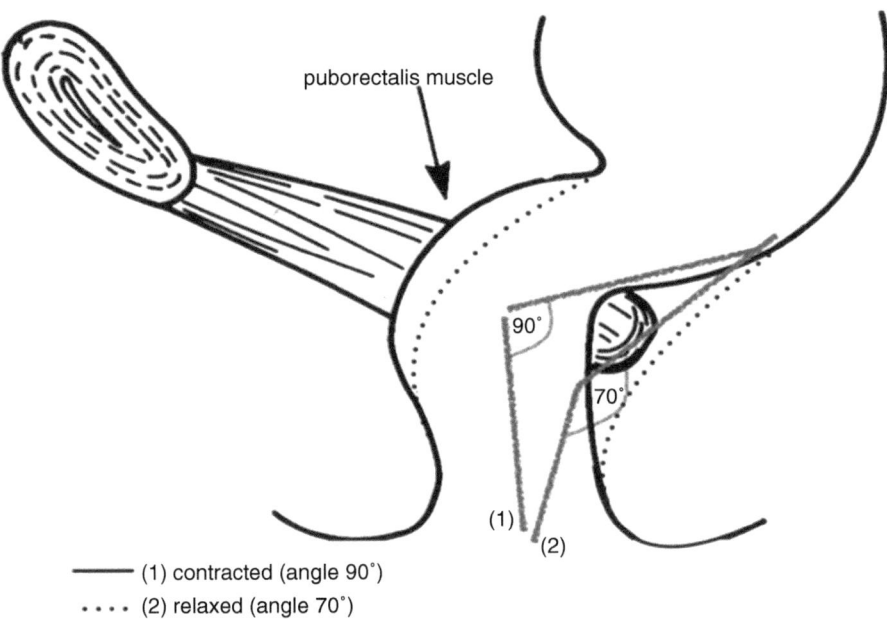

puborectalis muscle

90°

70°

(1)

(2)

———— (1) contracted (angle 90°)

· · · · (2) relaxed (angle 70°)

**Fig. 4.2** Anorectal angle during contraction and relaxation of puborectal and pelvic floor muscles

## 4.3.2   Internal Anal Sphincter Muscle

The internal anal sphincter is a circular muscle, located externally of the submucosa of the anal canal. It is formed by a caudal continuity of the inner circular layer of the rectum, reaching 2–5 mm of thickening and extending until about 1.5 cm below the pectinate line, where it ends in rounded edge. Being a smooth muscle, its involuntary permanent tonus accounts for 50–85% of the resting pressure of the anal canal (basal anal pressure) [4, 17] (see Fig. 4.3).

In resting conditions, the internal anal sphincter is the main occluder of the anal canal and exerts function in continence by performing transient periods of continence. In addition, its sensitive epithelium receives the analysis of rectal contents. This phenomenon, described as the anal sampling mechanism or rectoanal inhibitory reflex, contributes to the individual having the necessary discrimination, for example, for the release of gases without loss of fecal material [18–20].

## 4.3.3   External Anal Sphincter Muscle

The external anal sphincter is an expansion of the levator ani muscle and measures 0.6–1 cm in thickness. It surrounds the anal canal, internal anal sphincter, and conjoined longitudinal muscle in a cylindrical configuration. It is composed of striated muscles (see Fig. 4.3).

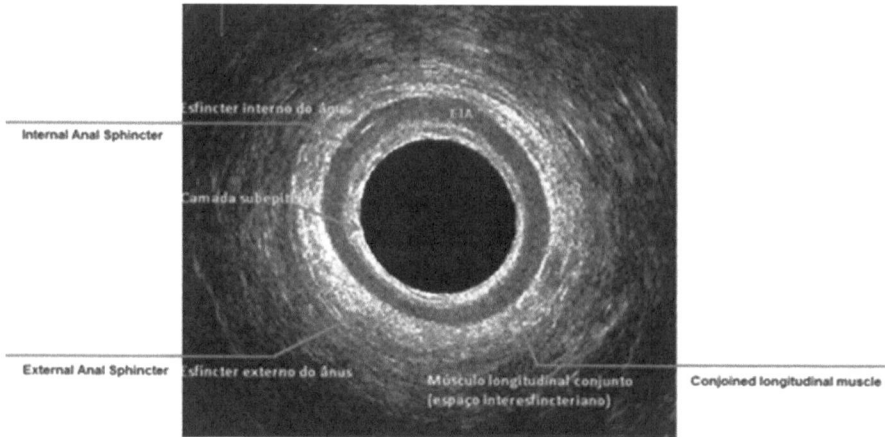

**Fig. 4.3** Anal sphincter on endoanal ultrasound. Internal anal sphincter (hypoechoic inner ring); 2, external anal sphincter (hyperechoic ring); 3, conjoined longitudinal muscle

Although with different innervations, the two sphincters act integrally on anal continence, both at rest and in situations where there is an increase in intrarectal pressure. The external anal sphincter complements the pressure exerted by the internal anal sphincter by means of a characteristic that distinguishes it from the rest of the striated muscles, which is the existence of a basal tonus. The external anal sphincter contains slow-twitch muscle fibers that can maintain contraction for long periods of time. These fibers generate 25–30% of the resting anal sphincter tone [4, 14].

When there is a distension of the rectum, it is up to the external anal sphincter to perform the contraction necessary to raise the pressure to the level of the anal canal, to avoid escape of the rectal contents, even in the event of reflex relaxation of the internal anal sphincter during sampling. This is due to a sacral reflex, which promotes involuntary contraction of the external anal sphincter as a response to distension of the rectum or abrupt increase in intra-abdominal pressure. This forced and voluntary contraction may occur until the intrarectal pressure is accommodated. It is estimated that the capacity of this contraction does not exceed approximately 3 min [18].

With voluntary squeeze of the external anal sphincter and puborectalis muscle, the anorectal angle becomes more acute (70°) in order to close off the anal canal and maintain continence [4] (see Fig. 4.2).

### 4.3.4   Longitudinal Anal Muscle

The longitudinal anal muscle is described as a vertical layer of muscular tissue interposed between the circular layers of the internal and external anal sphincters. From the anorectal junction, it extends along the anal canal, receives fibers from the innermost part of the puborectalis and the puboanalis muscles, and terminates with seven to nine fibroelastic septa. The septa traverse the subcutaneous part of the external anal sphincter, reaching the perianal dermis. The longitudinal anal muscle measures about 1.5–2 mm of thickness.

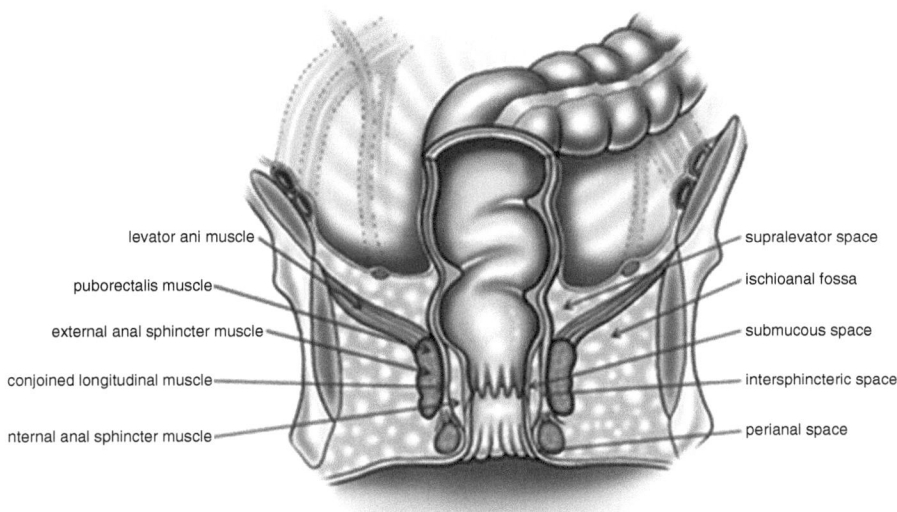

levator ani muscle

puborectalis muscle

external anal sphincter muscle

conjoined longitudinal muscle

nternal anal sphincter muscle

supralevator space

ischioanal fossa

submucous space

intersphincteric space

perianal space

**Fig. 4.4** Pelvic floor and the sphincterian apparatus

The longitudinal muscle fuses with striated fibers of the levator ani and puborectalis muscles at the level of the anorectal ring to form the conjoined longitudinal muscle [21] (see Fig. 4.4). The fibers descend between the internal and external anal sphincters and continue through the lower portion of the external sphincter composing the corrugator cutis ani, which inserts in the perianal skin [22].

Longitudinal anal muscle represents a strong muscular structure which connects the visceral and somatic parts of the anal sphincter complex contributing to the occlusion of the anal canal and exerting an important function in the continence.

## 4.4 Neural Control

### 4.4.1 Central Nervous System

The brain and spinal cord coordinate and integrate afferent signals from the anorectum and maintain continence until socially appropriate to defecate. The characterization of specific pathways involved in the central regulation of defecation is limited. In brain magnetic resonance imaging studies of healthy individuals subject to rectal distention, areas of the brain associated with sensation of rectal filling and urge to defecate include the anterior cingulate gyrus, insula, thalamus, and secondary somatosensory cortex [23]. Anal and rectal responses were observed at Brodmann area 4, part of the primary motor cortex, when cortical mapping with transcranial magnetic stimulation was performed [24]. The parasagittal motor cortex houses the upper motor neurons for the voluntary sphincter muscles, which communicate with Onuf's nucleus, located in the ventral horn gray matter of S2–S4 levels of the sacral spinal cord [25].

The conscious recognition of the need to defecate and the coordination of the proper social response are regulated by the frontal cortex [26]. A defecation center in the lumbosacral spinal cord, located in the second to fourth sacral segments, has also been described, through which the central nervous system can exert control over defecation by interacting with the enteric nervous system [27]. If an interruption in the spinal-cortical pathway to the defecation center occurs, such as in spinal cord injury, voluntary control of defecation is lost [27]. This results in fecal incontinence due to decreased anal sphincter resting tone, loss of voluntary control, and loss of anorectal reflexes [28]. Central control does not contribute significantly to baseline colonic tone but is important in effecting the voluntary relaxation of the external anal sphincter and contraction of abdominal muscles to facilitate defecation [29].

## 4.4.2   Peripheral Nervous System

Continence of stool involves both the autonomic nervous system, consisting of the sympathetic and parasympathetic nerves, and somatic nerves. Working in conjunction with these systems and unique to the gut is the enteric nervous system, a network of millions of interconnected ganglia responsible for carrying out the basic functions of the gut [4].

### 4.4.2.1 Autonomic Nervous System

The sympathetic and parasympathetic components of the autonomic innervation of the large intestine accompany their arterial irrigation. The sympathetic supply originates at the level of the first lumbar vertebrae—L1, L2, and L3. The preganglionic fibers through the sympathetic lumbar nerves make synapse in the preaortic plexus. The postganglionic fibers follow the branches of the mesenteric and upper rectal mesenteric arteries to the left and upper rectus colon. The lower rectum is innervated by the presacral plexuses, which are formed by fusion of the aortic plexus and lumbar splanchnic nerves. Bellow the promontory, the presacral nerves branch to form the right and left hypogastric nerves, which originate near the lateral wings of the rectum, the right and left pelvic plexus, or the lower hypogastric [14].

The parasympathetic supply originates from the second to the fourth sacral vertebrae—S2, S3, and S4—and constitutes the pelvic nerves. Its fibers emerge from the sacral foramen, pass laterally forward and upward, to join the sympathetic hypogastric nerves in the pelvic plexus. Postganglionic parasympathetic fibers are distributed to the left colon and upper rectum via the inferior mesenteric plexus and directly to the distal portion of the rectum and to the genitals [14].

The sympathetic (L5) and parasympathetic (S2, S3, S4) components of motor innervation of the internal anal sphincter follow the same route from the nerves to the rectum. The levator ani muscle is innervated by the sacral roots (S2, S3, and S4) on its pelvic surface and by the perineal branch of the pudendal nerve, on its underside. The puborectal receives additional innervation by the lower rectal nerves [30].

The external anal sphincter is innervated on each side by the lower rectal branch (S2 and S3) of the pudendal nerve and the perineal branch of S4. Despite some difference in innervation, the puborectal muscles and the external sphincter seem to act as a single unit [31].

The pudendal nerve is susceptible to stretch injury especially during vaginal delivery, which can compromise the ability of the puborectalis to close off the anorectal junction at rest resulting in fecal incontinence [10].

If there are impairments in mental function due to Alzheimer's disease, for example, the person may not be able to perform the various voluntary steps required to maintain continence. The impairments may range from lack of coordination of internal and external sphincters to not being able to find their way to the toilet.

## 4.5    Influence of Colonic Transit, Volume, and Consistency of Stool

Coordinated colonic motor activity drives transit, the rate at which colonic contents are delivered to the rectum, as well as the physical and chemical nature of feces itself. Stool volume and consistency are directly related to gastrointestinal transit time [32] and may also play a role in the pathogenesis of incontinence, besides the presence or absence of irritants in stool. As a general rule (though not absolute), loose stools are associated with more rapid gastrointestinal/colonic transit [33, 34], whereas constipation may be associated with slow gastrointestinal transit and reduced motility [35].

## 4.6    Continence and Defecation

Fecal continence is a complex function, sustained by the interaction of multiple mechanisms, including feces' consistency, colonic motility, rectal capacity and compliance, rectal and anal canal sensitivity, sphincter function, and muscle and nerves of the pelvic floor.

At rest, the anus remains occluded due to the tonic contraction of the internal anal sphincter, with reinforcement of the external anal sphincter and the puborectal handle, constituting the postural reflex [12].

Defecation involves the function of several integrated and complex mechanisms under the control of the central nervous system. The anal canal must open, and the intrarectal pressure must exceed that of the anal canal pressure. Inhibition of tonic pelvic floor activity allows relaxation of the puborectalis and straightening of the anorectal angle [4].

The filling of the rectum by the contents of the sigmoid triggers defecation. The distension of the rectum is consciously perceived as the desire to defecate by means of stretch receptors located in the pelvic floor muscles. Rectal distension also activates the rectoanal inhibitory reflex. Relaxation of the internal anal sphincter, by opening the superior anal canal, exposes the rectal contents to the highly sensitive mucosa of the anal canal, and then the differentiation between gases and feces can be made. This sampling mechanism determines the urgency of evacuation. Meanwhile, the simultaneous reflex contraction of the external sphincter of the anus maintains continence. If defecation is delayed, the conscious contraction of external anal sphincter allows the recovery of internal sphincter function.

If the call to defecation is answered, a sitting or squatting position is assumed, and with this, the anorectal angle tends to widen. Elevation of intrarectal and intra-abdominal pressures results in reflex relaxation of the external anal sphincter, internal anal sphincter, and puborectal muscles, and, at this point, defecation can occur effortlessly. However, some effort is usually needed to start evacuation of the rectum. The effort leads to an even greater relaxation of the sphincters and puborectal muscle, and the anorectal angle is even more obtuse. Consequently, the descent and tapering of the pelvic floor occur, and rectal contents are expelled by direct transmission of intra-abdominal pressure increased to the relaxed pelvic floor [36].

A combination of reflex and voluntary relaxation of the external anal sphincter with increasing rectal distension, prolonged relaxation of the internal anal sphincter, and "flattening" of the anal cushions due to the action of the conjoined muscle causes the anal pressure to fall [36].

After the evacuation of the rectum is completed, the transient contraction of the external anal sphincter and puborectal muscle, the so-called closing reflex, restores the tonus of the internal anal sphincter and closes the anal canal [4, 12].

The puborectalis and external anal sphincter temporarily contract and restore the anorectal angle, and the internal anal sphincter recovers its tone, which along with passive distension of the anal vascular cushions closes the anal canal [13].

The postural reflex is reinstated as a result of the decrease in intra-abdominal pressure, and the puborectalis sling returns to its contracted state to form an acute angle at the anorectal junction [12].

Table 4.1 shows a summary of the main anatomical structures involved in defecation and their respective contribution to the fecal continence.

**Table 4.1** Anatomical structures involved in defecation and respective contribution to fecal continence

| Structure, reflex, or function | Contribution toward continence |
| --- | --- |
| Anal canal | Stores feces until an acceptable place for defecation is found |
| Longitudinal anal muscle | Occludes the anal canal |
| Internal anal sphincter | Accounts for 50–85% of the resting sphincter pressure |
| External anal sphincter | Accounts for 25–30% of the resting anal sphincter pressure |
| Anal vascular cushions | Accounts for 15% of resting anal pressure |
| Rectoanal inhibitory reflex | Sampling mechanism that allows flatus to be expelled without feces |
| Rectal distension | Signals the central nervous system that defecation is needed and accommodates accumulation of feces until defecation |
| Postural reflex | Contraction of the puborectalis when sampling reflex occurs and when finishes defecation |
| Continence-preserving reflex | Contraction of the levator ani when a sudden urgency to evacuate occurs |

## 4.7    Fecal Incontinence

The maintenance of continence and defecation is determined by innumerable complex and multifactorial mechanisms, involving the integration of several functions and dependent on important factors [37].

There are a number of potential areas of injury or dysfunction in the complex mechanisms required for continence that might result in incontinence. Fecal incontinence occurs when one or more mechanisms that maintain continence are disrupted to an extent that other mechanisms are unable to compensate [38].

Perineal tears, even when carefully repaired, can be associated with incontinence, and patients may either present immediately or several years following delivery [39].

Fecal continence involves a complex interplay of sphincter and levator ani tone with pudendal nerve function. Risk factors for postpartum fecal incontinence include a history of operative delivery (forceps or vacuum) and an anal sphincter laceration. Third- and fourth-degree lacerations occur more frequently with macrosomic infants and the use of midline episiotomy. A prolonged second stage of labor may lead to an operative delivery and subsequent fecal incontinence [40]. Obstetric trauma is the most common cause of fecal incontinence in women, and symptoms of incontinence that persist for more than 6 months after delivery are reported by one-fourth of women [41].

Longer duration of defecation or incomplete emptying indicates constipation, as patients have to spend more time on the toilet. Constipation is also one of the significant risk factors related to fecal incontinence [42].

Fecal incontinence also may appear even after the simplest anal surgery. It may occur after hemorrhoidectomy as well as surgeries for anal fissures or fistulae. These procedures may result in the inability to discriminate between the contents of the rectum with resulting incontinence [43]. Hemorrhoidal vascular cushions and the anal canal mucosa support fecal continence, with the capacity of expansion to keep the anal canal closed and to prevent fecal incontinence when anal pressure decreases. The importance of cushions becomes obvious when patients present with fecal soiling after hemorrhoidectomy, even with normal sphincter pressure [37].

Fecal incontinence following anorectal surgery can result from several issues. In cases such as fistulotomy, sphincter muscle may have been intentionally divided with an underestimation of the functional consequence. At other times, damage to the anal sphincter or associated nerves occurs unintentionally. This has also been seen with intact sphincters, as the hemorrhoidal cushions are known to provide 15% of the patient's resting anal tone, and removal can unmask issues with incontinence that were being aided by these cushions [44].

Similar to obstetrical injuries, anorectal surgeries (hemorrhoidectomy, sphincterotomy, fistula surgeries) are frequently identified in patients with symptoms of incontinence. This is at variance with low percentages of incontinence when outcomes of such surgical series are reported. The explanation for this discrepancy may be found in the fact that such observational cohort studies frequently lack long-term follow-up of more than 10 years and hence fail to capture the delayed onset of symptoms to determine the true incidence of this long-term complication [1].

The major factors necessary for fecal continence are an enteric content that is substantially firm and bulky; a passively distensible, capacious, and evacuable reservoir; and an effective barrier to outflow. Therefore, changes in the quantity and/or quality of stool presented to the sphincter, the inability of the rectum to accommodate its contents, damage to or interference with the anal sphincter mechanism, and/or an impaired sensation can result in fecal incontinence. As a result, common causes of fecal incontinence include diarrhea, fecal impaction with overflow, impaired rectal storage, loss of rectal sensation to distension, rectal prolapse, and isolated or combined weakness/impairment of the internal anal sphincter, external anal sphincter, and puborectalis muscle. Frequently, it is a combination of more than one of these mechanisms [45].

Pelvic radiotherapy may lead to changes of anorectal function resulting in incontinence-related complaints. Low to moderate quality evidence indicates that radiotherapy reduces anal resting pressure, decreases rectal distensibility, and frequently induces telangiectasias of rectal mucosa. These changes may be associated with fecal incontinence, defecation urgency, and frequent bowel movements [46].

**Acknowledgments** To Dr. José Marcio Neves Jorge, Dr. Ilario Froehner Junior, and Dr. Afonso Henrique da Silva e Sousa Júnior for making available the figures used in this chapter, to Mr. Marcos Retzer (in memorium), the artist who created them and to Ms. Nádia Bollos Mosca Luque for formatting or modifying the figures and adding the English legends.

# References

1. Saldana Ruiz N, Kaiser AM. Fecal incontinence—challenges and solutions. World J Gastroenterol. 2017;23(1):11–24.
2. Sagar PM, Pemberton JH. Anorectal and pelvic floor function. Gastroenterol Clin. 1996;25(1):163–82.
3. Sun W, Donnelly T, Read N. Utility of a combined test of anorectal manometry, electromyography, and sensation in determining the mechanism of 'idiopathic' faecal incontinence. Gut. 1992;33(6):807–13.
4. Kadam-Halani PK, Arya LA, Andy UU. Clinical anatomy of fecal incontinence in women. Clin Anat. 2017;30(7):901–11.
5. Salvioli B, Bharucha AE, Rath-Harvey D, Pemberton JH, Phillips SF. Rectal compliance, capacity, and rectoanal sensation in fecal incontinence. Am J Gastroenterol. 2001;96(7):2158–68.
6. Siproudhis L, Bellissant E, Juguet F, Allain H, Bretagne J, Gosselin M. Perception of and adaptation to rectal isobaric distension in patients with faecal incontinence. Gut. 1999;44(5):687–92.
7. Siproudhis L, El Abkari M, El Alaoui M, Juguet F, Bretagne JF. Low rectal volumes in patients suffering from fecal incontinence: what does it mean? Aliment Pharmacol Ther. 2005;22(10):989–96.
8. Speakman C, Kamm M. Abnormal visceral autonomic innervation in neurogenic faecal incontinence. Gut. 1993;34(2):215–21.
9. Read N, Haynes W, Bartolo D, Hall J, Read M, Donnelly T, et al. Use of anorectal manometry during rectal infusion of saline to investigate sphincter function in incontinent patients. Gastroenterology. 1983;85(1):105–13.
10. Rao SSC. Pathophysiology of adult fecal incontinence. Gastroenterology. 2004;126:S14–22.
11. Campos F, Regadas F, Pinho M. Tratado de coloproctologia. São Paulo: Atheneu; 2012.
12. Palit S, Lunniss PJ, Scott SM. The physiology of human defecation. Dig Dis Sci. 2012;57(6):1445–64.

13. Thomson H. The anal cushions—a fresh concept in diagnosis. Postgrad Med J. 1979;55(644):403–5.
14. Kaiser AM, Ortega AE. Anorectal anatomy. Surg Clin North Am. 2002;82(6):1125–38.
15. Ashton-Miller JA, DeLancey J. Functional anatomy of the female pelvic floor. Ann N Y Acad Sci. 2007;1101(1):266–96.
16. Brookes S, Dinning P, Gladman M. Neuroanatomy and physiology of colorectal function and defaecation: from basic science to human clinical studies. Neurogastroenterol Motil. 2009;21(s2):9–19.
17. Frenckner B, Ihre T. Influence of autonomic nerves on the internal and sphincter in man. Gut. 1976;17(4):306–12.
18. Hoffman BL, Schorge JO, Bradshaw KD, Halvoroson LM, Schaffer JI, Corton MM, editors. Williams gynecology. 3rd ed. New York: McGraw-Hill; 2006.
19. Miller R, Lewis G, Bartolo D, Cervero F, Mortensen N. Sensory discrimination and dynamic activity in the anorectum: evidence using a new ambulatory technique. Br J Surg. 1988;75(10):1003–7.
20. Penninckx F, Lestar B, Kerremans R. The internal anal sphincter: mechanisms of control and its role in maintaining anal continence. Baillieres Clin Gastroenterol. 1992;6(1):193–214.
21. Lunniss P, Phillips R. Anatomy and function of the anal longitudinal muscle. Br J Surg. 1992;79(9):882–4.
22. Haas PA, Fox TA. The importance of the perianal connective tissue in the surgical anatomy and function of the anus. Dis Colon Rectum. 1977;20(4):303–13.
23. Bittorf B, Ringler R, Forster C, Hohenberger W, Matzel K. Cerebral representation of the anorectum using functional magnetic resonance imaging. Br J Surg. 2006;93(10):1251–7.
24. Turnbull GK, Hamdy S, Aziz Q, Singh KD, Thompson DG. The cortical topography of human anorectal musculature. Gastroenterology. 1999;117(1):32–9.
25. Bharucha AE. Pelvic floor: anatomy and function. Neurogastroenterol Motil. 2006;18(7):507–19.
26. Sultan AH, Nugent K. Pathophysiology and nonsurgical treatment of anal incontinence. BJOG. 2004;111(s1):84–90.
27. Furness JB, Callaghan BP, Rivera LR, Cho H-J. The enteric nervous system and gastrointestinal innervation: integrated local and central control. In: Lyte M, Cryan JF, editors. Microbial endocrinology: the microbiota-gut-brain axis in health and disease. Advances in experimental medicine and biology. New York, NY: Springer; 2014. p. 39–71.
28. Coggrave M, Norton C. Neurogenic bowel. Handb Clin Neurol. 2013;110:221–8.
29. Steele SR, Hull TL, Read TE, Saclarides TJ, Senagore AJ, Whitlow CB. The ASCRS textbook of colon and rectal surgery. 3rd ed. New York: Springer; 2016.
30. Tagliafico A, Perez MM, Martinoli C. High-resolution ultrasound of the pudendal nerve: normal anatomy. Muscle Nerve. 2013;47(3):403–8.
31. Shafik A. A concept of the anatomy of the anal sphincter mechanism and the physiology of defecation. Dis Colon Rectum. 1987;30(12):970–82.
32. Degen L, Phillips S. How well does stool form reflect colonic transit? Gut. 1996;39(1):109–13.
33. Davies G, Crowder M, Reid B, Dickerson J. Bowel function measurements of individuals with different eating patterns. Gut. 1986;27(2):164–9.
34. O'Donnell L, Virjee J, Heaton KW. Detection of pseudodiarrhoea by simple clinical assessment of intestinal transit rate. BMJ. 1990;300(6722):439.
35. Bharucha AE. Lower gastrointestinal functions. Neurogastroenterol Motil. 2008;20(s1):103–13.
36. Barleben A, Mills S. Anorectal anatomy and physiology. Surg Clin N Am. 2010;90(1):1–15.
37. Oliveira C. Fisiologia anorretal. 2nd ed. Rio de Janeiro: Editora Rubio; 2017.
38. Rao SSC. Diagnosis and management of fecal incontinence. Am J Gastroenterol. 2004;99(8):1585–604.
39. Sultan AH, Kamm MA, Hudson CN, Bartram CI. Third degree obstetric anal sphincter tears: risk factors and outcome of primary repair. BMJ. 1994;308(6933):887–91.
40. Chin K. Obstetrics and fecal incontinence. Clin Colon Rectal Surg. 2014;27(3):110–2.

41. Fitzpatrick M, O'Herlihy C. The effects of labour and delivery on the pelvic floor. Best Pract Res Clin Obstet Gynaecol. 2001;15(1):63–79.
42. Roslani AC, Ramakrishnan R, Azmi S, Arapoc DJ, Goh A. Prevalence of faecal incontinence and its related factors among patients in a Malaysian academic setting. BMC Gastroenterol. 2014;14(1):95.
43. Santos CRS, Lima TGS, Schmidt FMQ, Santos VLCG. Pelvic floor rehabilitation in analysis incontinence. In: Catto-Smith AG, editor. Fecal incontinence - Causes, Management and Outcome. Rijeka (Croatia): In-Tech. 2014:107–22. https://doi.org/10.5772/57364. ISBN 978-953-51-1241-9
44. Kunitake H, Poylin V. Complications following anorectal surgery. Clin Colon Rectal Surg. 2016;29(01):014–21.
45. Lazarescu A, Turnbull GK, Vanner S. Investigating and treating fecal incontinence: when and how. Can J Gastroenterol Hepatol. 2009;23(4):301–8.
46. Krol R, Smeenk RJ, Van Lin ENJT, Yeoh EEK, Hopman WPM. Systematic review: anal and rectal changes after radiotherapy for prostate cancer. Int J Color Dis. 2014;29(3):273–83.

# Clinical Assessment and Differential Diagnosis of Fecal Incontinence and Its Severity

5

Kathleen F. Hunter, Tamara Dickinson, and Veronica Haggar

**Abstract**

Assessment and diagnosis of fecal incontinence by the advanced practice nurse involve critical thinking in the process of differential diagnosis of fecal incontinence. Fecal incontinence is a stigmatized condition that requires the advanced practice nurse to approach the patient from a perspective of cultural competence, demonstrating respect and acknowledgment of the sensitive nature of the concern. History taking starts with symptom assessment, as well as gathering a comprehensive health history. The use of a standardized symptom assessment instrument, particularly one that includes quality of life, can be helpful. The physical examination includes abdominal examination, vaginal examination in women, assessment of pelvic muscles in both women and men, and rectal examination. Arriving at the differential diagnosis must take into account the data gathered in the history and physical exam, as well as consideration of the breadth of potential causes, including red flag symptoms and signs. Laboratory investigations for specific conditions that may contribute to fecal incontinence may include tests for suspected hypo- and hyperthyroidism, diabetes, celiac disease,

K. F. Hunter (✉)
Faculty of Nursing, University of Alberta, Edmonton, AB, Canada

Glenrose Hospital Continence Clinic, Edmonton, AB, Canada
e-mail: kathleen.hunter@ualberta.ca

T. Dickinson
Radiation Oncology, Southwestern Medical Center, Harold C. Simmons Comprehensive Cancer Center, Dallas, TX, USA
e-mail: tamara.dickinson@utsouthwestern.edu

V. Haggar
Homerton University Hospital, NHS Foundation Trust, London, UK
e-mail: v.haggar@nhs.net

© Springer International Publishing AG, part of Springer Nature 2018
D. Z. Bliss (ed.), *Management of Fecal Incontinence for the Advanced Practice Nurse*,
https://doi.org/10.1007/978-3-319-90704-8_5

colorectal cancer screening, and infection. Diagnostic imaging to further evaluate fecal incontinence may be ordered by the advanced practice nurse or be accessed through referral.

**Keywords**
Assessment · History taking · Rectal examination · Pelvic floor · Differential diagnosis

## 5.1    Introduction

The nursing process begins with assessment from which the advanced practice nurse initiates the critical thinking and differential diagnosis processes. Evidence-based clinical decision-making involves evidence-based research and theory, subjective and objective assessment, patient preferences and values, and clinical expertise [1]. Fecal incontinence management is often a collaborative process between the advanced practice nurse and patient/caregiver in which patient-centered expected outcomes are key to development of a comprehensive plan.

Unique to nursing is the holistic health model in which the person is seen and evaluated as a whole individual. For the advanced practice nurse to practice effectively, cultural competence is crucial. This concept may be even more important when sensitive topics such as fecal incontinence are discussed. It is important for the advanced practice nurse to provide effective care as well as respectful care within the framework of cultural competence [1, 2]. Cultural competence begins first and foremost with respect. In addition to cultural competence, the advanced practice nurse needs to understand the sensitivity of this issue and approach the interview and discussion with care. Research has shown that stigma is associated with incontinence [3]. The taboo of this issue has been a catalyst for work that includes anti-stigma awareness and education programs [4].

The 6th International Consultation on Incontinence identifies that initial clinical assessment of fecal incontinence should include history, physical examination, medication and diet review, and assessment on impact on quality of life [5]. Box 5.1 provides an overview of the steps in assessment of fecal incontinence. As many people may be reluctant to discuss this condition, active case finding is recommended and the advanced practice nurse should inquire about any problems patients experience with anal or fecal incontinence.

**Box 5.1: Steps in Assessment of Fecal Incontinence**
- Taking a thorough history allows the advanced practice nurse to understand the concern from the perspective of the patient.
    - The advanced practice nurse must demonstrate an open and respectful manner to build rapport about a sensitive topic.
- The focused interview should include:
    - Methodical symptom assessment including identification of stool consistency and use of a fecal incontinence scale that includes quality of life
    - A health history and review of systems including current pharmacological and non-pharmacological treatments
    - Functional assessment (activities of daily living, mobility, cognitive function)
    - Nutritional status (eating patterns, weight changes, appetite changes, food intolerances, non-prescription supplements)
- Physical examination should include:
    - A general survey and observation of mobility
    - Abdominal examination
    - Female pelvic/vaginal exam and assessment pelvic floor
    - Male assessment of pelvic floor
    - Rectal examination
- Other data to review:
    - Results of previous recent laboratory and diagnostics tests

## 5.2 Understanding the Concern: History Taking and Gaining the Patient Perspective

The interview is the process of obtaining the important subjective data from the patient. It is also the crucial point in which the advanced practice nurse can develop rapport with the patient. Rapport allows the patient to be able to openly share relevant information and to feel accepted [1]. Likewise, a good rapport allows the advanced practice nurse to build a continuing therapeutic relationship for future encounters for planning, treatment, and education. Important techniques of communication for the interview involve the ability to listen, ask open-ended and closed (or direct) questions as appropriate, facilitating the story, empathy, and clarification [1]. The patient interview should end smoothly and not abruptly. A summary of the focused concerns should likely be followed by giving the patient the opportunity to express any concluding thoughts [1].

The focused interview of the patient with fecal incontinence should include symptom assessment and health history. The health history includes review of systems to evaluate past and present health states and identify current pharmacological and non-pharmacological treatments. Particular attention should be paid to the gastrointestinal, reproductive, neurologic, and musculoskeletal systems. For women, obstetrical history should be included to identify potential risk of obstetrical anal injury. A functional assessment should be considered to evaluate for the ability to perform activities of daily living, mobility, cognitive function, and independence [1]. Questions about eating patterns, weight changes, appetite changes, food intolerances, and non-prescription supplements will add information about the patient's nutritional status [1].

## 5.2.1 Focused History Taking with the Patient Presenting with Fecal Incontinence

As with any patient concern, history taking begins with a methodical symptom assessment focused on the presenting concern. To ensure a thorough and systematic approach, many advanced practice nurses use a mnemonic such as OLDCARTS (onset, location, duration, character, aggravating/associated factors, relieving factors, temporal factors, severity) [6], PQRST (precipitating factors, quality, radiation, severity, timing [onset duration frequency]), or CLIENT OUTCOMES (character, location, impact, expectation, neglect, timing, other, understanding/ beliefs, treatment, complementary therapies, options, modulating factors, exposure, spirituality) [7]. Whatever the approach, the goal is to gain an in-depth understanding of the patient's perspective and symptom experience.

The symptom assessment in fecal incontinence can be augmented by use of a standardized assessment tool for assessing anal and fecal incontinence severity [8]. Symptoms included in the tools vary but most cover the nature of the incontinence (e.g., incontinence of feces and flatus), as well as awareness of the incontinence, frequency of loss, and consistency of stool. Some instruments have questions on accompanying complaints such as urgency and abdominal pain or incorporate a quality of life score with assessment of symptom severity. Examples of tools include the International Consultation on Incontinence Questionnaire-Bowel (ICIQ-B) module [9, 10], Revised Fecal Incontinence Scale [11], the Jorge-Wexner Incontinence Scale [12], Fecal Incontinence Quality of Life (FIQOL) scale [13], and St Mark's Incontinence Scale [14]. There is no tool currently available that assesses/scores the severity of fecal incontinence only, however. A detailed review of instruments for rating severity of fecal incontinence is available in Chap. 16 of the 6th International Consultation on Incontinence [5]. These tools are most often used for research but can be useful in clinical practice as well. The advanced practice nurse using a standardized instrument should be aware of what it measures in comparison to other tools in order to interpret its findings correctly and choose a tool suitable for their practice that is easy for their patients to complete.

Assessment should include determining the type of stool. There are several visual tools available. The Bristol stool chart [15] is a tool commonly used by clinicians or researchers in identifying types of stool form/consistency by using seven illustrations and descriptions of stool forms varying from hard to watery consistency. Another visual tool developed primarily for patient use by Bliss and colleagues [16] has illustrations and descriptions of four stool consistency types (hard and formed, soft but formed, loose and unformed, liquid) (see Fig. 5.1). It is also helpful to have the patient track their bowel movements 24 h a day for several days to determine the pattern of bowel movements and episodes of anal or fecal incontinence. See the example of a simple bowel record in Fig. 5.2. Stool consistency can be included in a bowel record. Assessment should also include questions about incomplete evacuation and constipation. These symptoms are addressed in Chap. 8 (about managing fecal incontinence in nursing home residents) and Chap. 9 (about neurogenic fecal incontinence).

| Hard and Formed | Soft but Formed | Loose and Unformed | Liquid |
|---|---|---|---|
| 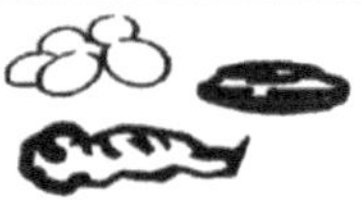 | 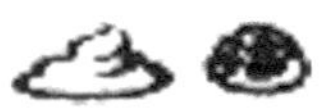 | 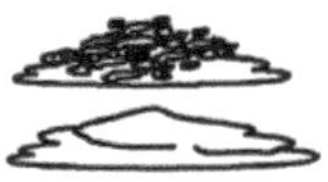 | 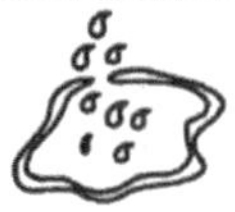 |
| Having a hard or firm texture & retaining a definite shape like a banana, cigar or marbles. | Retaining same general shape in the collection bag; does not spread all over the bottom of the bag or has a texture that appears like peanut butter. | Lacking any shape of its own; spreads over the bottom of the collection bag; having a texture that appears like hot cereal. | Like water. |

**Fig. 5.1** Example of a stool consistency system [16]. Reproduced with permission from copyright holder, D. Z. Bliss

| Bowel record Date: | | | |
|---|---|---|---|
| Time | Bowel movement | Stool consistency 1-4 | Bowel leak |
| 12:00 am Midnight | | | |
| 1:00 am | | | |
| 2:00am | | | |

**Fig. 5.2** Example of a simple bowel record

## 5.3    Physical Examination

### 5.3.1    General Survey/Mobility

As noted in the introduction, the physical examination begins with a general survey observation of the patient's mobility. People with impaired mobility may have difficulty accessing a toilet in a timely manner, compromising continence.

### 5.3.2    Abdominal Examination

With the patient lying supine, inspect the contour and symmetry of the abdomen noting if it is flat, scaphoid, rounded, or protuberant [1]. Distention can be marked in obstruction of the colon. Observe for scars, striae (stretch marks), and pulsations (in the thin person, normal pulsation of the aorta may be observed). Use the diaphragm of the stethoscope to auscultate the four quadrants for the normally high-pitched bowel sounds. The absence of bowel sounds (a silent abdomen) is established only after listening for 5 min. A silent abdomen may indicate intestinal obstruction, paralytic ileus, or peritonitis. Percuss the abdomen in all four quadrants. Normally, tympany should predominate due to gas in the gastrointestinal tract, with dullness over the liver and spleen. Perform light and deep palpation to assess for any areas of tenderness or for masses. Dilated loops of bowel may be palpable in fecal impaction or ileus.

### 5.3.3    Female Pelvic/Vaginal Exam and Assessment of the Pelvic Floor

Female pelvic examination should be undertaken with attention to assessment of any pelvic organ prolapse and pelvic floor strength and tone. The patient may have reported a bulge near the anus (anorectal prolapse). Higher stage prolapse (e.g., past the level of the hymen) can induce bladder symptoms as well as symptoms of anorectal dysfunction including constipation; incomplete bowel evacuation; the need to strain, splint, or digitally support or apply manual pressure to defecate; a sensation of anorectal blockage; fecal urgency; or soiling after defecation [17]. Higher stage posterior vaginal wall prolapse can involve a rectal protrusion into the vagina (rectocele).

Descent of the anterior or posterior vaginal walls or uterus (vaginal vault after hysterectomy) may be detected during inspection and palpation. With the patient in the dorsal lithotomy position, gently separate the labia and inspect the vaginal orifice for any bulge of tissue. Ask the patient to perform a Valsalva maneuver so the extent of the prolapse is evident. Insert the speculum to visualize the vaginal canal. In order to adequately assess the prolapse and identify if it involves the anterior or posterior walls (or both), the speculum must be split to a single blade or a single blade Breisky speculum must be used. The single blade is reinserted lifting the anterior wall and then reinserted to hold back the posterior wall [18]. The examiner inserts a gloved finger and again lets the patient do a Valsava maneuver to assess for apical (uterine or vault) prolapse.

The Pelvic Organ Prolapse Quantification System (POPQ) staging method is recommended for staging prolapse [17]. The POPQ is used to measure, describe, and stage pelvic organ prolapse. It uses anatomically specific points and their relationship to each other. There are six points that are measured, in centimeters, within the vagina in relationship to the hymen:

- Two points on the anterior vaginal wall
- The cervix or vaginal cuff scar (post-hysterectomy)
- Posterior fornix (not applicable post-hysterectomy)
- Two points on the posterior vaginal wall

Three other anatomical landmarks are also measured: total vaginal length, genital hiatus, and perineal body. The nine numbers are then presented in a grid. The numbers have positive or negative values depending on whether they are above or below the hymen. Negative numbers are within the vagina (or above the hymen), and positive numbers are external (or below the hymen). The greater the degree of positive numbers, the greater the genital prolapse external to the vagina. This number of measurements allows the individual variation of prolapse to be quantified and documented with accuracy. However, it may require additional education and skill building to use reliably.

For a less complex system, it is also possible to clinically stage the POP, looking at the most distal portion of the prolapse (anterior, posterior, or apical) in relation to the hymenal ring:

- Stage 0: No prolapse is demonstrated.
- Stage I: Most distal portion of the prolapse is more than 1 cm above the level of the hymen.
- Stage II: The most distal portion of the prolapse is situated between 1 cm above the hymen and 1 cm below the hymen.
- Stage III: The most distal portion of the prolapse is more than 1 cm beyond the plane of the hymen but everted at least 2 cm less than the total vaginal length.
- Stage IV: Complete eversion or eversion at least within 2 cm of the total length of the lower genital tract is demonstrated [17].

Keeping the finger in the vagina, the strength of the pelvic floor can be *estimated* using vaginal palpation. Have the patient contract the pelvic floor by squeezing the rectum as if they were trying to stop themselves from passing flatus. You may need to coach the patient not to contract the abdominal or buttocks muscles. Contraction and lift of pelvic floor are often graded on the modified Oxford scale developed by Laycock (1994) [19]. The contraction is scored from 0 to 5, with 0 being no contraction, 1 a flicker, 2 a weak squeeze without lift, 3 a fair squeeze with some lift, 4 a good squeeze with lift, and 5 a strong squeeze with lift. This scale is subjective and requires training and experience to use. Specialist nurses and physiotherapists may also employ other instruments to measure contraction more accurately and reliably. During contraction, the examiner should also palpate the puborectalis muscle (part of the levator ani muscle that forms a sling around the rectum and maintains the anorectal angle) for any defects that suggest previous injury [17]. This muscle can also be palpated rectally above the internal anal sphincter [20].

### 5.3.4  Male Assessment of Pelvic Floor

In the male, the pelvic floor strength can be assessed during rectal examination by palpating for contraction of the puborectalis muscle above the internal anal sphincter.

### 5.3.5  Rectal Examination

Assist the patient to take the left position with legs flexed and the right leg higher than the left (male or female), the lithotomy position (female), or standing position bent forward with arms resting on exam table with toes pointed in (male) [1]. The rectal examination begins with inspection of the perianal area and anus. Note any scarring, lesions, hemorrhoids, and rectal skin tags. Identify any erythema, rash, or excoriation of the perianal tissue or external presence of stool/smearing in undergarments. Normally, the anal opening is symmetrically round and closed tightly. Observe for any sphincter asymmetry, reduced or absent tissue in the perineal body, and a fibromuscular mass between the urogenital triangle and the anal triangle in both males and females. In the female, the perineal body is the tissue between the posterior border of the vagina and the rectum and can be damaged in childbirth. Potential abnormal findings are listed in Table 5.1. Describe the position of any abnormalities using clockface terminology (e.g., 12 o'clock is anterior toward the symphysis pubis, 6 o'clock toward the coccyx) [1].

With a gloved finger, apply gentle traction on the anal verge to further check for any gapping. To perform the digital rectal exam, lubricate the index finger and gently insert into the anus toward the umbilicus. You should feel the sphincter tighten then relax. Palpate the entire muscular ring of the sphincters (you may feel the intersphincteric grove between the internal and external sphincters). Press your thumb externally on the perineal body and palpate. Insert your finger further to assess the rectum, rotating gently. Have the patient voluntarily tighten the sphincter to assess tone, and perform a Valsalva maneuver to check for relaxation of the sphincter and pelvic floor muscles [20]. The advanced practice nurse can use the digital rectal examination scoring system (DRESS) to describe both resting and squeeze pressure [21]. The score ranges from 0 to 5 (0, no discernable pressure; 3, normal; 5, extremely tight). Normally the rectal tissue is smooth. In the male, the prostate gland is palpable on the anterior wall of the rectum and should be smooth and symmetrical. The cervix of the female may be palpable on the anterior wall.

**Table 5.1** Potential abnormal findings on inspection of the anus and DRE

| Appearance of the anus | Etiology | Further examination |
|---|---|---|
| Anus gapping or open at rest (patulous) | May be related to poor pelvic floor tone, rectal prolapse, or neurological damage | Have the patient perform a Valsalva maneuver to see if rectal mucosal walls prolapse. If a neurological component is suspected (e.g., poor tone), check sensation in the saddle area |
| Rectal prolapse | Rectal mucosa or full thickness of rectal walls protrude past the anal sphincters. Contributors may include weakened sphincter tone, poor pelvic floor tone (with or without concomitant pelvic organ prolapse in the female), or diastasis of the levator ani | May reduce spontaneously or manually. An incarcerated rectal prolapse that is edematous and nonreducible is a surgical emergency [22] |
| Thickened sphincter | May be associated with chronic constipation and straining | Have the patient sit on a commode and attempt to void, check the perineum for rectal prolapse [5] |
| Keyhole deformity | Indicative of a sphincter defect | Ensure entire sphincter is palpated during exam to identify location of any disruption in continuity of the sphincter or rectopubic diastasis |
| Anal fissures | Painful cracks in the walls of the anus, leading to pain with defecation. Chronic anal fissures may lead to hypertrophied anal papilla, a sentinel skin tag in the anal canal, and exposed internal anal sphincter muscle. A bleeding fissure may be misdiagnosed as hemorrhoids [23] | |
| Paradoxical puborectalis contraction (also called dyssynergia) | Persistent contraction of the sphincter/pelvic floor due to nonrelaxation during Valsava. Associated with retained stool and overflow incontinence | |

Abnormal findings include rectal masses or hard stool in the rectum. As you withdraw your finger, take note of any blood, stool, or mucous. Any stool on the glove should be soft and brown.

### 5.3.6   Neurological Exam

The cauda equina is the horse's tail, named as it includes the nerves with dorsal and ventral lumbar, sacral, and coccygeal roots that fan out. Sympathetic innervation of the rectum arises from T11 to L1 via hypogastric plexus and cause relaxation of the rectum and anal canal and contraction of the internal anal sphincter. Parasympathetic innervation arises from the second, third, and fourth sacral roots, with parasympathetic stimulation leading to relaxation of the internal anal sphincter. The external anal sphincter is innervated by the pudendal nerve (S2,3,4) and is a voluntary muscle [24]. If neurological involvement is suspected, the advanced practice nurse must assess the dermatomes in the saddle area. Sensation can be tested using sharp/dull differentiation and light touch in the areas of S2–S4. Stroking the area around the anus should normally elicit the anal reflex (anal wink). Acute onset of perianal (saddle) anesthesia with urinary retention and fecal incontinence may represent cauda equina syndrome. This syndrome is brought on by compression of the cauda equina by trauma, tumor, infection/inflammation, or herniated disc [25]. This condition requires immediate intervention to prevent long-term damage.

## 5.4 Diagnostic Reasoning and Differential Diagnosis of Fecal Incontinence

Diagnostic (clinical) reasoning involves the synthesis, interpretation and prioritization of the patient data from the history, physical exam and any existing laboratory, and diagnostic imaging results available. As with any condition, the advanced practice nurse must be careful not to close off diagnostic possibilities too soon and consider an array of possibilities that may explain the patient's fecal incontinence, including red flag symptoms that may indicate serious disease and acute conditions requiring immediate attention.

### 5.4.1 Common Conditions and Red Flags

Fecal incontinence can arise from a variety of etiological factors including diet and food intolerances, chronic diarrhea or impaction, functional and cognitive issues, inflammatory or infectious disease, congenital conditions, central or peripheral neurological conditions, colorectal cancer, obstetrical trauma, or postsurgical intervention. Many of these conditions are discussed in detail in subsequent chapters of this book. As fecal incontinence can be associated with a number of conditions from different body systems, it may be useful to use a mnemonic to assist in identification of potential conditions, followed by analysis and prioritization of the most likely conditions, and ruling out of those that are less likely. One tool is the mnemonic VINDICATED [26] (see Table 5.2).

Red flag symptoms requiring further investigation and referral include abdominal pain, rectal bleeding, unexplained anemia, blood mixed in stool, weight loss, change in stool caliber (e.g., ribbonlike stool suggestive of rectal obstruction from a mass), or any other recent, sudden change in bowel habits (diarrhea or constipation). In creating and validating an algorithm for identification of risk for colorectal cancer in primary care, Hippisley-Cox and Coupland (2012) [27] identified seven clinical variables for females (age, family history of gastrointestinal cancer, anemia,

**Table 5.2** Application of the VINDICATED mnemonic to fecal incontinence diagnostic reasoning

|  | Possible findings |
|---|---|
| V = vascular | Protruding internal hemorrhoids<br>Rectal ischemia |
| I = infectious/ inflammatory | Diarrhea from gut infection (e.g., *C. difficile*)<br>Perianal infections<br>Proctitis |
| N = neoplasm | Anal carcinoma<br>Rectal carcinoma |
| D = degenerative | Diseases of the central nervous system (e.g., cerebrovascular accident, dementia, multiple sclerosis)<br>Pelvic organ prolapse<br>Rectocele |
| I = iatrogenic/injury | Diarrhea from gut infection (e.g., *C. difficile*)<br>Obstetrical injury (forceps, episiotomy, perineal tears) leading to sphincter disruption or pudendal nerve injury<br>Spinal cord injury<br>Post colon/rectal resection or anorectal surgery<br>Anorectal trauma |
| C = congenital | Congenital abnormalities such as rectal sphincter malformation<br>Spinal bifida<br>Hirschsprung's disease |
| A = autoimmune | Inflammatory bowel disease |
| T = toxic | Constipation, fecal impaction, or diarrhea as medication side effects<br>Food intolerance or allergy (lactose intolerance, celiac disease) |
| E = endocrine | Diabetes, hypothyroidism |
| D = depression | Constipation associated with low activity/poor diet |

rectal bleeding, abdominal pain, appetite loss, and weight loss). For men, the risk variables also included alcohol use and change in bowel habit. Patients with suspected inflammatory bowel disease or malabsorption syndrome would benefit from referral to a gastroenterologist, although the advanced practice nurse may initiate investigations as a part of the referral. Findings on the physical examination that require surgical referral include a suspected rectovaginal fistula or pelvic organ prolapse beyond the introitus. Etiologies/causes of fecal incontinence can be multifactorial or unknown (i.e., idiopathic).

## 5.5    Diagnostic Investigation

### 5.5.1    Laboratory

There are a number of laboratory test that may be undertaken to exclude or monitor other pathologies that contribute to fecal incontinence. These include laboratory tests for hypo- or hyperthyroidism, diabetes, colorectal cancer screening, and celiac disease.

Hypo- or hyperthyroidism affects the body's metabolic rate (raising or lowering), consequently increasing or decreasing the number of bowel movements. An increased metabolism (hyperthyroidism) will increase the number and rate of bowel movement, which will decrease colonic transit time and create a softer stool and possible fecal urgency with fecal incontinence. Hypothyroidism will do the opposite, increasing the possibility of constipation and impaction. Thyroid function tests usually include thyroid-stimulating hormone (TSH), produced by the pituitary gland to stimulate the thyroid gland to produce thyroxine and thyroxine (T4). An elevated TSH and a low T4 are indicative of hypothyroidism, and a low TSH and elevated T4 are indicative of hyperthyroidism.

Uncontrolled diabetes can result in peripheral nerve damage which can in turn affect the nervous control and sensation of the bowel, resulting in changes to gastrointestinal motility and diabetes-related enteropathy and symptoms ranging from constipation, diarrhea, and potentially fecal incontinence [28]. A random blood glucose can be ordered, although more commonly hemoglobin A1c (HbA1c) is used to monitor diabetes as it measures glycated hemoglobin and reflects average blood glucose levels over a 3-month period.

The fecal immunochemical test is appropriate if there is any sign of gastrointestinal bleeding. It is a screening test for colorectal cancer that is specific for the globin portion of human hemoglobin. It does not require any dietary or medication restrictions and consequently has better patient compliance. False positives due to mucosal inflammation or medication are also reduced.

Patients with chronic diarrhea and signs of malabsorption suggestive of celiac disease should have an IgA anti-tissue transglutaminase antibody and total IgA blood test. IgA anti-tissue transglutaminase antibody is an antibody produced in response to the eating of gluten, common in those with celiac disease where diarrhea is a common symptom. This is the preferred test in primary care settings [29]. Those who are positive should be referred to a gastroenterologist for further evaluation including biopsy. Other relevant tests include stool studies to identify fecal parasites or microbial infection, such as *Clostridium difficile*. Stool osmolality is sometimes used in evaluation of chronic watery diarrhea.

## 5.5.2   Diagnostic Imaging

There is a wide variety of diagnostic imaging tools available to assist in the assessment of fecal incontinence. Although the advanced practice nurse may not be involved in interpretation of the test, she/he should have an understanding of the purpose and indications of investigative testing for appropriate ordering and referral, as well as explaining investigations to patients.

Proctoscopy (using a rigid scope) and sigmoidoscopy (with a flexible scope) are used to identify polyps, malignancy, and proctitis. This test is usually conducted by a gastroenterologist, colorectal surgeon, or other healthcare professional with specialized training.

Anorectal manometry measures the pressures in the anal canal and distal rectum including resting and maximal (squeeze) anal pressures, rectal compliance, and rectal sensitivity to distension [30]. Rectal compliance and sensitivity are measured by rectal balloon inflation, and probes can measure thermal and electrical sensitivity in the anal canal. Anal resting pressure is the combined pressure of the internal sphincter, the external sphincter, and the anal cushions. There is however, a lack of defined values for a normal range. Patients with fecal incontinence tend to have a lower anal resting tone than continent patients, though other factors contribute such as stool consistency and rectal compliance. The maximal pressure (squeeze pressure) is the increase in anal canal pressure with the contraction of the external anal sphincter, usually measured from resting pressure to maximal squeeze. Reduced maximal pressures are typically due to injury of the external anal sphincter, neurological conditions, poor patient compliance, or voluntary control. Rectal compliance and sensitivity are measured using rectal balloon inflation in the distal rectum with feedback from the patient regarding the first sensation, first urge to defecate, and the maximum tolerable volume. Hypersensitivity is a contributor to urgency fecal incontinence, while hyposensitivity results in passive or overflow fecal incontinence [5]. Recent advances in technology have allowed development of ambulatory monitoring [30], and high-resolution manometry using a catheter with over 200 miniature pressure sensors provides more detail of sphincter function [5].

Anorectal ultrasound and endoanal MRI measure sphincter muscle thickness and detect muscle defects from trauma or surgical injury. Endoanal ultrasound (EAUS) is the gold standard investigation for the structural assessment of the anal canal [5]. This test assesses the external sphincter and puborectalis muscle and can assist in differentiating incontinent patients with intact anal sphincters from those with defects, scarring, and atrophy due to vaginal delivery or anal surgery. It is also extremely useful prior to surgical repair and in the evaluation of treatments. Transperineal or transvaginal ultrasound can also be used. Endoanal ultrasound provides additional information on the condition of the pelvic floor muscles and levator hiatus. Endoanal magnetic resonance imaging (MRI) has been shown to be useful prior to sphincter repair and provides some prognostic information; however, this is more costly than ultrasound.

Defecography (defecating proctogram or evacuation proctography) involves the evacuation of a simulated stool (barium) and allows for both static and dynamic measurements of the pelvic floor, puborectalis function, and anorectal angle [30]. Although continence has been tested by infusing saline rectally or measuring the resistance to evacuation of a solid object [30], defecography has limited usefulness as a diagnostic test in the assessment of fecal incontinence but is useful in those undergoing laparoscopic ventral rectopexy or to identify rectal intussusception and rectocele [5].

Neurophysiological testing has a long history with assessment of incontinence but is used less frequently as the accuracy of imaging techniques has increased. It now tends to be used in complex cases that may be secondary to neurological disease and spinal injury. Electromyography assesses external sphincter and puborectalis muscle activity, although it is largely replaced now with more accurate sphincter imaging techniques [5]. Pudendal nerve conduction studies measure the nerve conduction velocity in the pudendal nerve, but there is little evidence that pudendal neuropathy correlates to incontinence [5].

## Conclusion

Assessment and diagnosis of fecal incontinence by the advanced practice nurse involve skills of history taking using an approach that is considerate of the sensitive nature of the problem and specialized physical examination techniques. Differential diagnosis must include thinking broadly of a wide variety of potential contributors and causes, and the advanced practice nurse must use the data from the history and physical exam to identify the most likely cause of the fecal incontinence and initiate any relevant investigations and referrals.

## References

1. Jarvis C. Physical examination and health assessment. Elsevier Health Sciences: St. Louis; 2016.
2. Stanhope M, Lancaster J. Public health nursing: population-centered health care in the community. 8th ed. Elsevier Mosby: Maryland Heights, MO; 2012.
3. Elstad EA, Taubenberger SP, Botelho EM, Tennstedt SL. Beyond incontinence: the stigma of other urinary symptoms. J Adv Nurs. 2010;66(11):2460–70.
4. The Simon Foundation for Continence. First International Conference on Stigma in Healthcare. http://simonfoundation.org/1st-conference-stigma-healthcare/.
5. Bliss DZ, Mimura T, Berghmans B, Bharucha A, Chiarioni G, Emmanuel A, et al. Assessment and conservative management of faecal incontinence and quality of life in adults. In: Abrams P, Cardozo L, Wagg A, Wein A, editors. Incontinence. 6th ed. Bristol: International Continence Society; 2017. p. 1993–2085.
6. Daines J, Baumann L, Scheibel P. Advanced health assessment and clinical diagnosis in primary care. 4th ed. St. Louis, MI: Elsevier Mosby; 2012.
7. Rhoads J, Petersen SW. Advanced health assessment and diagnostic reasoning. Burlington, MA: Jones & Bartlett Learning; 2016.
8. Nevler A. The epidemiology of anal incontinence and symptom severity scoring. Gastroenterol Rep (Oxf). 2014;2(2):79–84.
9. Cotterill N, Norton C, Avery KNL, Donovan JL. A patient-centered approach to developing a comprehensive symptom and quality of life assessment of anal incontinence. Dis Colon Rectum. 2008;51(1):82–7.
10. Cotterill N, Norton C, Avery KN, Abrams P, Donovan JL. Psychometric evaluation of a new patient-completed questionnaire for evaluating anal incontinence symptoms and impact on quality of life: the ICIQ-B. Dis Colon Rectum. 2011;54(10):1235–50.
11. Sansoni J, Hawthorne G, Fleming G, Marosszeky N. The revised faecal incontinence scale: a clinical validation of a new, short measure for assessment and outcomes evaluation. Dis Colon Rectum. 2013;56(5):652–9.
12. Jorge JMN, Wexner SD. Etiology and management of fecal incontinence. Dis Colon Rectum. 1993;36(1):77–97.
13. Rockwood TH, Church JM, Fleshman JW, Kane RL, Mavrantonis C, Thorson AG, et al. Fecal incontinence quality of life scale: a quality of life instrument for patients with fecal incontinence. Dis Colon Rectum. 2000;43:9–17.

14. Vaizey CJ, Carapeti E, Cahill JA, Kamm MA. Prospective comparison of faecal incontinence grading systems. Gut. 1999;44(1):77–80.
15. Lewis SJ, Heaton KW. Stool form scale as a useful guide to intestinal transit time. Scand J Gastroenterol. 1997;32(9):920–4.
16. Bliss DZ, Larson SJ, Burr JK, Savik K. Reliability of a stool consistency classification system. J Wound Ostomy Cont Nurs. 2001;28(6):305–13.
17. Haylen B, Maher C, Camargo S, Dandolu V, Withagen M. An International Urogynecological Association (IUGA)/International Continence Society (ICS) joint report on the terminology for female pelvic organ prolapse (POP). Neurourol Urodyn. 2016;35:137–68.
18. Riss P, Koch M. Evaluation of pelvic organ prolapse. In: Principles and practice of urogynaecology. New Delhi: Springer India; 2015. p. 107–14.
19. Laycock J. Pelvic muscle exercises: physiotherapy for the pelvic floor. Urol Nurs. 1994;14:136–40.
20. American Gastroenterological Association. American Gastroenterological Association Medical position statement on constipation. Gastroenterology. 2013;144:211–7.
21. Orkin BA, Sinykin SB, Lloyd PC. The digital rectal examination scoring system (DRESS). Dis Colon Rectum. 2010;53(12):1656–60.
22. Cannon JA. Evaluation, diagnosis, and medical management of rectal prolapse. Clin Colon Rectal Surg. 2017;30(01):016–21.
23. Stewart DB Sr, Gaertner W, Glasgow S, Migaly J, Feingold D, Steele SR. Clinical practice guideline for the management of anal fissures. Dis Colon Rectum. 2017;60(1):7–14.
24. Birnbaum E, editor. Surgical anatomy of the colon, rectum, and anus. Cham: Springer International; 2017.
25. Theys T, Kho KH. The saddle and the horse's tail: Cauda equina syndrome. JAMA Neurol. 2014;71(7):914–5.
26. Weinstein A, Pinto-Powell R. Introductory clinical reasoning curriculum. MedEdPortal. 2016.; https://doi.org/10.15766/mep_2374-8265.10370
27. Hippisley-Cox J, Coupland C. Identifying patients with suspected colorectal cancer in primary care: derivation and validation of an algorithm. Br J Gen Pract. 2012;62(594):e29–37. https://doi.org/10.3399/bjgp12X616346
28. Krishnan B, Babu S, Walker J, Walker AB, Pappachan JM. Gastrointestinal complications of diabetes mellitus. World J Diabetes. 2013;4(3):51–63.
29. Rubio-Tapia A, Hill ID, Kelly CP, Calderwood AH, Murray JA. ACG clinical guidelines: diagnosis and management of celiac disease. Am J Gastroenterol. 2013;108(5):656–76.
30. Yamada T, Inadomi J, Bhattacharya R, Dominitz J, Hwang J. Yamada's handbook of gastroenterology. 3rd ed. Hoboken, NJ: Wiley; 2013.

# Management of Fecal Incontinence in Community-Living Adults

6

Frankie Bates, Donna Z. Bliss, Alison Bardsely, and Winnie Ka Wai Yeung

**Abstract**

This chapter focuses on mainly independent, community-dwelling adults who have fecal incontinence. Included in this chapter is a review of factors associated with fecal incontinence, considerations for assessment in this population, and recommendation for management. Management may involve lifestyle changes including diet modifications; behavioral interventions such as pelvic floor exercises, biofeedback therapy, and electrical stimulation; and extracorporeal magnetic innervation. The chapter also addresses using medications and containment with devices and absorbent products.

**Keywords**

Incontinence management · Community-living adults · Self-management · Behavioral therapies · Absorbent products · Incontinence containment

F. Bates (✉)
Urology Wellness Clinic, St. Joseph's Hospital, Saint John, NB, Canada
e-mail: Frankie.Bates@Horizonnb.ca

D. Z. Bliss
University of Minnesota School of Nursing, Minneapolis, MN, USA
e-mail: bliss@umn.edu

A. Bardsely
School of Health and Life Sciences, Coventry University, Coventry, UK
e-mail: aa8538@coventry.ac.uk

W. K. W. Yeung
Pamela Youde Nethersole Eastern Hospital, Chai Wan, Hong Kong, China
e-mail: ykw377@ha.org.hk

© Springer International Publishing AG, part of Springer Nature 2018       93
D. Z. Bliss (ed.), *Management of Fecal Incontinence for the Advanced Practice Nurse*,
https://doi.org/10.1007/978-3-319-90704-8_6

## 6.1    Introduction

Fecal incontinence is a prevalent and often misunderstood problem [1] that is socially stigmatizing [2] and embarrassing to those suffering with it [3, 4]. Although not a life-threatening disorder, fecal incontinence negatively impacts quality of life and can be debilitating. It also has significant adverse medical, social, and economic consequences. There is a diversity of individuals in the community who suffer with fecal incontinence from young postpartum women to older adults and both sexes [5]. Conservative management approaches should always be the first-line treatment, targeting symptomatic relief [6]. This recommendation has been supported by an international group of experts [6]. Unfortunately due to the taboo nature of this topic, many individuals will suffer in silence and not seek medical intervention [2, 7, 8]. Both patient and caregiver often do not recognize fecal incontinence as a treatable condition [9, 10].

## 6.2    Management Overview

Management of patients with fecal incontinence will depend primarily on the underlying cause (if known), the functional aspects of continence involved, and the specific care setting. Individualized and patient-focused management, protection of patient privacy, and maintenance of patient dignity are key nursing responsibilities in all setting. Initial management should focus on correcting any reversible factors causing fecal incontinence and minimizing the physical and psychosocial impact (e.g., pain, skin damage, embarrassment) [11].

In the community, conservative management of fecal incontinence is reliant on the participation of the individual and self-management or caregiver supported management. There are a number of identified self-management strategies including modifications to diet and eating patterns, learning public restroom locations, taking antidiarrheal medications, and preparing hygiene kits with disposable wipes and a change of clothing [6] (see Chap. 1). Many strategies rely on trial and error [4, 12], and therefore support and education from a healthcare professional and fellow sufferers are vital to successful management. Management strategies also need to be sensitive to the cultural taboos and stigma associated with fecal incontinence and promote self-efficacy in self-management [2, 13]. It is important that healthcare professionals acknowledge and initiate discussions around assessment of symptoms, and impact on the individual as stigma may prevent an individual from communicating [1, 6, 14, 15].

Fecal/anal incontinence symptom severity scales and quality of life scales provide an estimated measure of the severity of fecal incontinence, frequency of leakage, urgency, use of pads, and impact on lifestyle/quality of life [6] (see Chap. 5). Although these scales are commonly used for research, utilizing them in clinical practice can provide an evaluation of the effectiveness of a treatment/management program. The Wexner [16] and St. Marks [17] anal incontinence scores are two scoring systems that have been utilized in practice [6].

Three subtypes of fecal incontinence are passive, urge, and functional incontinence (see Chap. 1) [6]. The severity of fecal incontinence is most often related to the frequency, consistency, and volume of fecal material lost [6]. Assessing fecal incontinence severity, the degree of bother to the patient, and any subtype present is important to understanding treatment approaches and patients' goals for management [6, 18].

## 6.3    Causes and Associated Factors of Fecal Incontinence in Community-Living Adults

There are a variety of problems, health conditions, and factors that influence the development of fecal incontinence in community-living individuals. Normal defecation and fecal continence require the intricate function of variety of structures and processes (see Chap. 4). Firstly, the individual must have sensory awareness of rectal distention, the ability to stop stool elimination via sphincter control, and the ability to store stool temporarily, which requires normal rectal capacity and compliance. These functions are orchestrated by voluntary and involuntary neural pathways that control peristalsis, the sphincters, and the pelvic floor musculature; critical structures and pathways include the central nervous system, autonomic nervous system, and enteric nervous system. Any intrinsic or extrinsic factor causing dysfunction of the gastrointestinal system can dramatically alter bowel function, continence, and ultimately quality of life [19]. Further, multiple mechanisms can be involved in the pathophysiology, such as altered stool consistency and delivery of stool to the rectum, abnormal rectal capacity or compliance, decreased anorectal sensation, and pelvic floor or anal sphincter dysfunction [16]. Therefore, initial assessment and physical exam are essential for a definitive diagnosis and to develop an individualized treatment plan.

The external anal sphincter is continuous with part of the pelvic floor (puborectalis muscle) and can also become weakened or even injured during labor allowing feces to escape. Men and women can equally be affected with certain medical conditions that are risks for fecal incontinence. These can include diabetic neuropathy; neurological disorders, such as MS and Parkinson's disease; and spinal cord injury [20]. Age is also a factor in community-dwelling individuals, and fecal incontinence is more commonly seen in both sexes as age progresses [21]. Lactose intolerance and previous history of colorectal cancer can be precursors to fecal incontinence [22]. It is very important for the advanced practice nurse to obtain a detailed history and physical exam from patients. Adequate assessment leads to accurate diagnosis and ultimately successful treatment (see Chap. 5).

Community-living older adults with dementia can develop fecal incontinence as the disease worsens (see Chap. 7). Drennan observed that management guidelines for incontinence in older adults with dementia in residential care cannot simply be transposed into the home setting, and yet, research findings, reviews, and clinical guidelines often fail to make a clear differentiation between the two settings [23].

Individuals living in the community with presenile dementia or mild cognitive impairment are more prone to both urinary and fecal incontinence due to multifaceted reasons. Often the individual is unable to recognize the signals that their rectum needs emptying, resulting in both fecal staining and incontinence. In more severe cases, the individual is unable to even comprehend the need to defecate and is unable to locate the toilet in a timely fashion, especially when away from their own environment [24]. Cognitive impairment can also affect the person's ability to defecate in a socially acceptable place or time [25].

Functional incontinence can also occur in those individuals unable to reach the bathroom in a timely fashion. Mobility is an influential cause of fecal incontinence. Although the individual is able to recognize their signals to defecate and locate the toilet, their functional disability restricts them from reaching the toilet. These functional disabilities could arise from a stroke, arthritis, fractures, depression, cardiac disease, emphysema, and other breathing disorders, just to name a few. Certainly many comorbidities can contribute to fecal incontinence, and this list is not exhaustive. Individuals often have to live alone with limited assistance from caregivers and family and so can find coping mechanisms difficult. This is covered more extensively in the chapter on frail older adults. Box 6.1 describes the general recommendations for the advanced practice nurse for managing fecal incontinence in the community-living adult.

---

**Box 6.1: General Management Recommendations for Community-Living Adults**
- Conduct a history and physical examination.
- Make an appropriate differential diagnosis.
- Assess severity of fecal incontinence.
- Elicit patients' initial complaints about fecal incontinence and symptoms that are most troubling.
- Discuss priorities for short- and long-term goals of management with patient.
- Target recommendations for therapy to achieve priority goals, particularly short-term ones.
- Set realistic outcomes, and schedule follow-up appointments to monitor progress or need for modification of the management plan.

---

## 6.4    Assessment Considerations for Community-Living Adults

Fecal incontinence is often a symptom or sign of an underlying disease or condition rather than a diagnosis [6, 26] but can also be idiopathic. Therefore, an assessment is important to diagnose the cause and contributing factors for each individual. A holistic and patient-centered approach to assessment is required to elicit the amount, pattern, and duration of incontinence as well as the impact on the individual's quality of life (see Box 6.2).

Most individuals do not need to undergo formal testing of anorectal function and can be managed within a primary/community care setting. As there is little research that examines the initial assessment of fecal incontinence, expert consensus was used to determine international and national guidance. A thorough history and physical examination, differential diagnosis, and accurate assessment of fecal incontinence severity by the advanced practice nurse (see Chap. 7) are critical to develop an appropriate individualized management plan. Double incontinence is often related to a severe form of pelvic floor dysfunction, and needless to say, it is associated with a greater negative effect on the patients' quality of life [27, 28] (also see Chap. 14).

## 6.4.1  Identifying Patient Goals of Management

Initial management of fecal incontinence in adults living in the community includes discussion of the patient's goals for desired outcomes [6]. The initial complaint of the patient may provide cues to symptoms of fecal incontinence that are most troubling and an initial focus for improvement. The advanced practice nurse should confirm these observations and engage the patient in identifying preferences for short- and long-term outcomes of management.

Although elimination of fecal incontinence is likely the ultimate desire of most patients, this goal may not always be feasible or may take some time to achieve. Success in reducing the severity of some incontinence symptoms may be a satisfactory outcome or a motivation for continued efforts toward long-term goals. When asked about their top goals of management, if cure is not possible, community-living men and women identified the following: a decrease in the leakage of loose or liquid feces, a decrease in the number leaks, and greater confidence in controlling fecal incontinence [18]. These same goals were determined to be of the greatest importance as well [18].

---

**Box 6.2: Special Considerations for Assessment of Community-Living Adults**
- Any functional impairment
  - For example, can the individual sit on the toilet and adopt the correct position (see Fig. 6.1) without support or is assistance or a frame required?
- Any cognitive impairment
  - For example, does the individual recognize the correct place to defecate and/or are they able to recognize the signals telling them they need to defecate?
- The environment
  - Is the environment suitable, i.e., warm, well-lit, and private? Most of us are unable to defecate in what is considered a public place (e.g., on a commode next to their bed in hospital) for fear of creating a noise or odor.

- Underlying medical conditions
- Self-management
  - What the patient has already tried to relieve their fecal incontinence, including over-the-counter medications or complementary/herbal remedies.

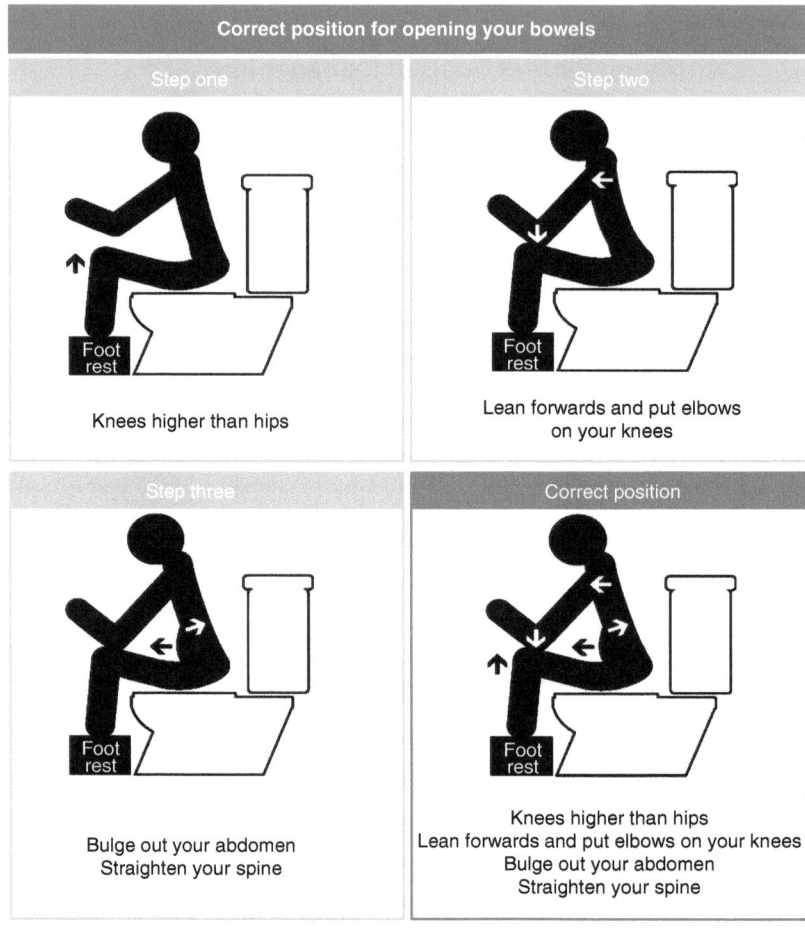

**Fig. 6.1** Correct position for opening your bowels. (Reprinted with permission from Norgine Ltd. who has reproduced and distributed the image with the kind permission of the co-authors including Wendy Ness, Colorectal nurse specialist. Produced as a service to the medical profession by Norgine Ltd. ©2017 Norgine group of companies. UK/COR/0118/0855. Date of preparation: January 2018)

## 6.5 Caregiver Considerations

Even patients who are fairly independent in living in the community may receive periodic assistance from family members with their daily care. As advanced practice nurses, it is important we include these caregivers, whether they are family members or general healthcare providers (see Chap. 7).

For patients with neurogenic causes of fecal incontinence, such as multiple sclerosis, Parkinson's disease or spinal cord injuries, and varied levels of independence, informal caregivers may have been participating in their care (often for many years), prior to the onset of fecal incontinence. The caregivers may be involved with assisting the patient in mobilizing, transferring, and toileting prior to ever being seen by a healthcare professional. They may be capable assistants and should not be underestimated in their importance and value in care planning. For example, the caregiver may help with toileting records and bowel diaries and describe activities that may have precipitated fecal incontinence episodes. This information will benefit the advance practice nurse in forming a more accurate diagnosis. However, considering and respecting the patient's privacy, level of independence, and perspective are essential. The advance practice nurse must develop communication skills that facilitate a satisfactory encounter with patients and caregivers.

## 6.6 Modification of Diet and Eating Patterns

### 6.6.1 Foods and Fluids Contributing to Fecal Incontinence

Conservative management of fecal incontinence includes assessing and possibly recommending modifications of their intake of foods and fluids [6]. Problems associated with diet intake are worsening of the severity of symptoms of fecal incontinence, precipitation of leakage or defecation urgency, or gastrointestinal discomfort and cramping. Dietary intake can result in flatus (or intestinal gas) that in turn causes involuntary expulsion of feces from the rectum [12, 29–32].

A list of common foods and fluids aggravating fecal incontinence has begun to emerge (see Table 6.1). A few points to note are that the list may not be all-inclusive, and not all of the foods on the list are bothersome to all persons with fecal incontinence. Diet intake and tolerance may differ by regional and cultural diets as well as individual preferences. There has not yet been a large survey of the international population of individuals with fecal incontinence that has examined associations of diet components and fecal incontinence.

Foods and fluids thought to worsen fecal incontinence are listed in Table 6.1. Some of the foods on the list, such as onions, beans, cabbage, and broccoli, are associated with increased flatus [4, 12, 30, 33]. Other aggravating foods are nuts, foods with small seeds or hulls such as strawberries or popcorn, and raw salad ingredients such as lettuce. A variety of herbs and seasonings that are used to make foods taste peppery or spicy or associated with ethnic cooking (e.g., Italian sauce, Mexican chili, etc.) can be bothersome. Some patients attribute eating fried or

**Table 6.1** Foods avoided or restricted to prevent or lessen fecal incontinence

| Food type | Example |
| --- | --- |
| Fatty, greasy foods | Sausage, bacon, ribs, fried foods, fast food |
| Gas-producing foods | Onions, beans, broccoli, cabbage, cauliflower, radishes, apricots |
| Spicy foods, rubs | Various ethnic peppery/hot spices |
| Nuts, foods with seeds, hulls | Nuts, seeds, popcorn, strawberries, watermelon |
| Dairy products | Milk, cheese |
| Eggs | |
| Caffeinated beverages and foods | Coffee, chocolate, colas |
| Raw fruits (especially citrus) and raw vegetables | Oranges, grapefruit and juices, apples and pears Lettuce, cucumbers |
| Alcohol | Beer, red wine |
| Foods and beverages with artificial sweeteners | Low-calorie/diet sodas |

"fatty" foods, dairy products, or "acidic" citrus fruits or juices with fecal incontinence. Ingesting drinks and foods containing caffeine, such as coffee and chocolate, and alcoholic beverages, beer in particular, is also associated with fecal incontinence [12, 30]. As many foods are complex in their nutrient composition and preparation, more than one aggravating characteristic may be present (e.g., spare ribs may have a high-fat content and may also be prepared as spicy; dairy products such as cheese or whole milk may have a fat and lactose content that are less tolerated). There have been few studies examining diet modification as a treatment for fecal incontinence.

In self-managing fecal incontinence, some patients have modified their diets prior to seeking clinical care, while others have not given thought to an association of diet intake [12, 30, 34]. Although the aim of reducing or avoiding intake is to avoid accidental fecal leakage, patients may decide to ingest favorite foods or drinks on a special occasion, because they crave them, or as a "reward" or celebration, and "deal with the consequences" of potential fecal leakage afterward [4, 12].

Ingestion of a supplement of psyllium fiber has been shown to reduce the frequency of fecal incontinence in community-living patients in randomized clinical trials [35–37]. Doses ranged from a total of approximately 3 g per day to 16 g per day. More than a 50% reduction in the frequency of fecal incontinence, a measure considered to be clinically significant, was reported. As part of their self-management of fecal incontinence, patients have reported adding supplements of psyllium fiber available in over-the-counter products to their diets [12].

Supplemental psyllium fiber has also been included in a management plan along with transrectal irrigation with positive results but with a less robust research design [38]. Results of one study suggested that the addition of psyllium supplement while taking anti-motility medication such as loperamide did not decrease fecal incontinence more than the medication alone [39]. Some patients eat foods, such as cooked or dried prunes, or take supplements, such as senna [12, 30], which can have a mild laxative effect to assist in stimulating rectal emptying to prevent leakage. Amounts taken are adjusted by patients until the desired effect is achieved.

Patients eat yogurt containing active bacterial cultures or take a probiotic supplement with the aim of promoting a more beneficial profile of colonic bacteria and a more regular bowel pattern [12]. Inquiring about use of complementary diet therapies is recommended as a published case study has shown that a probiotic preparation containing a *Lactobacillus* strain and an herbal preparation have been used to manage fecal incontinence [40]. Section 6.6.2 explains the focused history taking and assessment of diet intake of a patient with fecal incontinence. Section 6.6.4 describes recommendations for diet modification that the advanced practice nurse can make.

## 6.6.2   Management Recommendations for History and Assessment of Diet Intake

- Inquire if the patient has associated their diet intake with any of the following: the occurrence of episodes of fecal incontinence, worsening of symptoms (i.e., frequency, softer or more liquid consistency, or greater amount), more flatus, or urgency.
- Inquire about the type of foods, fluids, or supplements that are thought to worsen leakage; refer to the common list of bothersome foods (see Table 6.1) as needed to assist the patient in recall.
- Inquire if the patient has self-restricted or removed aggravating foods or fluids from their diet, how long and to what degree they have maintained the restriction, and its effectiveness.
- Inquire if the patient has associated diet intake with improvement in fecal incontinence and the type of foods, fluids, or supplements (e.g., dietary fiber) with this effect. Inquire if the patient has associated diet intake with improvement in fecal incontinence and the type of foods, fluids, or supplements (e.g., dietary fiber) with this effect.
- Inquire about ingestion of probiotics, herbal preparations, or complementary therapy supplements and their side effects on fecal incontinence.
- Assess risks of any diet modification in terms of nutritional status/malnutrition potential.
- Explain interactions of supplements or complementary therapy preparations with medications taken and side effects.

## 6.6.3   Modifying Eating Patterns

In addition to modifying dietary intake, individuals with fecal incontinence may have to modify their eating patterns, especially before social gatherings or public events, to reduce chances of accidental leakage. Example of these strategies includes eating smaller amounts or skipping a meal before the event [4, 29, 30].

When eating at restaurants or social gatherings, individuals may need to be selective to avoid foods or alcoholic drinks known to aggravate fecal incontinence and perhaps limiting the amount eaten. Some individuals find that having a set or a regular time for meals or snacks helps establish a regular pattern of bowel elimination, lessening the unpredictability of incontinence episodes.

### 6.6.4 Management Recommendations for Modifying Diet and Eating Patterns

- If diet restrictions or additions have improved fecal incontinence, symptoms without adverse risks recommend continuation; if diet modifications are not effective, recommend discontinuation to lessen burden of self-management.
  - Support times when patient feels periodic need to loosen restrictions and can cope with possible leakage.
- If the patient is unsure of a possible association between diet and fecal incontinence, recommend that they record a daily diary of diet intake and incontinence episodes for a period of time during which they would usually have an incontinence episode (e.g., for a week and a weekend if they leak once or more per week).
  - Review diet and incontinence records with the patient at a follow-up visit to identify possible associations and diet modifications such as reducing fried foods or eliminating certain spices.
- If the patient has not tried a dietary fiber supplement, recommend a psyllium supplement.
  - Suggest taking the supplement twice per day with meals. Start with a lower amount of 2–3 g per day divided into two equal amounts and increase as needed. Higher amounts of psyllium may need to be prepared in a baked product such as a muffin.
  - The fiber should be mix in enough fluid to allow easy swallowing and reduce risk of choking.
- Recommend discontinuation of supplements or complementary therapy preparations that interfere with actions of other medications.
- Inquire about patient's knowledge and use of modifications in eating patterns.
- Discuss common eating pattern modifications.
- Evaluate effectiveness of modifications; discontinue those without benefit.

### 6.7 Environmental Modification

Home assessments are required at times, especially if the patient has a functional disability. An occupational therapist will be beneficial for assessment and environmental manipulation and can often assist the patient in correct sitting techniques (see Fig. 6.1). An elevated toilet seat for independent toileting or the use of a bedside commode can often help the individual attain continence [41]. Assistive products, such as a commode, should be evaluated in terms of safety, stability, fit, and comfort for the patient. The location and visibility of the commode should be considered. A commode also may be appropriate if the patient only has a bathroom on an upper level, requiring climbing a flight of stairs. The caregiver needs to be included in this assessment as they will ultimately be emptying the device of stool and/or urine. Appropriate walking aids such as canes, tripods and walkers, as well as clear markings for the location of a toilet can be very helpful. Some older adults have a lot of "clutter" in their homes. Clearing away clutter and allowing easy access to the toilet (particularly at night) are essential to prevent falls and promote continence. Lighted hallways and nightlights will also assist with this.

Education for the patient and caregiver regarding looser clothing, elasticated waistbands, Velcro closures, and reducing "layers" of clothing will help the patient facilitate a speedier and more successful toilet visit.

Bowel movements are associated with the ability to sit well supported on the toilet with knees higher than hips and lean slightly forward in order to raise intra-abdominal pressure and utilize abdominal effort if needed (see Fig. 6.1). Physical disabilities may therefore impair an individual's ability to maintain continence. Healthcare professionals and care providers should ensure that the environment provided for toileting is as private as possible. Environmental obstacles, such as stairs, distance, and requiring money for public toilet access, can also hinder continence.

## 6.8    Establishing Regular Bowel Habits

Measures to normalize bowel movements and habits will help the patient restore continence [42]. Diet is one of the most influential factors of bowel consistency and is covered as a special consideration in this chapter. Defecation and fecal incontinence are complex, interrelated processes that depend primarily on the interactions among the pelvic floor, the anal sphincters, the rectum, the anal canal, and the colon [43]. Alterations in sensory awareness (feeling of rectal fullness) or lack of sphincter control can result in fecal incontinence. Patients with chronic constipation often have fecal loading which leads, over time, to loss of rectal sensation of fullness.

Constipation is one of the most chronic causes of fecal incontinence in the elderly population. Establishing soft movements with dietary modifications, increasing mobility, and listening to body signals will improve symptoms. Individuals living in the community often live alone and do not eat healthy diets or exercise adequately, increasing the risk of constipation. Monitoring stool consistency using one of the charts described in Chap. 5 will help to inform the patient, caregiver, and healthcare provider. Constipation may present as infrequent movements, straining, or hard consistency. Normal stool should appear as soft sausage-shaped logs, easy to pass without straining.

Evaluation of patterns of normal defecation and leakage using a bowel diary organized as a table/chart should be conducted by the patient for a 1–2-week period before any treatment plan is implemented. The bowel diary typically records information about the frequency and amount of normal bowel movements and leakage episodes and includes a standard scale of stool consistency/form [44, 45] (see Chap. 5). It may also allow notes about medications or other self-management interventions taken (see Table 6.2).

A bowel diary can assist in establishing if there is any pattern to the incontinence and how frequently incontinence occurs. It can also be used to monitor progress and assess the effectiveness of any treatment measures. In addition, a food diary can be used to identify any dietary-related contributory factors. Table 6.3 provides an example of a diet and fluid intake diary.

Studies have shown that eating increases the electrical and motor activity in the colon, resulting in a decrease in colonic transit time and increased stool frequency. Exercise has a similar effect [46]. To establish a "normal" bowel pattern, recommend the patient eat at regular times, avoid aggravating foods, attempt a bowel movement after eating, and exercise regularly. Once established, changes can be made if necessary to their usual eating habits, especially promoting a high-fiber diet and encouraging high water intake. Educating the patient regarding rectal fullness, listening to body signals indicating the need to defecate (so as not to "miss the moment"), and adopting satisfactory toileting routines can promote more normal bowel habits.

Often, individuals are apprehensive about having a bowel movement in a public place due to fear of odors, noise, flatulence, etc. Odor eliminators/reducers that neutralize the smells associated with defection can encourage individuals to use public toilets. These products are available in either odorless or scented sprays or drops that can be placed in the toilet bowl before a bowel movement.

With increasing volume in the rectum, an urge to defecate occurs. If this initial signal of rectal fullness is ignored, it can lead the patient to miss their bowel movement completely that day. The urge may disappear as accommodation occurs. Liquid stool can be very hard to control as it will rapidly transit through the intestine into the rectum. The rectal sphincter mechanism can also find it very difficult to hold liquid stool for the time it takes to get to the toilet. Changing the consistency of the stool away from the liquid form is paramount. A study by Collins, Hibberts et al. [47] showed that 81% of patients completing a program of therapy by a specialist physiotherapy or nurse improved symptoms (per the St. Mark's anal incontinence score). The program consisted of a median of three visits with these specialists.

### 6.8.1 Management Recommendations for Regular Bowel Habits

- Teach the patient the recommended position on toilet as needed.
- Advise the patient to eat meals, sleep, and rise at regular times.
- Advise the patient to defecate about 30 min. after meals and before bed.
- Advise the patient to avoid foods that aggravate fecal incontinence and drink recommended amounts of fluid, considering any health conditions.
- Teach the patient to complete a bowel diary/chart for 1–2 weeks and evaluate their report at a follow-up visit to inform treatment plan.

**Table 6.2** Example chart from a bowel diary for fecal incontinence

| Date and time | Form or consistency of stool | Quantity of stool | Soiled underwear or pad | Type of soiling | Type and dose of medication taken |
|---|---|---|---|---|---|
| | Refer to stool chart | Large (L) Medium (M) Small (S) | Yes or no | (a) None (b) Stain on clothing (c) Loose stool (d) Liquid stool (e) Solid stool | |

**Table 6.3** Example diet and fluid intake diary

| Day | Meal 1 Type of food and How prepared (e.g., baked, fried, raw) | Meal 2 | Meal 3 | Other meal or snacks | Nonalcoholic drinks, number of cups/glasses, and size of cup/glass | Alcohol, number of glasses and size of glass, and any mixers | Other comments (e.g., if meals were not typical, eaten in a restaurant) |
|---|---|---|---|---|---|---|---|
| Monday | | | | | | | |
| Tuesday | | | | | | | |

## 6.9    Taking Control: Rectal Evacuation

Patients with fecal incontinence often feel that they have no control over their bowels, and this transfers to feeling as if they have no control in their lives [4, 6] (see Chap. 1). They will often describe how they are unable to leave their homes until "their bowels are empty" for fear of having an accident. They may describe devastating outings during which they had an episode of fecal incontinence while running their errands [4].

Advising and educating patients about how to evacuate their rectum completely, prior to any outings and in the comfort of their own home environment, may help to give them a better sense of control. Suggesting interventions to empty their bowel such as the use of a glycerine or bisacodyl suppository per rectum upon arising and following their first meal/drink of the day will help them to evacuate most of their rectal contents. This should prevent accidents and enable them to exercise, socialize, work, and manage their daily chores with less worry. If a glycerine suppository is ineffective for rectal evacuation, the patient may need to use a small enema. This can be conducted independently or by the caregiver. These enemas come in disposable units and should not cause the patient a lot of discomfort. Trans-anal irrigation is another option to use to evacuate the bowel.

### 6.9.1    Trans-Anal Irrigation

Trans-anal irrigation has been used by patients with neurogenic bowel problems for many years to manage both fecal incontinence and constipation (see Chap. 9). Additionally, other patients, especially those with passive fecal incontinence or incomplete evacuation, may find performing trans-anal irrigation using mini-irrigation devices helpful [48, 49]. Two examples of these irrigation devices are the Qufora® (MBH International A/S, Allerod, Denmark) and Peristeen® (Coloplast A/S, Humblebak, Denmark devices) (see Chap. 9).

The use of trans-anal irrigation by community-living adults with fecal incontinence is increasing as it can provide individuals with some control over their bowel motions. Trans-anal irrigation is described in detail in Chap. 9. Briefly, it is used to empty the contents of the large bowel in a place and at a time convenient to the individual. While seated on the toilet, the individual slowly instills water through a small external catheter into the rectum through the anus. When the catheter is removed, the water and fecal matter are emptied from the bowel into the toilet. Most individuals will irrigate on alternate days; however, the volume of water required and frequency of use vary between individuals. The procedure is designed to be self-administered, but carers/healthcare professionals can also be utilized to assist. Careful selection of suitable individuals is important to maximize effectiveness and prevent complications [50].

### 6.9.2    Management Recommendations for Bowel Evacuation

- Assess the potential capability of performing and benefit of rectal evacuation.
- Teach patient and/or caregiver appropriate procedures (for using a suppository, mini-irrigation system, etc.).

## 6.10   Practical Coping Strategies

Coping with fecal incontinence is enhanced for some patients by a sense of control and preparedness for preventing accidental leakage or managing it if it occurs [4]. A common coping strategy is knowledge of where the location of the closest toilet when in public places [4, 30]. This knowledge can prevent leakage especially when there is urgency. There are mobile applications such as "Sit or Squat" or "Flush" that can assist in locating toilets and in mapping routes while traveling short or long distances. In restaurants, a request can be made for seating at tables nearer the toilet/restroom without divulging the reason for the table selection [30]. Awareness of typical times of leakage, often by keeping a bowel diary, can be helpful for scheduling appointments outside the home around these times. Women report that carrying a small kit in their purse containing moist wipes for cleansing, an absorbent pad, pair of underwear, and plastic bag for soiled items increases their feelings of security [4]. Women and men feel that they can provide advice and support to others with fecal incontinence after gaining experience and developing confidence in self-managing their own condition over years [6, 51, 52].

### 6.10.1   Management Recommendations to Promote Practical Coping

- Inquire about the patent's current level of coping and strategies used.
- Share practical strategies for coping with fecal incontinence used by other patients to increase a sense of control.
- Suggest participation in a support group if available.

## 6.11   Medications

### 6.11.1   Medication Review

There are a number of medications that can exacerbate fecal incontinence, and so a medication review should form part of the clinical assessment (see Chap. 5). A medication review should take into account any prescribed medication as well as over-the-counter medications, herbal remedies, and recreational drugs, as these may have unintended side effects which can aggravate or cause fecal incontinence. Nitrates and calcium channel blockers can decrease sphincter tone, whereas metformin and some antacids (e.g., those containing magnesium) can lead to loose stools. Excess vitamin and mineral supplementation can loosen stools. Long-term laxative use can lead to incontinence in some patients. Box 6.3 lists some of the medications that can exacerbate fecal incontinence.

**Box 6.3: Medications That Can Exacerbate Fecal Incontinence**
- Medications that alter sphincter tone: nitrates, calcium channel antagonists, β-blockers, sildenafil, and selective serotonin reuptake inhibitors
- Broad-spectrum antibiotics (multiple mechanisms): cephalosporins, penicillins, and macrolides
- Topical anal medications: glyceryl trinitrate ointment, diltiazem gel, bethanechol cream, and botulinum A toxin
- Medications causing profuse loose stools: laxatives, metformin, orlistat, selective serotonin reuptake inhibitors, antacids containing magnesium, and digoxin
- Constipating medications: loperamide, opioids, tricyclic antidepressants, antacids containing aluminum, and codeine
- Tranquillizers or hypnotics (reduce alertness): benzodiazepines, tricyclic antidepressants, selective serotonin reuptake inhibitors, and antipsychotics

## 6.11.2 Medication Treatment

Many individuals will use a combined approach for managing fecal incontinence, for example, diet and fluid modification, medications, and behavioral therapy. The use of medication focuses on three main aspects: the reduction of diarrhea, increasing resting anal canal pressure, and treatment and/or prevention of constipation [53]. Medications used to treat diarrhea act to improve stool consistency by slowing intestinal transit or optimizing fluid reabsorption, thereby increasing the viscosity and overall volume of the stool. About 8–10 L of fluid enters the small intestine daily. The majority of this is reabsorbed in the small intestine and the colon.

Three medications used to treat fecal incontinence are synthetic opioid derivatives, loperamide, codeine phosphate, and co-phenotrope. Opioids produce an agonist effect on m or d opioid receptors on the enteric nerves, epithelial cells, and muscle. The effects of opioids include decreased intestinal motility (m receptors) and decreased intestinal secretion (d receptors) and increased absorption (m and d receptors) [54]. Loperamide, codeine phosphate, and co-phenotrope act primarily by peripheral m opioid receptors and have minimal central nervous system (CNS) effects. Loperamide hydrochloride can be used in doses from 0.5 to 16 mg per day long term. Loperamide is an opiate derivative which acts by increasing the transit time through the small intestine and proximal colon, which promotes water reabsorption and improves stool consistency [39, 53]. Loperamide also impairs the recto-anal inhibitory reflex and increases anal resting pressure and reduces secretion in the bowel [55, 56]. Loperamide has a good safety record with a low side effect profile. The main disadvantage of loperamide is that it can cause constipation and abdominal pain and as such should be started at low doses and titrated as required.

Patients who are unable to tolerate loperamide hydrochloride can be offered codeine phosphate or co-phenotrope [6, 26]. Codeine phosphate acts in a similar way to loperamide, although it has a greater side effect profile in long-term use. Codeine phosphate can cause side effects such as constipation and drowsiness, which limit its use. Combining the use of both loperamide and codeine phosphate may be useful. Co-phenotrope (a proprietary mixture of diphenoxylate and atropine) acts on the smooth muscle of the intestinal tract inhibiting gut motility and excessive gut propulsion. However, as it can cross the blood-brain barrier, it can cause euphoria and dependence in long-term use [29].

An alternative medication is topical phenylephrine gel that has selective α-1 adrenergic agonist that resembles naturally occurring catecholamines in the intestine and which can produce sympathomimetic effect on the internal and external anal sphincters [29]. Phenylephrine aims to modulate the extrinsic innervation of the internal anal sphincter muscle, increasing tone and resting anal canal pressure [54]. Outcomes of this medication for fecal incontinence are mixed and its effects are considered moderate [6].

As noted earlier in this chapter, individuals with complete evacuation difficulty or post-defecation fecal incontinence may benefit from using suppositories, mini-enemas or trans-anal irrigation to empty the rectum of fecal contents or provide a regular bowel evacuation.

### 6.11.3  Medications for Impaction/Constipation-Related Fecal Incontinence

Suspected impaction or constipation as a cause of fecal incontinence should be identified and treated before initiating treatment specific to fecal incontinence. Constipation is treated with diet, fluid, and lifestyle modifications such as increasing physical activity as previously discussed. However, for those individuals for whom this is ineffective or inappropriate, stool softening and stimulant laxatives should be the first choice. A regime should start with regularly administered osmotic agents (e.g., polyethylene glycol), with the addition of a stimulant laxative such as senna on an as-required basis [57]. Polyethylene glycols (macrogol laxatives) are increasingly being used for chronic constipation [58], and there is clear evidence that these are superior to lactulose and ispaghula husk [59, 60]. Table 6.4 lists oral laxatives for fecal impaction or constipation. Although oral medication is always preferable, a combination of oral laxatives and rectal interventions (enemas or suppositories) may be required initially [61]. Rectal stimulants include bisacodyl and glycerine suppositories. Rectal stimulants can be used alone or in combination with digital stimulation and digital removal of feces.

### 6.12    Behavioral Therapies

### 6.12.1  Pelvic Floor Muscle Training

Pelvic floor muscle training is recommended as a second-line therapy for managing fecal incontinence when initial interventions previously described are inadequate [6]. Pelvic floor muscle training is helpful to restore pelvic floor muscle function for both urinary and fecal incontinence. The pelvic floor muscle consists of

**Table 6.4** Oral laxatives for fecal impaction or constipation

| Type of laxative | Name | Action | Considerations |
|---|---|---|---|
| Stimulant | Senna®, bisacodyl®, co-danthramer®, co-danthrasate®, dioctyl®, docusol®, dantron® | Stimulate an increase in colonic motility (peristalsis) and mucus secretion | Stimulant laxatives are rapid acting, usually taking effect in 8–12 h<br>They are best taken in evening or at bedtime<br>Stimulant laxatives are effective when used with bowel management programs, where predictable rectal contents are required prior to performing digital stimulation or digital removal of feces<br>Prolonged use can be justified for some patients, but monitoring of potassium and electrolytes may be required<br>Dantron should only be prescribed for terminally ill patients<br>Patients should be made aware that dantron can change the color of their urine |
| Osmotic | Lactulose ® and magnesium salts | Osmotic laxatives act by drawing fluid from the body into the bowel by osmosis. This increases the water content of the feces making it softer and easier to pass | Can take 2–3 days to take effect<br>Can lead to dehydration when given in larger doses |
| Isoosmotic | Macrogol oral powder compound (3350) (polyethylene glycol, PEG) Cosmocol®, Laxido®, Movicol® | Macrogol laxatives increase stool water content and directly trigger colonic propulsive activity and defecation. This has a four in one mode of action: bulks, softens, stimulates, and lubricates | Macrogols are licensed for fecal impaction and can be used for chronic constipation |

approximately 70% slow-twitch (type 1) and 30% fast-twitch (type 2) muscle fibers [62]. Pelvic floor muscle weakness is recognized as one of the problems encountered in patients with incontinence, and reeducation should address the perceived deficit.

The aim of pelvic floor muscle training is to teach the patient to isolate and correctly contract the pelvic floor muscles to increase strength, endurance, and coordination of sphincter function. Repeated contractions are thought to improve continence through increased support for the pelvic organs [63]. Thoracoabdominal pelvic muscle training has also been advocated, as it has been theorized that training all core muscles to work in tandem may be more effective than a narrow focus on the pelvic floor muscles alone [64].

Instruction can be simple verbal education although many individuals will tend to use incorrect muscles (such as gluteal and abdominal muscles) to extenuate their pelvic floor contraction. A finger digit placed vaginally or rectally by the practitioner as well as a hand placed externally on the perineum will often help to instruct the patient to isolate the pelvic floor muscles. This technique will also enable the practitioner to feel the strength and endurance of the patients' pelvic floor muscle contraction as well as assess rectal tone and the presence of any prolapses.

## 6.12.2  Biofeedback Therapy

Biofeedback therapy is an effective way of increasing proprioception of the location of the pelvic floor muscles, thereby improving treatment outcomes for fecal incontinence. Biofeedback therapy is a term that can be used to describe many different types of training regimens for different muscle groups, including the pelvic floor. It is defined as the process of gaining greater awareness of many physiological functions, primarily using instruments that provide information on the activity of those functions with a goal of being able to manipulate them by the patient themselves [65]. Biofeedback can be used to gain awareness of the pelvic floor muscles group by using striated muscles that are under voluntary control. Since many patients have difficulty in identifying, controlling, and coordinating the function of the pelvic floor muscle group, patients may perform them ineffectively if the practitioners give only verbal instruction for pelvic floor muscle exercises.

Biofeedback can help to increase strength and endurance of the pelvic floor and/ or anal sphincter. The biofeedback apparatus gives information about how strongly the muscles are being contracted, whereby the patient can use that information to learn how to do the pelvic floor exercises more effectively. It is also thought that biofeedback motivates the patient to improve by giving information on performance and progress. The theory behind strength and endurance training of the sphincter muscles or the detrusor muscle is that the patient will be able to hold in the stool or urine for a longer period of time and enable them to make it to the toilet with fewer accidents.

Biofeedback can range in varying degrees from simplistic to more complex therapies. Simple techniques range from telephone discussions to face office visits with verbal education only [66]. More complex therapies include medical grade equipment, ranging from a simple pelvic floor home exercisers (similar to that used by Dr. Arnold Kegel over 50 years ago) to more complex models. These modules give the patient a visual representation of how well they are contracting their pelvic floor, showing both strength and endurance. Pressure probes can be used either vaginally or rectally or for less invasive treatments; EMG electrodes can be applied. Surface electrodes are also placed on the gluteal or abdominal accessories to ensure the patient does not use their accessory muscle to help extenuate their pelvic floor contraction. Box 6.4 describes an example biofeedback protocol.

Biofeedback therapy can also be utilized for dyssynergic-type evacuation of stool and enhance relaxation of the external anal sphincter [67]. This should be combined with learned techniques of correct positioning on the toilet and relaxation to defecate as discussed earlier in the chapter.

Biofeedback treatment should always be as an adjunct to other conservative therapies (including diet and fluid modifications, techniques to improve evacuation, bowel training programs, management of stool consistency, and review and modification of medications if necessary). These will benefit approximately 25% of patients and should be the first line of treatment [68]. Home exercise programs of specific regimes of repetitions and development of an individualized pelvic floor muscle training program are essential in order for biofeedback to be effective. Biofeedback treatments regimens vary from 6 to 12 weekly or biweekly treatments, and no standardization is seen in the literature.

Most of the data in the literature relate to biofeedback to treat urinary incontinence, and certainly more studies need to be conducted for the treatment of fecal incontinence. The 5th International Consultation on Incontinence (ICI) [69] concluded that "manometric biofeedback training is possibly effective but the variability between studies suggests that results may be dependent on the training and experience of the therapist." The authors of this chapter agree, and this is true of other therapies.

Heymen et al. [70] reported that patients treated with biofeedback and pelvic floor muscle training were significantly more likely than patients treated with pelvic floor muscle training alone to report adequate relief (76% vs. 41%.)

---

**Box 6.4: Example Biofeedback Protocol**

A protocol used in a clinic in Canada tailors the treatment regime to the client's progress. Six weekly treatments are given initially, and if the patient requires further time management, this will be evaluated. Treatment is conducted using pressure probes either vaginally or rectally and surface electrodes either on the abdominal muscles or the gluteal muscles (dependent upon which accessories the patient is using when the initial assessment is performed). The patient receives visual cues to start and stop their pelvic floor contraction, and they are able to visualize their strength and their endurance with a graphic representation of their contraction. The patient is also able to visualize if they are using their accessory muscles and, over time, try to use them less.

The treatment paradigm is structured specifically to the patient. If they have a weak contraction of 1–3 $\mu V$ and poor endurance of 2 s, then the patient needs to be encouraged to isolate their pelvic floor muscle and hold for a longer period of the time. Goal lines can be added to the biofeedback treatment graph to help the patient.

Initially the patient is taught slow-twitch exercises to increase strength and endurance in the slow-twitch muscle fibers of the pelvic floor. The treatment duration is 15 min. Once the patient has shown that they can isolate well, without the use of any accessory muscles, and their strength and endurance is improving, they are then taught fast-twitch exercises. They are taught to do 10 quick repetitions of their pelvic floor muscle (described as "flicks") in 10 s. This will help them to be able to recruit their pelvic floor muscle more readily when they use their pelvic floor muscle appropriately to suppress a bowel movement or to defer their urge to defecate until reaching the toilet.

Over the 6-week period, depending on how the patient progresses, the goal lines can be increased to help the patient hold their contraction longer or increase their strength.

The advanced practice nurse needs to ensure that the patient is compliant with their daily home program in between weekly sessions. The patient should be started on an individualized pelvic floor muscle training program. This would typically be three sets of ten exercises three times a day [29]. If the patient is found to tire easily, this routine can be reduced. The patient is instructed to hold for 5 s and rest for 5 s and gradually increase the time to 10 s. Written instruction has been found to be valuable to patients to remember their routines.

For pelvic floor rehabilitation purposes, the most common types of biofeedback use electromyography (EMG) and biofeedback therapy. However, other forms of pelvic floor biofeedback include the use of ultrasound (either intrarectal, intravaginal, or perineal), rectal balloons, digital guidance (the use of an intrarectal/intravaginal finger or hand placed on the perineum), and anorectal manometry [71, 72].

For fecal incontinence, biofeedback therapy can also be used to improve rectal sensitivity and/or compliance. This type of treatment has also been termed volumetric rehabilitation or discrimination training and is typically done with rectal balloons [73]. The balloon is inflated with air or water to determine the first sensation of rectal filling. It is then gradually inflated with decreased amounts of air or water, to teach the patient to sense stool in the rectal vault at progressively lower volumes. Normally, as the rectum fills up, the rectal walls expand. Stretch receptors in the rectal walls stimulate the desire to defecate. If the person does not defecate on feeling this urge, the stools may return to the colon, where more water is absorbed. The rectal balloon allows for the patient to have more time to perform a voluntary anal sphincter contraction before the volume of stool in the rectal vault overwhelms the patient's ability to hold it inside. Rectal balloons can also be used on patients with fecal urgency and rectal hypersensitivity; in those cases, the balloons are simply inflated to progressively larger volumes, which the patient is then coached to tolerate without feeling the need to expel the rectal contents [71].

### 6.12.3 Trans-anal Electrical Stimulation Therapy

Electrical stimulation is another second-line management modality that has been proposed for the rehabilitation of fecal and urinary incontinence. It was reported that pelvic floor electrical stimulation achieves a cure rate of 30–60% and an improvement rate of 74% in those with stress urinary incontinence (SUI) [74]. However, for fecal incontinence, success is lower [6]. Electrical stimulation can be delivered to the pelvic floor and sphincters in many different forms, including via surface electrodes or intrarectal probes.

One of the postulated mechanisms of electrical stimulation in urinary incontinence is that it increases the level of transforming growth factor-$\beta$1 (TGF-$\beta$1) which is a pleiotropic cytokine that plays important roles in many physiological and pathological processes [75]. It has unique and widespread actions in the remodeling of the extracellular matrix and is critical for tissue integrity. Recent studies have reported that the TGF-$\beta$1 pathway is activated, and expression of collagens I and III is significantly decreased in stress urinary incontinence [76]. Electrical stimulation therapy potentially causes T-type calcium channels to open and subsequently activates a TGF-$\beta$1-protein pathway. This encourages collagen deposition, which restores tissues' tensile strength and mechanical stability as well as pelvic tissue structure and function, producing a therapeutic effect for stress urinary incontinence [77]. These effects also related to pelvic tissue when working on coordination of anal sphincter activity and working to isolate a contraction of the anal sphincter [78].

The goal of electrical stimulation is to enhance the strength and/or endurance of striated muscle contraction; the target is typically the external anal sphincter in the case of fecal incontinence. Another goal is for patients with decreased kinesthetic awareness to become more cognizant of where their pelvic floor muscles are in space and what it feels like when the muscles and sphincter are contracting. Electrical stimulation has been shown to transform fast-twitch muscle fibers to slow-twitch muscle fibers, which is thought to help with improving endurance [79]. It also increases capillary density, allowing more blood flow to the oxidative slow-twitch fibers [80].

Norton et al. in 2006 compared daily anal electrical stimulation of two different frequencies—35 Hz versus 1 Hz—and there were no differences between the groups in terms of any outcome measures, and 63% of patients who completed treatment felt that electrical stimulation had improved their symptoms at least somewhat. They speculated that improvements in both groups were possibly related to improved rectal sensation rather than direct muscle strengthening, or alternatively, a placebo effect.

Healy et al. [81] randomized 48 patients to endo-anal electrical stimulation with a home unit versus endo-anal electrical stimulation plus augmented biofeedback under supervision of a physical therapist [81]. Both groups improved in terms of continence scores, manometric pressure readings in posttreatment, and quality of life. However, this study had no control group. A "triple therapy" approach using medium frequency electrical stimulation (3000 Hz, 500 mV) via a plug electrode and EMG biofeedback twice per day has had better results, reducing anal incontinence compared to EMG biofeedback alone. The protocol, however, may be complex and intensive for some patients to follow or sustain. More research is needed to further ascertain the most efficacious treatment protocols [82].

**Box 6.5: Examples of Electrical Stimulation Protocols**
Treatment modalities will certainly vary locally, nationally, and globally. One center in Hong Kong, China (the Urology Centre of Pamela Youde Nethersole Eastern Hospital), uses an intravaginal electrical probe to deliver stimulation to the pelvic floor for patients with urinary or double incontinence. The protocol consists of two 20-min sessions per week over a 6-week period. The electrical parameters used in all sessions were frequency of 30–60 Hz; pulse time of 500 μs, with a continuous stimulation; and the intensity varied according to each patient's tolerability. All patients receive a combination of intravaginal electro-stimulation and home pelvic floor muscle exercise which was taught by the urology advanced practice nurse. Results from that center on intravaginal electro-stimulation showed that it was especially effective for poor responders to pelvic floor exercise monotherapy [83]. In addition, the actual number of pads used showed a significant decline [83].

Another center in Canada (St. Joseph's Hospital, St. John, NB) uses a different protocol of 6 weekly treatments with biofeedback and electrical stimulation. Most of the literature will site between 8 and 12 weekly treatments. This can be rather time intensive, and the advance practice nurses at this center have found 6 weekly treatments suffice as long as the patient is committed and is compliant with practicing their pelvic floor exercise routine between appointments. For the electrical stimulation therapy, this center uses a protocol of 50 Hz for stress incontinence with pulse width of 1.0 ms, ramping of 20%, and a biphasic wave. The optimal protocol for electrical stimulation has not been established.

## 6.12.4   Extracorporeal Magnetic Innervation

The initial clinical application of extracorporeal magnetic innervation technology was for the treatment of urinary incontinence. Pulsed magnetic technology has been developed for pelvic floor therapy. The magnetic field generator (therapy head) is contained in the middle of the seat of the neocontrol system using an external power unit (Neotonus, Inc., Marietta, Ga). The output of the power unit consists of magnetic pulses, and the amplitude can be adjusted by the advanced practice nurse. It is the amplitude that determines the volume of the field needed to generate stimulation strong enough to induce a nerve impulse. This application relies on the basic principle of physics that a changing magnetic field will induce a flow of electrons within the field triggering a nerve stimulation [84]. However, there are no randomized controlled studies on using extracorporeal magnetic innervation therapy to treat fecal incontinence alone.

A pilot study by an advance practice nurse in Pamela Youde Nethersole Eastern Hospital, Hong Kong, China, using extracellular matrix therapy for the treatment of double incontinence observed positive results [85]. Patients who had a modified Oxford score grade 0–1 and failed pelvic floor muscle training for 6 months were treated with extracorporeal magnetic innervation therapy. Ten adult female patients (age range from 44 to 77 years) were studied. Patients were seated fully clothed in a neocontrol chair. Each treatment sessions lasted for 20 min and conducted twice a week for 6 weeks. The frequency of the pulsed magnetic field was 5 Hz, intermittently for 10 min, followed by a rest period of 1–5 min and a second treatment at 50 Hz intermittently for 10 min. The treatment intervals were intermittent (5 s on and 5 s off) to avoid muscle fatigue. Validated quality of life surveys were used (e.g., UDI-6 IIQ-7, FIQOL) at the beginning of treatment and again at 3 months. A 3-day bladder diary was used to assess frequency, urgency, urge incontinence, bladder capacity, and fluid intake. The number of pads used was also counted.

The results [85] showed a signification decrease in both fecal and urinary incontinence per day; pad used decreased from 2.8 to 1.4 ($p < 0.05$). The mean UDI-6 score decreased from 2.5 to 1.5 ($p < 0.05$); the mean IIQ-7 score decreased from 4.5 to 5.5 ($p < 0.05$). The FIQOL subscale scores improved. Limitations of the study were the small sample size and lack of random assignment to a control or comparison group and self-reported measures. There were no complications or adverse events during or after the treatment. Long-term follow up and randomized controlled studies are crucial to properly evaluate the efficacy of this treatment for fecal incontinence.

## 6.13 Devices and Products for Containment of Fecal Incontinence

Not all people with fecal incontinence can be cured with conservative or surgical treatment, and they may need to rely on containment products and devices. Several containment devices offer options for preventing leakage from the rectum. These devices include anal plugs, anal inserts, and vaginal bowel devices.

The anal plug and anal insert function are similar but have different designs. The anal plug is made of soft foamlike material which is inserted in a partially collapsed state into the rectum and then expands like a tampon (Fig. 6.2a). Once inside the rectum, the anal plug blocks the passage of feces around it. It is removed by using the "string" that is securely attached to the plug or pushed out during defecation. Anal plugs come in different sizes and designs. Because of the materials used in the plug, it is not flushable, which can make its use difficult for male patients as male public toilet stalls do not have sanitary bins for their discrete disposal.

The anal insert has a spindle shape with a top and bottom disk and an applicator for insertion into the rectum (Fig. 6.2b). The top disk is inserted into the rectum to seal the outlet to the anus and is available in two diameters. The bottom disk remains outside the anus to avoid displacement into the rectum and facilitates easier manual removal. The anal insert is made of soft silicone, is single-use, and can be expelled with a bowel movement.

Anal plugs and inserts have been shown to be effective in preventing leakage and are usually used on an as-needed basis [42, 86, 87]. Reviews by the Cochrane group [86] and the International Consultation on Incontinence [69] suggested that anal plugs can be uncomfortable and therefore difficult to tolerate. Therefore, anal plugs are recommended to be placed at the upper end of the anal canal to reduce discomfort. Educating the patient how to position and use these devices (building up the time of inter-rectal use of these plugs gradually) may help improve tolerance. Although Fox et al. stated that "Anal plugs are a last resort" [88], anal plugs can be useful in a selected group of people either as a substitute for other forms of management or as an adjuvant treatment option. Some individuals may need time to adjust to this device similar to a young woman getting used to wearing a tampon vaginally.

A vaginal bowl device uses a different approach than the plug and insert for occluding the rectum. It is inserted into the vagina after which its balloon is inflated by the patient using an external hand pump. The inflated balloon presses against the adjacent wall of the rectum to prevent feces from leaking out of the rectum (see Fig. 6.3). The insert is then deflated for removal. An insert lasts about 1 year [42].

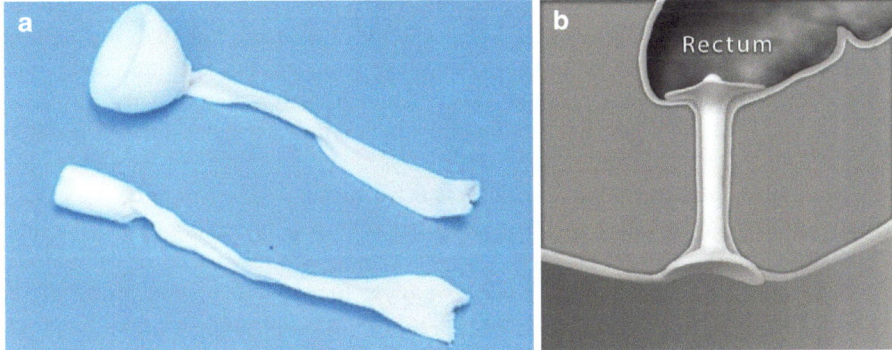

**Fig. 6.2** (**a**) Anal plug. (Reprinted with permission from Coloplast, the International Continence Society, and the Continence Products Advisor [89]). (**b**) Anal insert. (Reprinted with permission from Renew Medical Inc., the International Continence Society [42] and the Continence Products Advisor [89])

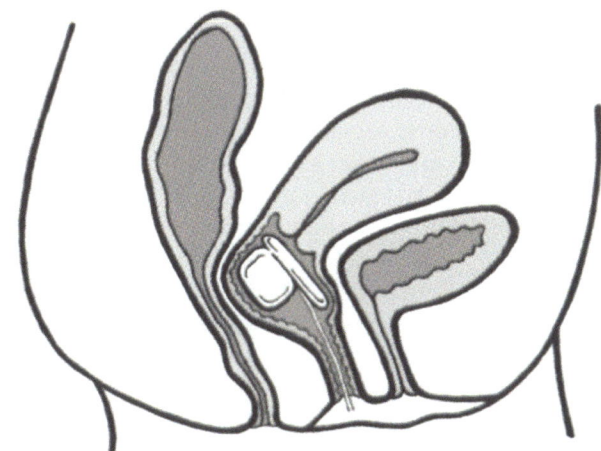

**Fig. 6.3** Vaginal bowel device. Reprinted with permission from the International Continence Society [42]

The vaginal bowel device seems to be well tolerated by many women [90]. Adverse effects are cramping, discomfort, urinary incontinence, and vaginal spotting [90]. A clinician needs to fit the patient with the correct size of the insert for comfort and effectiveness.

### 6.13.1 Absorbent Products

Absorbent products are a part of the management plan for fecal incontinence. They are useful as an adjunct to other therapeutic options or as an option when intractable incontinence continues despite active treatment modalities. Body-worn absorbent products can promote socialization in public, assist in protecting skin integrity, and maintain a person's dignity. An individual's preference should always be taken into account.

There are a variety of absorbent products available differing in design, shape, size, and degrees of absorbency. Some are body-worn products, while others are pads for bedding and furnishings [42, 91]. Body-worn products are available in disposable and washable versions. Styles range from full briefs to thin small ones that line underpants. Many patients "mix and match" different body-worn absorbent products to meet their needs depending on whether they are worn during the day or night and the degree of their leakage [89, 92].

Most absorbent products are designed for urinary incontinence. An exception is a small insert that can be placed between the buttocks against the anus to absorb small leakages of feces [42, 93]. Unfortunately there are few absorbent products designed specifically for fecal incontinence, and many of the characteristics of those for urinary incontinence are not optimal for fecal incontinence. Community-living individuals with fecal incontinence identified needed improvements for absorbent products including being made of materials that can protect skin from more solid/softer feces or particulate irritants in liquid feces and that are flushable, better/more absorption toward the back without increasing bulkiness, better control of odor, capability of placing them on or taking them off without removing outer pants, and better protection against larger leaks [94].

Many patients with fecal incontinence need advice for selecting among the many types of absorbent products available from the advanced practice nurse (see Box 6.5). An interactive continence products advisor website is available to assist advanced practice nurses as well as patients in reviewing the features and selecting absorbent or containment products [89]. In many countries, the costs of many of these absorbent products are not covered by many governmental programs or private insurance policies for those living in the community with fecal incontinence. These out-of-pocket costs of absorbent products add to the burden and stress for patients and their families. Case studies illustrating conservative management of fecal incontinence in community-living adults by the advanced practice nurse are described in Boxes 6.6 and 6.7.

## 6.13.2  Management Recommendations Regarding Absorbent Products

- Recommend use of containment or absorbent products as needed to support other conservative management approaches and facilitate public/social activities.
- Review options for styles, sizes, and levels of absorption of absorptive products.
- Teach patients how to use an anal, plug, insert, or a vaginal bowel device if they opt to use one of these devices.
- Make follow-up appointments to assess patient's ability to use them, satisfaction, effectiveness, and complications.
- Refer patients interested in a vaginal bowel device to an appropriate healthcare practitioner for a prescription and fitting as needed.
- Apprise patients of the lack of healthcare insurance coverage of these products.

---

**Box 6.6: Case Study 1**

A 48- year-old male presented with fecal incontinence complaining of "No control over his bowels at times." He works in the pulp and paper industry in the fields and often has no access to a public toilet. History taking revealed that he had mild asthma, hypertension, and hypocholesteremia and a recent hemorrhoidectomy. He had previous surgeries related to hemorrhoids and had no significant problems postoperatively. The patient had a history of constipation since a young child. He described having diarrhea at times after not having a movement for many days with what he described as "explosive diarrhea."

Over the last 2 years, he complained of increasing symptoms with his bowels, again ranging from constipation to very loose and even liquid stool. He said he was diagnosed with irritable bowel syndrome. He had been given a diet sheet by his family doctor but felt it wasn't clear exactly what foods he should eliminate or change. The patient would have two or three bowel evacuations daily, sometimes incontinent and loose. He appeared to have fairly normal sensations for stool but did have urgency at times with very little warning. He then had gradual onset of urinary and fecal incontinence and lost more control over time. He wore a full brief but said it made him feel "infantile." The brief felt sweaty and was noisy, and he felt that he "smelled bad all the time." His worst fear was losing stool at work as he was out in the field with no facilities for cleaning himself up and/or changing.

His anorectal exam showed that his internal and external sphincters were weak with reduced resting and squeezing anal pressures. There was some mild diminished sensory awareness. His 2-week bowel chart showed days with no movements at all and then other days with very loose stools which he couldn't control. His incontinent episodes occurred only when the stool was very loose. If he was having a formed stool, he could get to the bathroom in a timely fashion. On digital rectal exam, he had a weak pelvic floor contraction of 1/5 on the modified Oxford scale and poor endurance of 3 s.

*Treatment Plan*

The advanced practice nurse developed a treatment plan with the patient and discussed dietary modifications. She gave the patient a chart of "aggravating" foods and explained that all of these would not necessarily apply to him. The nurse instructed him to take one specific food item and eliminate it from his diet. This may be in the form of acidic products, for example, to start with. He was to record his movements with a bowel chart over 2 weeks during this diet change and see if there was any noticeable improvement. If this did not make a difference to his bowel symptoms, he could then continue to have acidic foods but eliminate another product for 2 weeks such as spicy foods.

The advanced practice nurse taught the patient pelvic floor exercises and placed him on a home routine three times a day. She taught him appropriate use of his pelvic floor muscles using quick-twitch exercises for urge suppression. The nurse suggested that the patient start on psyllium fiber on a daily basis to bulk up his stool. It was explained that this would help to form his loose stool while adding bulk and preventing constipation. His water intake was poor, and so he was educated on the importance of drinking adequate amounts of water as well as other fluids to help soften his stool and move it through the bowel.

The nurse showed the patient how to use an anal plug and gave him samples of a few different products and sizes. The nurse explained to him that an anal plug could be somewhat uncomfortable initially, and he should start using one for short periods around the house so he could get used to it. He was instructed to place the plug higher up in the anal canal for improved comfort. After he became used to the device, he could wear one when working in the field. The nurse also suggested that he use a glycerine suppository in the morning if he had not evacuated his bowels prior to going to work. This would give him control when his movement would occur.

The advanced practice nurse followed the patient over the next several months. While on the elimination diet, he found that two particular foods worsened his fecal leakage. He completely eliminated these foods from his diet and found an improvement in his symptoms and particularly in the consistency of his stools. He initially found the anal plug extremely uncomfortable. He was brought into the clinic to show him correct placement, and over time, it became more tolerable, albeit only for short periods of time. As his symptoms improved, he found he needed to use the plug less often. He could use a glycerine suppository with good results and felt he had more control, particularly at work when he went with an empty rectum.

He had very few episodes of fecal incontinence now as his stools were almost always soft and formed. The psyllium had also reduced his constipation and bulked up his stool. The patient was faithful with his pelvic floor exercise routine two to three times a day. He was using fast-twitch exercises for urge suppression and was able to ward off the urge for approximately 15 min now. He was no longer using full briefs but a smaller thinner product that was black in color. He found it much more comfortable and noticed less of the smearing and leakage as the pad was not white. At his last appointment, he was pleased with his progress to date, particularly when he was able to empty his rectum before going to work. The advanced practice nurse continued to work with him to achieve a gradual increase in his improvement over time.

---

**Box 6.7: Case Study 2**

Mrs. Jones is a 45-year-old lady who is referred to the community nursing team with a long-standing history of fecal incontinence. Until recently Mrs. Jones has been managing her incontinence by wearing pads and reducing her working hours (she only works in the afternoons as the problem is worse in the morning). Mrs. Jones had started to avoid exercise classes and the gym which she had previously enjoyed and was worrying that she was starting to put on weight. This was also affecting her mental health as she had always enjoyed swimming and playing with her children. Mrs. Jones is wishing to explore alternatives that would allow her to return to a normal work and activity routine.

Mrs. Jones developed fecal incontinence following the birth of her second child, and the problem then worsened after the birth of her third child 5 years ago. Mrs. Jones has no other relevant medical or surgical history. The birth of Mrs. Jones' second child was a natural birth with a prolonged second stage of labor. Unfortunately during the birth, she sustained a perineal tear that required suturing. Mrs. Jones developed fecal incontinence and could not control the passage of flatus, which she found very embarrassing. Mrs. Jones avoided highly spiced foods and had reduced her fiber intake, meaning that she was also prone to constipation, which meant that when the incontinence occurred, it was often worse.

*Treatment Plan*

Mrs. Jones was referred to the physiotherapist for pelvic floor exercises. The physiotherapist discussed diet and lifestyle modifications along with teaching Mrs. Jones pelvic floor exercises. Although pelvic floor exercises and dietary modifications enabled Mrs. Jones to control her flatus, the fecal incontinence did not resolve, and she became more anxious about having accidents while out in public. She discussed the problem with her primary care physician who prescribed loperamide up to 10 mg per day as needed. Although initially this enabled Mrs. Jones to feel more confident when out in public, this was not an absolute resolution of the problem and left her more prone to constipation. After a particularly embarrassing accident while shopping with friends, Mrs. Jones returned to her physiotherapist who referred her to the bladder and bowel specialist nurse of the continence advisory service.

The advanced practice nurse discussed the option of trans-anal irrigation with Mrs. Jones, who felt that this may be an option to avoid future accidents. Mrs. Jones was initially taught to irrigate three to four times a week with 300–400 mL of water depending on what she could tolerate. On review Mrs. Jones had experienced no accidents or incontinence in between irrigations and felt happy with the procedure and technique. She was performing irrigation in the mornings three times a week prior to going to work and found this was suiting her lifestyle well. After 3 months Mrs. Jones felt confident enough to return to work again in the mornings and was starting to return to the gym and was hoping to feel confident to take some exercise classes in the near future.

## References

1. Bliss DZ, Rolnick C, Jackson J, Arntson C, Mullins J, Hepburn K. Health literacy needs related to incontinence and skin damage among family and friend caregivers of individuals with dementia. J Wound Ostomy Cont Nurs. 2013;40(5):515–23.
2. Garcia JA, Crocker J, Wyman JF, Krissovich M. Breaking the cycle of stigmatization: managing the stigma of incontinence in social interactions. J Wound Ostomy Cont Nurs. 2005;32(1):38–52.
3. Chelvanayagam S, Norton C. Quality of life with faecal continence problems. Nurs Times. 2000;96(31 Suppl):15–7.
4. Peden-McAlpine C, Bliss DZ, Hill J. The experience of community-living women managing fecal incontinence. West J Nurs Res. 2008;30(7):817–35.
5. Milsom I, Altman D, Cartwright R, Lapitan MC, Nelson R, Sjostrom S, et al. Epidemiology of urinary incontinence (UI) and other lower urinary tract symptoms (LUTS), pelvic organ prolapse (POP) and anal incontinence (AI) adults. In: Abrams P, Cardozo L, Wagg A, Wein A, editors. Incontinence. 6th ed. Bristol: International Continence Society; 2017. p. 1–142.
6. Bliss DZ, Mimura T, Berghmans B, Bharucha A, Chiarioni G, Emmanuel A, et al. Assessment and conservative management of faecal incontinence and quality of life in adults. In: Abrams P, Cardozo L, Wagg A, Wein A, editors. Incontinence. 6th ed. Bristol: International Continence Society; 2017. p. 1993–2085.
7. Johanson JF, Lafferty J. Epidemiology of fecal incontinence: the silent affliction. Am J Gastroenterol. 1996;91(1):33–6.
8. Norton C, Dibley L. Help-seeking for fecal incontinence in people with inflammatory bowel disease. J Wound Ostomy Cont Nurs. 2013;40(6):631–8.
9. Peden-McAlpine C, Bliss DZ, Becker B, Sherman S. The experience of community-living men managing fecal incontinence. Rehabil Nurs. 2012;37(6):298–306.
10. Klingele CJ, Pettit PD. Mayo clinic on managing incontinence. Mayo Found Med Educ Res. 2014;2(9):2074.
11. Wishin J, Gallagher TJ, McCann E. Emerging options for the management of fecal incontinence in hospitalized patients. J Wound Ostomy Cont Nurs. 2008;35(1):104–10.

12. Hansen JL, Bliss DZ, Peden-McAlpine C. Diet strategies used by women to manage fecal incontinence. J Wound Ostomy Cont Nurs. 2006;33(1):52–61.
13. Kılıç SP, Sevinç S. The relationship between cultural sensitivity and assertiveness in nursing students from Turkey. J Transcult Nurs. 2017; https://doi.org/10.1177/1043659617716518.
14. Mullins J, Bliss DZ, Rolnick S, Henre CA, Jackson J. Barriers to communication with a health-care provider and health literacy about incontinence among informal caregivers of individuals with dementia. J Wound Ostomy Cont Nurs. 2016;43(5):539–44.
15. Rolnick SJ, Bliss DZ, Jackson JM. Healthcare providers' perspectives for promoting communication with family caregivers and patients with dementia about incontinence and skin damage. Ostomy Wound Manage. 2013;59(4):62–7.
16. Jorge JMN, Wexner SD. Etiology and management of fecal incontinence. Dis Colon Rectum. 1993;36(1):77–97.
17. Vaizey CJ, Carapeti E, Cahill JA, Kamm MA. Prospective comparison of faecal incontinence grading systems. Gut. 1999;44(1):77–80.
18. Manthey A, Bliss DZ, Savik K, Lowry A, Whitebird R. Goals of fecal incontinence management identified by community-living incontinent adults. West J Nurs Res. 2010; 32(5):644–61.
19. Reed KK, Wickham R. Review of the gastrointestinal tract: from macro to micro. Semin Oncol Nurs. 2009;25(1):3–14.
20. Park SE, Elliott S, Noonan VK, Thorogood NP, Fallah N, Aludino A, et al. Impact of bladder, bowel and sexual dysfunction on health status of people with thoracolumbar spinal cord injuries living in the community. J Spinal Cord Med. 2017;40(5):548–59.
21. Shamliyan T, Wyman J, Bliss DZ, Kane RL, Wilt TJ. Prevention of urinary and fecal incontinence in adults. Evid Rep Technol Assess. 2007;161:1–379.
22. Norton C, Whitehead WE, Bliss DZ. Management of fecal incontinence in adults: reports from the 4th international consultation on incontinence. Neurourol Urodyn. 2010;29(1):199–206.
23. Drennan VM, Greenwood N, Cole L, Fader M, Grant R, Rait G, et al. Conservative interventions for incontinence in people with dementia or cognitive impairment, living at home: a systematic review. BMC Geriatr. 2012;12(1):77.
24. Harari D, Igbedioh C. Restoring continence in frail older people living in the community: what factors influence successful treatment outcomes? Age Ageing. 2008;38(2):228–33.
25. Ayers T, Wells M. Incontinence after stroke: guidance to overcome shortcomings in management. Br J Neurosci Nurs. 2007;3(10):468–71.
26. The National Institute for Health and Care Excellence (NICE). Faecal incontinence (bowel control problems). London: Royal College of Obstetricians and Gynaecologists Press; 2007.
27. Jelovsek JE, Barber MD. Women seeking treatment for advanced pelvic organ prolapse have decreased body image and quality of life. Am J Obstet Gynecol. 2006;194(5):1455–61.
28. Memon HU, Handa VL. Vaginal childbirth and pelvic floor disorders. Womens Health. 2013;9(3):265–77.
29. Carter D. Conservative treatment for anal incontinence. Gastroenterol Rep. 2014;2(2):85–91.
30. Croswell E, Bliss DZ, Savik K. Diet and eating pattern modifications used by community-living adults to manage their fecal incontinence. J Wound Ostomy Cont Nurs. 2010;37(6):677–82.
31. Dancey CP, Backhouse S. Towards a better understanding of patients with irritable bowel syndrome. J Adv Nurs. 1993;18(9):1443–50.
32. Martini MC, Kukielka D, Savaiano DA. Lactose digestion from yogurt: influence of a meal and additional lactose. Am J Clin Nutr. 1991;53(5):1253–8.
33. WebMD. Gas (Flatus). https://www.webmd.com/digestive-disorders/tc/gas-flatus-topic-overview.
34. Bliss DZ, Fischer LR, Savik K. Self-care practices of the elderly to manage fecal incontinence. J Gerontol Nurs. 2005;31(7):35–44.
35. Bliss DZ, Jung HJ, Savik K, Lowry A, LeMoine M, Jensen L, et al. Supplementation with dietary fiber improves fecal incontinence. Nurs Res. 2001;50(4):203–13.
36. Bliss DZ, Savik K, Jung HJG, Whitebird R, Lowry A, Sheng X. Dietary fiber supplementation for fecal incontinence: a randomized clinical trial. Res Nurs Health. 2014;37(5):367–78.
37. Markland AD, Burgio KL, Whitehead WE, Richter HE, Wilcox CM, Redden DT, et al. Loperamide versus psyllium fiber for treatment of fecal incontinence: the fecal incontinence

prescription (Rx) management (FIRM) randomized clinical trial. Dis Colon Rectum. 2015;58(10):983–93.

38. van der Hagen SJ, Soeters PB, Baeten CG, van Gemert WG. Conservative treatment of patients with faecal soiling. Tech Coloproctol. 2011;15(3):291–5.
39. Lauti M, Scott D, Thompson-Fawcett MW. Fibre supplementation in addition to loperamide for faecal incontinence in adults: a randomized trial. Colorectal Dis. 2008;10(6):553–62.
40. Lorback S. Naturopathic treatment for bowel incontinence in a patient with multiple sclerosis: a case study. Aus J Herbal Med. 2015;27(2):62–6.
41. Cottenden A, Bliss DZ, Buckley B, Fader M, Getliffe K, Paterson J, et al. Management using continence products. In: Abrams P, Cardozo L, Khoury S, Wein A, editors. Incontinence. 4th ed. Paris: Health Publication Ltd; 2009. p. 1519–642.
42. Cottenden A, Fader M, Beeckman D, Buckley B, Kitson-Reynolds E, Moore K, et al. Management using continence products. In: Abrams P, Cardozo L, Wagg A, Wein A, editors. Incontinence. 6th ed. Bristol: International Continence Society; 2017. p. 2303–426.
43. Doughty D. A physiologic approach to bowel training. J Wound Ostomy Continence Nurs. 1996;23(1):46–56.
44. Heaton K, Lewis S. Stool form scale as a useful guide to intestinal transit time. Scand J Gastroenterol. 1997;32(9):920–4.
45. Bliss DZ, Larson SJ, Burr JK, Savik K. Reliability of a stool consistency classification system. J Wound Ostomy Cont Nurs. 2001;28(6):305–13.
46. Holdstock DJ, Misiewicz JJ, Smith T, Rowlands EN. Propulsion (mass movements) in the human colon and its relationship to meals and somatic activity. Gut. 1970;11(2):91–9.
47. Collins E, Hibberts F, Lyons M, Williams AB, Schizas AM. Outcomes in non-surgical management for bowel dysfunction. Br J Nurs. 2014;23(14):776–80.
48. Collins B, Norton C. Managing passive incontinence and incomplete evacuation. Br J Nurs. 2013;22(10):575–9.
49. Rosen H, Robert-Yap J, Tentschert G, Lechner M, Roche B. Transanal irrigation improves quality of life in patients with low anterior resection syndrome. Colorectal Dis. 2011;13(10):e335–8.
50. McWilliams D. Rectal irrigation for patients with functional bowel disorders. Nurs Stand. 2010;24(26):42–7.
51. Wilson M. Living with faecal incontinence: a 10-year follow-up study. Br J Nurs. 2015;24(5):268–74.
52. Wilson M, McColl E. The experience of living with faecal incontinence. Nurs Times. 2007;103(14):46–9.
53. Duelund-Jakobsen J, Worsoe J, Lundby L, Christensen P, Krogh K. Management of patients with faecal incontinence. Ther Adv Gastroenterol. 2016;9(1):86–97.
54. Halverson AL. Nonoperative management of fecal incontinence. Clin Colon Rectal Surg. 2005;18(1):17–21.
55. Omar MI, Alexander CE. Drug treatment for faecal incontinence in adults. Cochrane Database Syst Rev. 2013;6:CD002116. https://doi.org/10.1002/14651858.CD002116.pub2.
56. Ooms LA, Degryse AD, Janssen PA. Mechanisms of action of loperamide. Scand J Gastroenterol Suppl. 1984;96:145–55.
57. Prichard D, Norton C, Bharucha AE. Management of opioid-induced constipation. Br J Nurs. 2016;25(10):S4–5. S8–11
58. Ramkumar D, Rao SSC. Efficacy and safety of traditional medical therapies for chronic constipation: systematic review. Am J Gastroenterol. 2005;100(4):936–71.
59. Lee-Robichaud H, Thomas K, Morgan J, Nelson RL. Lactulose versus polyethylene glycol for chronic constipation. Cochrane Database Syst Rev. 2009;7:CD007570. https://doi.org/10.1002/14651858.CD007570.pub2.
60. Wang H-J, Liang X-M, Yu Z-L, Zhou L-Y, Lin S-R, Geraint M. A randomised, controlled comparison of low-dose polyethylene glycol 3350 plus electrolytes with ispaghula husk in the treatment of adults with chronic functional constipation. Clin Drug Investig. 2004;24(10):569–76.
61. Larkin P, Sykes N, Centeno C, Ellershaw J, Elsner F, Eugene B, et al. The management of constipation in palliative care: clinical practice recommendations. Palliat Med. 2008;22(7):796–807.

62. Gilpin SA, Gosling JA, Smith AR, Warrell DW. The pathogenesis of genitourinary prolapse and stress incontinence of urine. A histological and histochemical study. BJOG. 1989;96(1):15–23.
63. Bø K. Pelvic floor muscle training is effective in treatment of female stress urinary incontinence, but how does it work? Int Urogynecol J Pelvic Floor Dysfunct. 2004;15(2):76–84.
64. Bartlett L, Sloots K, Nowak M, Ho Y-H. Biofeedback for fecal incontinence: a randomized study comparing exercise regimens. Dis Colon Rectum. 2011;54(7):846–56.
65. Durand VM, Barlow D. Abnormal psychology: an integrative approach. Belmont, CA: Wadsworth Cengage Learning; 2009.
66. Young CJ, Zahid A, Koh CE, Young JM, Byrne C, Solomon MJ, et al. A randomised control trial of four different regimes of biofeedback program in the treatment of faecal incontinence. Colorectal Dis. 2017;20(4):312–20. https://doi.org/10.1111/codi.13932
67. Vivas CG, Moya JM, Roldán PS, Granero CR, Vinuesa SJ, López AM. Home training as a treatment of faecal incontinence and sphincter dyssynergia. Cir Pediatr. 2017;30(1):28–32.
68. Bharucha AE, Rao SS, Shin AS. Surgical interventions and the use of device-aided therapy for the treatment of fecal incontinence and defecatory disorders. Clin Gastroenterol Hepatol. 2017;15(12):1844–54.
69. Bliss DZ, Mellgren A, Whitehead W, Chiarioni G, Emmanuel A, Santoro G, et al. Assessment and conservative management of faecal incontinence and quality of life in adults. In: Abrams P, Cardozo L, Khoury S, Wein A, editors. Incontinence. 5th ed. Arnhem: ICUD-EAU; 2013. p. 1444–85.
70. Heymen S, Scarlett Y, Jones K, Ringel Y, Drossman D, Whitehead WE. Randomized controlled trial shows biofeedback to be superior to pelvic floor exercises for fecal incontinence. Dis Colon Rectum. 2009;52(10):1730–7.
71. Norton C, Cody JD. Biofeedback and/or sphincter exercises for the treatment of faecal incontinence in adults. Cochrane Database Syst Rev. 2012;7:CD002111. https://doi.org/10.1002/14651858.CD002111.pub3.
72. Enck P, Van der Voort IR, Klosterhalfen S. Biofeedback therapy in fecal incontinence and constipation. Neurogastroenterol Motil. 2009;21(11):1133–41.
73. Chiarioni G, Whitehead WE. The role of biofeedback in the treatment of gastrointestinal disorders. Nat Rev Gastroenterol Hepatol. 2008;5(7):371–82.
74. Shamliyan TA, Kane RL, Wyman J, Wilt TJ. Systematic review: randomized, controlled trials of nonsurgical treatments for urinary incontinence in women. Ann Intern Med. 2008;148(6):459–73.
75. Heldin CH, Miyazono K, ten Dijke P. TGF-beta signalling from cell membrane to nucleus through SMAD proteins. Nature. 1997;390(6659):465–71.
76. Wang H, Liu J, Zeng J, Zeng C, Zhou Y. Expression of TβR-2, Smad3 and Smad7 in the vaginal anterior wall of postpartum rats with stress urinary incontinence. Arch Gynecol Obstet. 2015;291(4):869–76.
77. Min J, Li B, Liu C, Hong S, Tang J, Hu M, et al. Therapeutic effect and mechanism of electrical stimulation in female stress urinary incontinence. Urology. 2017;104(Suppl C):45–51.
78. Norton C, Chelvanayagam S, Wilson-Barnett J, Redfern S, Kamm MA. Randomized controlled trial of biofeedback for fecal incontinence. Gastroenterology. 2003;125(5):1320–9.
79. Salmons S, Vrbová G. The influence of activity on some contractile characteristics of mammalian fast and slow muscles. J Physiol. 1969;201(3):535–49.
80. Hudlická O, Dodd L, Renkin EM, Gray SD. Early changes in fiber profile and capillary density in long-term stimulated muscles. Am J Physiol Heart Circ Physiol. 1982;243(4):H528–35.
81. Healy CF, Brannigan AE, Connolly EM, Eng M, O'Sullivan MJ, McNamara DA, et al. The effects of low-frequency endo-anal electrical stimulation on faecal incontinence: a prospective study. Int J Colorectal Dis. 2006;21(8):802–6.
82. Schwandner T, Konig IR, Heimerl T, Kierer W, Roblick M, Bouchard R, et al. Triple target treatment (3T) is more effective than biofeedback alone for anal incontinence: the 3T-AI study. Dis Colon Rectum. 2010;53:1007–16.
83. Yeung W. Evaluation of treatment outcomes in pelvic floor muscle training with biofeedback versus intra-vaginal electrical stimulation in women with urinary incontinence in Hong Kong. Hong Kong: Abstract presented at Hospital Authority Convention; 2016.

84. Galloway NT, El-Galley R, Sand PK, Appell RA, Russell H, Carlin S. Update on extra corporeal magnetic innervation (EXMI) therapy for stress urinary incontinence. Urology. 2000;56(6:82–6.

85. Yeung W. The most updated treatment in urinary incontinence. China: Abstract presented at CUAN Conference; 2015.

86. Deutekom M, Dobben AC. Plugs for containing faecal incontinence. Cochrane Database Syst Rev. 2015;7:CD005086. https://doi.org/10.1002/14651858.CD005086.pub4.

87. Lukacz ES, Segall MM, Wexner SD. Evaluation of an anal insert device for the conservative management of fecal incontinence. Dis Colon Rectum. 2015;58(9):892–8.

88. Fox A, Tietze PH, Ramakrishnan K. Anorectal conditions: Fecal incontinence. FP Essent. 2014;419:35–47.

89. Continence Products Advisor. International Continence Society, International Consultation on Incontinence, University College London, University of Southampton. https://www.continenceproductadvisor.org/.

90. Richter HE, Matthews CA, Muir T, MM TS, Hale DS, Van Drie D, Varma MG. A vaginal bowel-control system for the treatment of fecal incontinence. Obstet Gynecol. 2015;125(3):540–7.

91. Canadian Nurse Continence Advisors. http://www.cnca.ca.

92. Cottenden A, Bliss DZ, Buckley B, Fader M, Gartley C, Hayder D, et al. Management using continence products. In: Abrams P, Cardozo L, Khoury S, Wein A, editors. Incontinence. 5th ed. Arnhem: ICUD-EAU; 2013. p. 1651–786.

93. Bliss DZ, Savik K. Use of an absorbent dressing specifically for fecal incontinence. J Wound Ostomy Cont Nurs. 2008;35(2):221–8.

94. Bliss DZ, Lewis J, Hasselman K, Savik K, Lowry A, Whitebird R. Use and evaluation of disposable absorbent products for managing fecal incontinence by community-living people. J Wound Ostomy Continence Nurs. 2011;38(3):289–97. https://doi.org/10.1097/WON.0b013e31821530ca.

# Management of Fecal Incontinence in Frail Older Adults Living in the Community

7

Kathleen F. Hunter, Melissa Northwood, Veronica Haggar, and Frankie Bates

**Abstract**

Most older adults live in the community either alone or in a family arrangement. Community-living older adults are diverse, and the health status of some is characterized by complexity related to having multiple morbidities and possibly frailty. Assessment and management of fecal incontinence in frail community-dwelling older adults with health-related complexity may be enhanced using a complexity framework that accounts for social, environmental, and political contextual factors as well as health/medical concerns. This chapter will explain common problems that contribute to fecal incontinence in these older adults such as impaction with overflow, constipation, diarrhea, and mild to moderate cognitive impairment. It will address special considerations that the advanced practice nurse must take into account including hearing and vision impairment, physical limitations, the physical environment and toilet access in the home, diet and

K. F. Hunter (✉)
Faculty of Nursing, University of Alberta, Edmonton, AB, Canada

Glenrose Hospital Continence Clinic, Edmonton, AB, Canada
e-mail: kathleen.hunter@ualberta.ca

M. Northwood
Saint Elizabeth Health Care, Hamilton, ON, Canada

Aging, Community and Health Research Unit, School of Nursing, McMaster University, Hamilton, ON, Canada
e-mail: northwm@mcmaster.ca

V. Haggar
Homerton University Hospital NHS Foundation Trust, London, UK
e-mail: v.haggar@nhs.net

F. Bates
Urology Wellness Clinic, St. Joseph's Hospital, Saint John, NB, Canada
e-mail: Frankie.Bates@Horizonnb.ca

© Springer International Publishing AG, part of Springer Nature 2018
D. Z. Bliss (ed.), *Management of Fecal Incontinence for the Advanced Practice Nurse*,
https://doi.org/10.1007/978-3-319-90704-8_7

hydration, and the role of the caregiver. The chapter will then discuss appropriate management interventions. Interventions highlight the importance of a holistic approach, client and caregiver engagement and education, and referral to other healthcare professionals and community services.

**Keywords**
Fecal incontinence · Frailty · Older adult · Community-living · Health complexity

## 7.1 Introduction

The demographic shift and population aging in most countries of the world is well recognized. However, the tremendous diversity in aging is not always appreciated, with variation in physical and cognitive function among individuals of similar ages. Worldwide, most older people live in the community in their own home on their own, with a spouse or other family members, rather than in long-term care or nursing homes. Living in the community in an extended family arrangement is more common in some traditional cultures, although this pattern is changing [1].

Just as there is diversity in aging, there is diversity among older adults regarding etiology of fecal incontinence, ranging from acquired neurological disease (e.g., Parkinson's, multiple sclerosis), life-long congenital conditions, and, for women, childbirth years earlier resulting in pelvic floor or rectal trauma in later life. This chapter focuses on advanced practice nursing management of common types of problems that could lead to fecal incontinence in community-living older adults (see Box 7.1) whose health status has complexity due to multiple morbidities and who could potentially be frail.

---

**Box 7.1: Common Problems Contributing to Fecal Incontinence in Frail Older Adults in the Community**
- Overflow from constipation or fecal impaction
- Adverse side effects of medications
- Polypharmacy due to relief of cyclical symptoms
- Inadequate fluid and diet/fiber intake
- Effects of multiple morbidities
- Reduced sensorimotor function

## 7.2   The Concept of Frailty

Some view aging from a deficit perspective, a period of decline and dependency, while others advocate for a perspective of active and successful aging that challenges stereotypes [1]. With greater recognition and appreciation of the heterogeneity in aging, being able to distinguish the frail from the non-frail has become an important concept for advanced practice nurses and other healthcare professionals to take into consideration in planning and delivery of health services. While many definitions of frailty exist, there is general agreement that loss of physiologic reserve capacity and resistance to stressors is involved, and that frailty is a multidimensional concept with physical, psychological, and social dimensions, not just a biological or physiological state [2]. Frailty is complex, not static, and there is potential for improvement or worsening through modifying influencing factors and putting interventions in place [3].

Similar to estimates of fecal incontinence in community-dwelling older persons, prevalence of frailty among this population varies by country and definition used. Between 7% and 27% of community older adults 65 years of age and older are frail, and another 10–40% are pre-frail [4, 5]. The risk of becoming frail rises with increasing aging, and frail older adults often exhibit geriatric or frailty syndromes. These are multifactorial conditions that include impairment of cognition and/or mobility, falls, and incontinence [3]. Frail older adults are more frequent users of the healthcare system and have higher rates of institutionalization, stimulating recent interest in prevention and treatment of frailty.

There are two competing models of frailty and multiple approaches to measure the phenomena. The first of the definitions is the phenotype model, exemplified by the work of Fried and colleagues [6]. It is based on physiological indicators including unintended loss of weight, reduced muscle strength and gait speed, and low energy expenditure. The second is the cumulated deficit model, described by Rockwood and Mitnitski [7]. This model takes into account physical, mental, and psychosocial health status, noting frailty to be highly age associated and reflective of multisystem change. This group has developed a clinically friendly tool, the Clinical Frailty Scale, based on a fitness-frailty model that emphasizes function and acknowledges the diversity among older adults. The assessor can also take into account the presence of dementia, which may interfere with the person's ability to remain continent independently. Frailty, along with multimorbidity, leads to complexity.

## 7.3   A Conceptual Framework of Complexity

Conceptual frameworks can facilitate an advanced practice nursing approach to care of patient populations with diverse and complex needs [8]. For older adults with frailty and fecal incontinence, where empirical evidence regarding complex interventions is lacking, employing a framework to guide assessment and intervention selection is even more important and useful [9]. A complexity framework was developed following a scoping review of the literature by Schaink and colleagues [10] to understand the nature of complexity in older persons with multiple chronic conditions. This framework includes five health dimensions (demographics, mental health, social capital, medical and physical health, health and social experiences) occurring in the context of sociopolitical and physical environment [10]. Considering all of these dimensions provides a comprehensive perspective to approach the challenges, goals, and care needs of older adults and is useful to inform interventions for fecal incontinence for this population [10]. This complexity framework addresses the shortcomings of previous frameworks that included only a few indications of complexity, such as medical complexity, and did not contain social, environmental, and political contextual factors [10, 11]. The framework has been evaluated in an ongoing program of research with community-dwelling older adults with multimorbidities receiving primary care [12].

## 7.4 Common Problems Contributing to Fecal Incontinence in Frail Older Adults in the Community

### 7.4.1 Overflow Fecal Incontinence

Overflow incontinence is often secondary to fecal impaction and rectal loading that result from similar causes as constipation. Although these conditions are not a physiological consequence of normal aging, the prevalence increases significantly with age, particularly in care facilities [13]. The management of fecal impaction in older adults living in nursing homes is addressed in Chap. 8. For older adults living in the community, the contributing factors to fecal incontinence caused by constipation and fecal impaction or rectal loading are multifactorial, including polypharmacy, dehydration, reduced dietary fiber, multiple comorbidities, decreased mobility, and rectal sensory motor dysfunction.

- *Polypharmacy.* Medications can contribute to constipation in older adults (e.g., anticholinergics, opioids, tricyclic antidepressants, calcium channel blockers, calcium supplements [14], high-dose laxatives) [15]. Medications can also contribute to diarrhea/loose stool in older adults (such as antibiotics, proton pump inhibitors, allopurinol, selective serotonin reuptake inhibitors, angiotensin II receptor blockers, psycholeptics (anxiolytics, antipsychotics)) [14]. Polypharmacy is a pressing concern and consideration for older adults as 23% are taking ten or more medications [14]. This polypharmacy translates to adverse events requiring medical attention and a "pill burden" where the total number of pills the older adult has to swallow in 1 day contributes to not eating due to feeling full, complicated medication scheduling, and poor compliance [14]. Polypharmacy is an issue for the advanced practice nurse when evaluating fecal incontinence in the frail older adult. For example, the advanced practice nurse needs to assess whether the self-administration of antimotility agents to prevent loose overflow bowel movements associated with rectal loading or fecal impaction is followed by laxative medications to treat the resultant worsening of constipation and/or impaction. This can create a cycle of over-the-counter symptom relief medication use without addressing the underlying cause of constipation.

- *Dehydration due to decreased fluid intake.* Often self-induced to reduce the number of trips to the toilet but also sometimes enforced due to the lack of caregivers to assist with drinking. Those living alone at home may be at higher risk.
- *Reduced dietary fiber intake.* Poor teeth and ill-fitting dentures can lead older people to choose a reduced fiber diet. This can go along with a decreasing ability to prepare meals for themselves and result in an increased use of convenience foods that lack adequate fiber and further the risk of impaction.
- *Multiple chronic conditions.* Older people often have multiple chronic conditions including dementia, metabolic disorders (e.g., hypothyroidism), anatomical defects such as pelvic organ prolapse or intussusception, neuropathy as a result of diabetes mellitus or stroke, or neurological disease such as multiple sclerosis and Parkinson's disease.
- *Decreased mobility.* Decreased mobility reduces colonic mass movement [16], thereby increasing transit times. Reduced mobility also makes transferring to the toilet more difficult, resulting in the use of bedpans or bedside commodes, and consequently correct anatomical positioning for defecation does not occur.
- *Rectal sensorimotor function*, which encompasses sensation and motility, as well as biomechanical components (compliance, capacity), is now strongly implicated in the disease process of constipation.

### 7.4.2   Diarrhea

Diarrhea is defined as the passage of loose or liquid stool that can often result in fecal incontinence. The causes of diarrhea vary and can range from infection (e.g., *Clostridium difficile* and *Salmonella*), inflammation (e.g., colitis and diverticulitis), medications such as laxatives, tube feeding, and constipation/impaction with overflow. Polypharmacy and interactions with the healthcare system put older adults more at risk for an infective process that would alter stool consistency [9, 14]. Patients with fecal incontinence may inaccurately report diarrhea rather than fecal incontinence as the presenting problem due to embarrassment, which can mislead the healthcare practitioner to mislabel the diarrhea as the primary cause [17]. It is very important to get an accurate measure of the degree of looseness of the stool as the definition of diarrhea can vary from person to person. A stool consistency chart is a very useful aid in this situation for the client or caregiver to use at home.

### 7.4.3   Mild-Moderate Cognitive Impairment

Cognitive impairment may not necessarily meet criteria for diagnosis of dementia but can result from any neurological impairments that occur as a result of brain damage/injury or disease. Mild cognitive impairment has been conceptualized as an "intermediate stage of cognitive impairment that is often, but not always, a transitional phase from cognitive changes in normal aging to those typically found in dementia" [18] (p. 214). In addition to those with mild cognitive impairment, worldwide, the majority of older people who have progressed to dementia live in the community [19]. People with cognitive difficulties may experience challenges that lead to fecal incontinence such as:

- *Visuospatial problems in finding the toilet.* These visual disturbances and disorientation can be reduced by using plain colors to identify and differentiate between the toilet and other bathroom furniture. A black toilet seat and white china toilet can make the toilet easier to see. Mirrors can also confuse people with dementia as they may think there is someone else in the bathroom.
- *Agnosia* (difficulty with object recognition). Clear visible signs with a picture can aid people to identify the toilet, as well as leaving the toilet door open when not in use.
- *Apraxia* (difficulty performing tasks, e.g., clothes off to toilet, toileting tasks, e.g., wiping/cleaning, dressing). Consider altering clothing—increasing the length of the opening and replacing zips and buttons with Velcro (hook-and-loop fastening) to make clothes quick and easy to remove or adding loops of thread to a zipper to aid opening and closure.

## 7.5    Special Considerations for Assessment and Diagnosis

The goals and outcomes of addressing fecal incontinence in community-dwelling older adults should focus on maximizing function and independence. Thus, assessment of fecal incontinence in this population by the advanced practice nurse should include the standard elements of assessment outlined in Chap. 5, as well as strategies to assess hearing and vision, physical/cognitive function, the physical environment, access to toilet in the home, diet and hydration, and the role of the caregiver/care partner in continence. These special considerations are listed in Box 7.2. These considerations correspond with the conceptual model of complexity health dimensions of mental health, social capital, medical and physical health, health and social experiences in the context of the physical environment of the home, and sociopolitical context of available assistance through formal and informal caregivers [10].

---

**Box 7.2: Special Considerations for Assessment and Diagnosis for the Frail Older Adult in the Community**
- Demographic considerations: age, gender, ethnicity, education, and frailty mental health concerns such as depression and dementia
- Social capital including social support, caregiver presence and strain, socioeconomic status, relationships, and leisure activities
- Medical and physical health considerations including the impact of multiple chronic conditions impacting fecal incontinence
- Health and social experience considerations such as healthcare utilization and access, quality of life, self-management support, and healthcare system navigation

## 7.5.1  Hearing and Vision

Sensory loss, and particularly dual sensory loss, is associated with functional impairment in older people. Guthrie and colleagues [20] reported that among older persons living in the community and receiving home care, those with dual sensory loss were more likely to have impairments in many aspects of functional ability, including bladder and bowel incontinence, than those without hearing and vision deficits. Sensory loss can adversely affect independent way finding and communication of toileting needs. Otoscopic examination of the ear canal to assess for abnormalities and cerumen impaction, along with a screening test for auditory acuity such as whispered voice test [21], can provide the advanced practice nurse with insight into hearing impairment. To screen for visual impairment, an ophthalmoscope examination and screening of visual acuity using the Snellen chart and visual fields testing [21] can be undertaken.

## 7.5.2  Physical and Cognitive Function

Both basic activities of daily living (e.g., bathing, dressing, eating, toileting, transferring) and instrumental activities of daily living (e.g., meal preparation, shopping, managing money, transportation) should be assessed using a standardized assessment tool. Physical ability and cognitive ability affect performance. People with mild cognitive impairment often have difficulty with instrumental activities of daily living, but their ability to perform basic activities of daily living remains intact. [18]. Those living with dementia have increasing difficulty with both, requiring assistance and support. Common assessment tools for basic activities of daily living include the Modified Barthel Index [22] and Katz Index [23]. An example instrument for assessing instrumental activities of daily living is the Lawton Scale [24].

There are many cognitive screening and assessment tools. The Montreal Cognitive Assessment (MoCA) is useful for screening for both mild cognitive impairment and dementia and was designed to take only 10 min to administer [25]. This tool is easily accessible to clinicians through the website www.moca.org and has been translated into many languages.

## 7.5.3  Physical Environment and Access to Toilet in the Home

Easy access to the toilet is important for those with mobility limitations, and additional equipment such as a commode or raised toilet seat may be needed. Wheelchair accessibility to the toilet may also be important in supporting continence and maximizing independent function. The advanced practice nurse can consult with an occupational therapist in cases where specialty equipment or home modifications are needed.

## 7.5.4  Diet and Hydration

Due to increased risk of poor nutrition and dehydration in frail older individuals, attention to dietary and fluid intake is needed. Whenever possible, the older person should be engaged in completing their own diet and fluid diary, with caregiver assistance only when needed.

## 7.5.5 Role of the Caregiver

The family caregiver may have an important role in promoting and maintaining continence in the frail older person. When assessing how toileting is approached in the home, the advanced practice nurse needs to include how the family care approaches assist with managing any episodes of fecal incontinence. Fecal incontinence can add to caregiver burden and increase workload for formal caregiving services [26]. Even patients who are fairly independent in living in the community may receive periodic assistance from family members with daily care. Guidelines for educating caregivers of frail older people with dementia and incontinence are lacking [27]. Challenges in continence care for people with dementia living at home include perceptions about dementia, availability of support, financial costs, and emotions such as shame on the part of the person with dementia and their caregiver.

To promote successful outcomes, the advanced practice nurse can inquire if the patient wishes to have a family member/or other caregivers present during the nursing assessment visit and subsequent follow-up appointments. Mullins et al. [28] reported that distant relatives or friends (versus immediate family members) who assist an individual to manage fecal incontinence are often overlooked and excluded from clinic visits. These caregivers believe their participation in the plan of care may be beneficial. Often, it is these individuals that are going to be toileting their family member/care recipient, reminding them to toilet, implementing any treatments, changing their products, and helping with any environmental challenges. Bringing the family member/caregiver into the nursing assessment visit and subsequent follow-up appointments will help them feel included and will contribute to the success of the management plan for fecal incontinence.

It can be very frustrating for the caregiver to manage an individual with fecal incontinence as the patient will often use inappropriate places to defecate, refuse to be wiped or cleaned, and react aggressively to the offer of help, especially those with dementia. Also the caregivers are often uncomfortable handling feces.

Caregivers have suggested there is a need for healthcare professionals to have a better understanding of treating patients in the community with issues related to continence care [29]. Santini et al. [30] found that in some parts of Europe, the main provider, both from a psychological and practical point of view, was the family. In other countries, the family provided mainly emotional support, and the formal care sector delivered the practical needs. Some countries may have better support services and more specialized healthcare professionals to treat fecal incontinence. Availability of family and other support services within a healthcare system needs to be taken into consideration [27, 30].

Caregivers can find that dealing with how to manage fecal incontinence can be overwhelming. Lack of understanding and education on the topic makes it frustrating for them. Sometimes just listening to the family member/caregiver and providing simple advice or helping to refer them to a multidisciplinary team can be extremely effective. Gove et al. [27] found that care and support are often inadequate or inappropriate for community-dwelling individuals suffering with incontinence.

For clients with a chronic condition and varied levels of independence, informal caregivers may have been participating in their care for years prior to the onset of fecal incontinence. The caregivers may be involved with assisting the patient in mobilizing, transferring, and toileting prior to being seen by a healthcare professional. This makes them very capable, and they should not be underestimated in their importance and value in care planning. The caregiver may help with toileting records and bowel diaries and describe activities that may have precipitated fecal incontinence episodes. This information will benefit the provider from a more accurate diagnosis. However, considering and respecting the patient's privacy, level of independence, and perspective are essential. The advance practice nurse should develop the tact and communication that facilitate a satisfactory encounter with these patients and caregivers.

Mullins et al. [28] examined barriers to communicating with healthcare professionals as well as health literacy about incontinence among different types of informal caregivers of individuals with Alzheimer disease. They concluded that specialist continence nurses have an important role in improving health literacy around incontinence and its management for informal caregivers. Interventions must be tailored to the caregiving situation to improve the continence care of those receiving care. Educating both the patient and their caregiver will improve treatment outcomes and provide accurate measurability and successful communication.

## 7.6    Initial Interventions of Management

The advanced nursing practice approach to the management of fecal incontinence in older adults with frailty and multiple chronic conditions living in the community requires a comprehensive approach. This approach must attend to the multiple dimensions of complexity and frailty that influence patient and advanced practice nurse goals, the selection of appropriate interventions, and patient outcomes [10].

Boxes 7.4 and 7.5 present case studies highlighting how the advanced practice nurse assesses and treats fecal incontinence in community dwelling older adults.

### 7.6.1    Specific Considerations

The advanced nursing practice approach to the management of fecal incontinence in older, frail adults living in the community requires specific considerations beyond those addressed in Chap. 6 regarding younger adults. These specific considerations can be categorized by the five health dimensions of the complexity framework (demographics, mental health, social capital, medical and physical health, health and social experiences) and the sociopolitical and physical context [10].

### 7.6.1.1 Demographic Considerations

Interventions for older adults with fecal incontinence will necessarily vary based on their age, gender, ethnicity, education, and frailty [10]. For example, interventions must be tailored to accommodate different age-related changes by gender, such as pelvic organ prolapse in older women. Furthermore, culturally sensitive care extends to interventions for fecal incontinence, such as ensuring the availability of educational materials in multiple languages. See, for example, the patient education publications available on the Australian Continence Foundation in 30 different written languages (https://www.continence.org.au/other-languages.php).

### 7.6.1.2 Mental Health Considerations

Approaching fecal incontinence in community-dwelling older adults living must attend to mental health [10]. Persons with fecal incontinence describe feelings of worthlessness, poor mood, and low self-esteem [31]. Introducing any strategies that require a self-management component, where the patient is implementing and monitoring their response to behavioral changes, will not be successful unless underlying depression is identified and treated [32]. Depression is also common in older adults managing multiple chronic conditions and experiencing functional decline and frailty [33]. Additionally, older adults with fecal incontinence may be experiencing cognitive changes, including dementia, as these conditions tend to occur together [15]. Thus, optimizing cognitive function in persons with dementia has potential to improve fecal incontinence [15].

### 7.6.1.3 Social Capital Considerations

The advance practice nursing approach to fecal incontinence must consider the older adult's social capital [10]. Social capital refers to the older adult's social support, caregiver presence and strain, socioeconomic status, relationships, and leisure activities [10]. In relation to interventions for fecal incontinence, the advanced practice nurse must provide care that is inclusive and responsive to the caregiver's understanding and needs. In the home environment, this could involve education and support to formal caregivers, such as personal support workers, to assist in meal preparation or toileting assistance. Informal caregiver needs and burden must be managed by the advanced practice nurse as informal caregivers are providing the majority of instrumental support for older adults with personal care needs, in particular for persons with dementia [34]. Additionally, the advanced practice nurse needs to consider the environmental safety of the home, in particular, related to bathroom accessibility. The financial resources of the older adult are an important aspect in planning the intervention, as many older adults are living on fixed incomes [35]. Internationally, there is variable governmental funding for conservative treatment of fecal incontinence (e.g., medications) and incontinence products.

#### 7.6.1.4 Medical and Physical Health Considerations

Consideration of medical and physical health is integral to the treatment of fecal incontinence, but for older adults, the impact and interplay of multiple chronic conditions need to be addressed [15, 36]. For example, in a Pan-European investigation of older adults receiving home care services, those with diarrhea were 4.37 times more likely to have fecal incontinence than those without diarrhea [36]. These loose bowel movements could be related to poorly controlled diabetes, for example, and further aggravated by impaired rectal sensitivity and rectal weakness associated with diabetes in older adults [9]. Older adults who have had a stroke will also likely experience activity of daily living and cognitive deficits that could contribute to the development of fecal incontinence [9]. Thus, interventions to promote function in this population have the potential to improve fecal incontinence [9, 15]. Conversely, interventions to improve mobility and, thereby, daily function could be challenging in the presence of painful arthritis, so individualization of interventions is critical. Constipation-induced fecal incontinence has particular importance and urgency for treatment in older adults with Parkinson's disease as it can negatively affect absorption of antiparkinsonian medications [37].

#### 7.6.1.5 Health and Social Experience Considerations

Health and social experiences that influence patient complexity include healthcare utilization and access, quality of life, self-management support, and healthcare system navigation. The use of home healthcare services alone is an indicator of complexity. For example, older adults receiving home care services have a higher prevalence of fecal incontinence—ranging from 9% to 13% depending on the study—than those who live independently [9, 15, 36]. Also in the home care context, ADL function and cognitive function are more important predictors of fecal incontinence than would be seen in independently living older adults [9, 36]. Experiences of healthcare are also affected by the complexity of the system itself for older adults. Older adults with multiple chronic conditions routinely require care from multiple providers in different settings, for example, primary and specialist care in both community and hospital settings [38]. The advanced practice nurse has the requisite skill set to lead and coordinate a team approach to treat fecal incontinence across these types of complex networks of healthcare providers.

### 7.7    Other Interventions

### 7.7.1    Address Reversible Causes

With the special considerations in mind, the advanced practice nurse must first address any reversible cause of fecal incontinence in the older adult.

#### 7.7.1.1 Medications

As discussed earlier, assessing polypharmacy is an important part of caring for an older adult with fecal incontinence, and de-prescribing is an intervention [39]. The advanced practice nurse must consider if a "prescribing cascade" was involved [14]. For example, a narcotic could have been prescribed for pain, which resulted in constipation, which was treated with sennosides, but the sennosides caused diarrhea and fecal incontinence, so loperamide was added, which could worsen constipation [14].

### 7.7.1.2 Toilet Access and Abilities
Based on the assessment of the home environment, functional ability, and presence of caregiver support, a determination must be made in regard to whether the fecal incontinence is related to not accessing the toilet in a timely manner [40]. If so, the advanced practice nurse can intervene to discuss strategies such as prompting, timed defecation, adaptive clothing, and adaptive devices to get on and off the toilet easily (e.g., grab bars).

### 7.7.1.3 Infection
Treatment for *Clostridium difficile*-associated diarrhea is discussed in Chap. 10. In regard to care in the community, the advanced practice nurse must first determine if the older adult was diagnosed and treated for *Clostridium difficile* during a hospital stay. Older adults are at risk of a *Clostridium difficile* recurrence [41]. There is a strong evidence that two probiotics (*Lactobacillus rhamnosus* GG and *Saccharomyces boulardii*) can decrease the incidence of antibiotic-associated diarrhea [41].

### 7.7.1.4 Rectal Loading/Fecal Impaction
As impaction can be a common and reversible cause of fecal incontinence in older adults, the advanced practice nurse should include this management in her treatment plan [9, 40]. Treatment for rectal loading and fecal impaction in an institutional setting, such as a nursing home, is addressed in Chap. 8. In the community environment, if the older adult requires support, the advanced practice nurse can coordinate home care nursing support to administer and monitor outcomes, as jurisdictional services and funding permits. Older adults with multiple chronic conditions and frailty frequently experience constipation [42]. Clinical experience with older adults has revealed that constipation has the real potential to translate into impaction and fecal incontinence. Thus, the prevention and management of constipation is a proactive advanced practice nurse intervention in preventing this condition worsening into episodes of fecal incontinence in community-based frail older adults (see Chap. 6).

### 7.7.1.5 Dietary and Fluid Intake
The maintenance of adequate hydration and fiber intake is critical to prevent constipation [40, 42, 43]. For older adults, eating meals and snacks at regular times promotes bowel regularity [42]. Troubleshooting how to achieve these goals is part of the advanced practice nurse role. Income, energy level, function, and tolerance are all factors for a frail older adult in enacting these self-care activities. The advanced practice nurse can connect clients to community support services, such as subsidized home delivery meal programs (i.e., meals-on-wheels) or food banks. She/he can also initiate referrals to home support services and develop meal plans for the personal support workers to prepare with or for the client.

### 7.7.1.6 **Exercise**

Regular activity through exercise is a foundational component of constipation treatments as it is believed to improve peristalsis and colonic transit time [44]. Also, any activity to improve mobility will improve fecal continence by preventing functional decline and incontinence [15]. The advanced practice nurse should suggest walking as a treatment for constipation based on the client's ability and energy levels [44]. Walking for 15–20 min once or twice a day or 30–60 min daily or three to five times per week is optimal [42, 44]. For older adults with more limited mobility or energy resources, ambulating at least 50 feet twice a day is recommended [44]. These recommendations are based on expert clinical opinion [44].

### 7.7.1.7 **Pharmacological Treatment of Constipation**

Constipation cannot always be effectively treated with fluid, fiber, and fitness, particularly in older adults with polypharmacy or chronic conditions that cause constipation. In these situations, the advanced practice nurse must consider the addition of laxatives. First line would be the addition of a psyllium supplement to bulk up stool by adding fiber and drawing in moisture [9, 45, 46] with the aim of stimulating defecation and softening stool that may be hard. However, psyllium supplementation must be accompanied by adequate fluid intake, or it can alter the stool consistency making it more difficult to pass. Osmotic laxatives, which also draw fluid into the stool, are the next line of treatment, and the product choice depends on client preference and reimbursement rules of different private and public drug benefit plans. Finally, stimulant laxatives and enemas are reserved for occasional use or "rescue" if the regular treatment is intermittently not effective [46]. Refer to Fig. 7.1 for a medication management pyramid. Although commonly prescribed for older adults, the use of surfactant is not recommended due to the lack of high-quality evidence of its effectiveness [46].

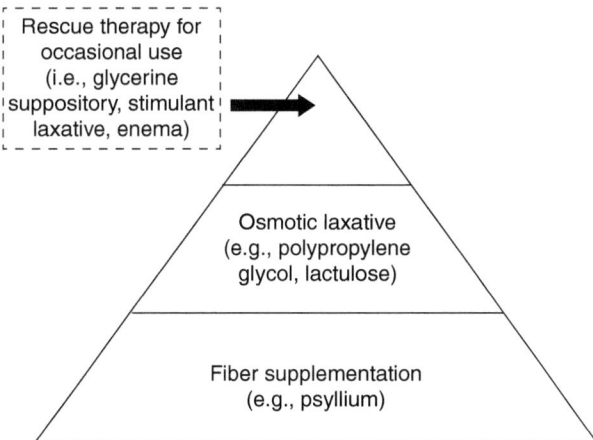

**Fig. 7.1**  Medication management pyramid for treatment of constipation in older adults. Adapted from Liu 2011 [46] and Wagg et al., 2017 [9]

#### 7.7.1.8 Hemorrhoids

Hemorrhoids are caused by chronic straining due to hard stool and constipation and are also associated with fecal incontinence in older adults [9]. While the advanced practice nurse is working with the client on treating and resolving constipation, the pain and swelling of hemorrhoids must also be addressed. Clients should be advised to cleanse hemorrhoids gently with moistened wipes that do not contain perfume or alcohol or a cotton pad dampened with witch hazel. Topical treatments that can be purchased over the counter containing lidocaine and hydrocortisone can also be recommended for short-term use.

#### 7.7.1.9 Rectocele

A rectocele is the herniation or bulging of the posterior vaginal wall from the rectum pushing anteriorly into the vagina [47]. Rectoceles are associated with fecal incontinence in older women [9] and can contribute to constipation and an incomplete evacuation of the bowel. The best treatment for a rectocele is prevention of hard stool and straining to have a bowel movement, which can worsen the degree of prolapse. The advanced practice nurse can also instruct the client on techniques, such as using the first and second fingers together as a brace to support the rectocele external to the vagina when bearing down. Alternatively, the advanced practice nurse can instruct the client to insert her finger into the vagina to exert pressure on the back wall to facilitate bowel emptying. These techniques rely on clinical expertise. For some clients, with some types of rectocele, there is some evidence that a pessary could provide the necessary support [48]. For older women, the success of a pessary is enhanced when local hormone replacement therapy is used to treat vaginal atrophic changes [48].

#### 7.7.1.10  Abdominal Massage

For older adults with fecal incontinence related to constipation, self-massage of the abdomen, which involves applying firm pressure in the direction of stool movement, could facilitate movement of stool through the bowel [40, 49]. Although there are no empirical studies with an older adult population, some evidence exists that this is effective for younger adults with multiple sclerosis [49]. Yet, having multiple techniques to try to improve bowel function can bolster clients' feelings of self-efficacy and is worth considering by the advanced practice nurse with willing clients.

### 7.7.2   Establishing Regular Bowel Habits

The advanced practice nurse works with the client to establish a regular bowel elimination pattern (see Chap. 6). Of particular importance for the older adult is to take advantage of the gastrocolic reflex (which results in increased peristalsis) that occurs after the first meal of the day and to plan for defecation at this time [40, 42]. The advanced practice nurse might need to work with the client in troubleshooting and planning related to the client's regular schedule in order to account for disruptions, such as doctor's appointments or visits from community healthcare providers.

### 7.7.2.1 Positioning on Toilet

Comfort and position on the toilet are a component of establishing regular bowel habits for the older adult. Adaptive aids in the home, such as a raised toilet seat or poorly fitting over-the-seat commode, may make sitting comfortably and properly on the toilet a challenge. Refer to Fig. 7.2 for the correct position to sit on the toilet to effectively evacuate the bowels. This image is also a helpful teaching tool. As can be seen in the images, if a raised toilet seat is in place, assuming the squat position is not possible. In this case, the advanced practice nurse would suggest a small

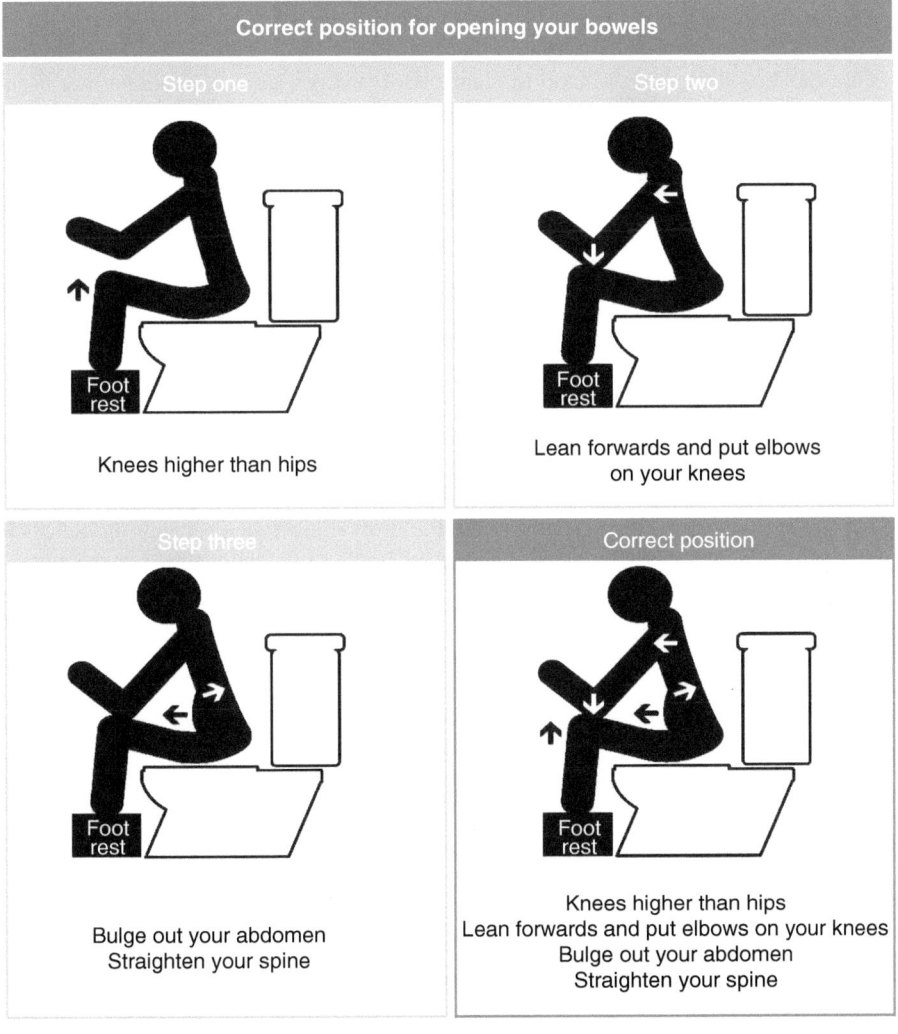

**Fig. 7.2** Correct position for opening your bowels. (Reprinted with permission from Norgine Ltd. who has reproduced and distributed the image with the kind permission of the co-authors including Wendy Ness, Colorectal nurse specialist. Produced as a service to the medical profession by Norgine Ltd. ©2017 Norgine group of companies. UK/COR/0118/0855. Date of preparation: January 2018)

footstool be available in the bathroom so that the client can bring their knees higher. The client should be instructed to bulge out the abdomen, rather than contracting, in order to more effectively open the bowel [50, 51].

#### 7.7.2.2 Adaptive Aids

Adaptive aids to promote fecal continence can be useful for older adults. The advanced practice nurse's role with her/his older adult client can be to collaborate with other members of the interdisciplinary team to assess for and recommend adaptive aids. For example, in the community, the advanced practice nurse could initiate a referral to an occupational therapist for an assessment of bathroom safety.

#### 7.7.2.3 Privacy and Dignity

This topic is discussed in detail in Chap. 10. However, older adults residing in the community may be supported by a caregiver. Defecation is intimately private, and fecal incontinence is socially stigmatized [51]. The advanced practice nurse must consider this when planning interventions for the older adult client that involve enlisting the assistance of a formal or informal caregiver [9]. The advanced practice nurse can suggest practical strategies to the client such as the use of a deodorizing spray to use in the bathroom before summoning help for those concerned about odor [51]. Also, the advanced practice nurse should work with the caregiver to ensure client privacy (both auditory and visual) during toileting.

### 7.7.3  Improve Stool Consistency

#### 7.7.3.1  Loose Stool/Diarrhea

Loose stools and long-term diarrhea are the most important contributing factors to fecal incontinence in older adults [9]. Loose stools overwhelm the anal sphincter's ability to maintain continence due to the challenge of differentiating loose stool from gas [40]. In older adults, a change in stool consistency and pattern signals a need to consider the risk for colorectal cancer if other warning signs are present (e.g., weight loss, blood in stool, pain) [9]. In this situation, the advanced practice nurse would collaborate with the client's primary care provider and/or medical specialist.

Once the advanced practice nurse has determined the cause of the loose stool, they must work with the older adult client to implement a variety of strategies to improve stool consistency. As discussed in the reversible causes section, the impact of medication or an infective process must first be ruled out [9]. Diet modifications are negotiated with the client (see Chap. 6) with special attention paid to foods that can contribute to loose stools. The advanced practice nurse may also recommend the supplementation of soluble, moderately fermentable dietary fiber such as psyllium [40]. This type of fiber firms stool consistency, likely by forming a gel in feces reducing the free water content in stool [40, 52]. Food sources of dietary fiber include oats, barley, oranges, dried beans, and lentils [44]. For some older adult clients, meeting these nutritional goals by eating more fiber-containing foods could be challenging, and the advanced practice nurse can recommend a fiber supplement, such as psyllium [40]. The advanced practice nurse must discuss the need for adequate fluid intake (1500–2000 mL per day of water) when taking a fiber supplement and how to dilute and prepare a powder-based supplement [40, 44].

### 7.7.3.2 Medication Management

Antimotility or antidiarrheal medications are useful treatments for fecal incontinence in older adults where the stool consistency cannot be modified, for example, in an older adult with prior surgical removal of part of the bowel for cancer or with diabetes-related neuropathic changes [9]. The strongest evidence is for loperamide, which can reduce the frequency of fecal incontinence in older adults [9]. Loperamide must be used with caution in older adults as it could inadvertently cause constipation [9]. As loperamide can be titrated from a very small dose (1 mg) to higher doses, the advanced practice nurse must support the older adult in making small, incremental changes to achieve the desired stool consistency, frequency, and absence of incontinent episodes [40].

## 7.7.4   Containment

Containment products and skin care are discussed in detail in Chap. 13; however a few key points related to the older adult are considered here.

### 7.7.4.1 Incontinence Products

When working with a frail older adult to select the best incontinence product, consideration must be given to the client's dexterity, mobility, and balance. For example, a pull-up style may not work if the client is not able to undress and redress his or her lower body when the pull-up is soiled. Alternatively, a pad and pant system may be superior, so the soiled pad can be more easily removed and replaced. As urinary incontinence is often present with fecal incontinence in older adults with multiple chronic conditions, the product must also be adequate for that purpose [9]. Finally, the advanced practice nurse must consider the cost impact and potential sources of funding, such as private insurance, municipal special support funds, or even food banks or other community programs.

### 7.7.4.2 Skin Care

The perineal skin of older adults is more sensitive and vulnerable due to the normal age-related changes of thinning of the skin, loss of elasticity, and atrophic changes in women. The advanced practice nurse must also assess and make recommendations on cleansing and wiping after a bowel movement or a fecal incontinence episode, as some older adults do not have the range of motion or dexterity to reach and adequately clean around their rectum. The advanced practice nurse can suggest devices, such as a "reacher" designed for wiping or a spray bottle. Working with an occupational therapist skilled in adaptive aides can enhance the advanced practice nurse's practice in this regard.

### 7.7.5 Education and Teaching

Education and teaching are integrated into all of the interventions that the advanced practice nurse plans with her clients. Quite often, older adults have had fecal incontinence for a long period and have not sought treatment due to embarrassment, so they need education and reassurance that resolving the problem will take time. The advanced practice nurse must work with the client to set reasonable goals and timeframes for evaluation [46].

## 7.8 Expected Outcomes and Evaluation

The expected primary outcome of involvement of the advanced practice nurse is reduction in episodes of fecal incontinence or, if this is not feasible, appropriate containment and prevention of adverse secondary conditions including incontinence-associated dermatitis. Evaluation should include the five health dimensions in the complexity model (demographics, mental health, social capital, medical and physical health, health and social experiences) and contextual features of the sociopolitical and physical environment that may affect outcomes [10].

### 7.8.1 Follow-Up

Follow-up will depend on the role played by the advanced practice nurse and the severity of the problem. If the advanced practice nurse is part of a primary team or attached to home care services, long-term follow-up will be required as long as the frail person remains supported in the community. For the advanced practice nurse in a consulting role, follow-up will be more limited, ending with resolution or effective management of the fecal incontinence to the satisfaction of the client and family caregiver.

### 7.8.2 Team Work/Interprofessional Consultation

Holistic, integrated approach to management of fecal incontinence is needed in the community [27]. The community-based advanced practice nurse caring for the frail older person with fecal incontinence enacts the consultation role through various channels. They may consult with the primary care provider about health concerns and medications contributing to fecal incontinence if they are not in that role themselves or with a specialist physician such as a geriatrician for comprehensive geriatric assessment and recommendations stemming from that assessment. The advanced practice nurse may be a part of a home care service or access home care services on behalf of the client for home modification and equipment recommendations from an occupational therapist or for interventions to maintain or restore mobility from a physical therapist. The advanced practice nurse may work with the home care case manager (often a nurse) and facilitate access to assistance from healthcare aides for toileting and hygiene or reimbursement for containment products.

**Box 7.3: Key Points for Managing Fecal Incontinence in Frail Community-Dwelling Older Adults**

- Involve the client and caregiver in development of the management plan with realistic goals in the home setting. Education of both the client and caregiver is key.
- Address reversible causes of fecal incontinence, including intervening in a prescribing cascade that results in inappropriate polypharmacy or teaching the client and family about risks of over-the-counter antidiarrheal agents and laxatives.
- Address toilet access and environmental barriers in the home environment of the frail older person.
- Promote and facilitate access to mobility aids as well as adaptive clothing and devices. Devices can include a stool at the toilet to promote proper position for defecation.
- Assess for risk of *Clostridium difficile*-associated diarrhea, particularly post hospitalization.
- Address constipation to avoid rectal loading and fecal impaction. In the community, this could include access to meal services and other community supports and promotion of exercise within the tolerance of the older person.
- Judiciously use antimotility agents if the fecal incontinence is related to loose stool and not due to infection and not modified with diet changes.
- Refer to other healthcare professionals and community services as needed.

**Box 7.4: Case Study 1**

Mr. S is a 79-year-old male living at home with his wife, his main family caregiver. He has mild to moderate stage dementia, and Mrs. S is highly motivated to keep him at home rather than having him go to an institution such as a nursing home. She presents to the advanced practice nurse in a continence clinic with a concern that he is having daily fecal incontinence occurring when they are out walking.

The advanced practice nurse conducted an assessment including a history and physical exam. The physical exam was normal, but the symptom assessment portion of the history revealed that they were walking in the morning right after breakfast. Knowledge of the caregiver was also assessed. Mrs. S was unaware of the gastrocolic reflex and had not tied the fecal incontinence to the physiological phenomena.

The recommended intervention was to change the time of day they took their daily walk to late morning or afternoon, so that Mr. S could easily access the toilet after breakfast. The incontinence episodes resolved to the satisfaction of the client and caregiver.

**Box 7.5: Case Study 2**

Mrs. Z is an 83-year-old woman who was referred to the home care advanced practice nurse with frequently loose stool that is difficult to control, resulting in episodes of fecal incontinence. History reveals issues of chronic pain related to arthritis in the knees, hips, and lower back, spinal stenosis, hypertension, and COPD.

Medications include candesartan (angiotensin II receptor blocker) for hypertension, a tiotropium bromide (anticholinergic bronchodilator) inhaler for COPD, and acetaminophen with codeine (analgesic with opioid) for pain. She also identified taking over-the-counter Lomotil (diphenoxylate, a weak opioid, and atropine) for loose stool every 2–3 days when she felt the stool was too loose to control.

Physical exam revealed a moderately distended abdomen with palpable bowel loops and hard stool in the rectum.

The advanced practice nurse ordered an abdominal flat plate, which showed fecal impaction. Disimpaction was achieved using daily enemas for 3 days with the assistance of the home care service staff. The advanced practice nurse was a prescriber and weaned down the acetaminophen with codeine, replacing it with plain acetaminophen supplemented with 10% diclofenac gel topically twice daily to knees and lower back for pain management. X-rays of the knees and lower back were ordered, and a referral was made to the orthopedic service for further assessment.

Referrals were also made to the home care occupational therapist for a home environment assessment and physical therapist for maintenance of mobility.

# References

1. World Health Organization. World report on ageing and health. Geneva: WHO; 2015.
2. De Vries N, Staal J, Van Ravensberg C, Hobbelen J, Rikkert MO, Nijhuis-Van der Sanden M. Outcome instruments to measure frailty: a systematic review. Ageing Res Rev. 2011;10(1):104–14.
3. British Geriatric Society. Fit for frailty: consensus best practice guidance for the care of older people living with frailty in community and outpatient settings. London. London: British Geriatric Society; 2014. http://www.bgs.org.uk/campaigns/fff/fff_full.pdf
4. Santos-Eggimann B, Cuénoud P, Spagnoli J, Junod J. Prevalence of frailty in middle-aged and older community-dwelling Europeans living in 10 countries. J Gerontol A Biol Sci Med Sci. 2009;64(6):675–81.
5. Song X, Mitnitski A, Rockwood K. Prevalence and 10-year outcomes of frailty in older adults in relation to deficit accumulation. J Am Geriatr Soc. 2010;58(4):681–7.
6. Fried LP, Tangen CM, Walston J, Newman AB, Hirsch C, Gottdiener J, et al. Frailty in older adults: evidence for a phenotype. J Gerontol Ser A Biol Med Sci. 2001;56(3):M146–M57.
7. Rockwood K, Mitnitski A. Frailty in relation to the accumulation of deficits. J Gerontol Ser A Biol Med Sci. 2007;62(7):722–7.
8. Schober M. Introduction to advanced nursing practice: an international focus. Cham: Springer; 2016.

9. Wagg A, Chen LK, Johnson IIT, Kirschner-Hermanns R, Kuchel G, Markland A, et al. Incontinence in frail older persons. In: Abrams P, Cardozo L, Wagg A, Wein A, editors. Incontinence. 6th ed. Bristol: International Continence Society; 2017. p. 1309–441.
10. Schaink AK, Kuluski K, Lyons RF, Fortin M, Jadad AR, Upshur R, et al. A scoping review and thematic classification of patient complexity: offering a unifying framework. J Comorb. 2012;2:1):1–9.
11. Zullig LL, Whitson HE, Hastings SN, Beadles C, Kravchenko J, Akushevich I, et al. A systematic review of conceptual frameworks of medical complexity and new model development. J Gen Intern Med. 2015;31(3):329–37.
12. Kuluski K, Gill A, Naganathan G, Upshur R, Jaakkimainen RL, Wodchis WP. A qualitative descriptive study on the alignment of care goals between older persons with multi-morbidities, their family physicians and informal caregivers. BMC Fam Pract. 2013;14(1):133.
13. De Giorgio R, Ruggeri E, Stanghellini V, Eusebi LH, Bazzoli F, Chiarioni G. Chronic constipation in the elderly: a primer for the gastroenterologist. BMC Gastroenterol. 2015;15(1):130.
14. Kwan D, Farell B. Polypharmacy: optimizing medication use in elderly patients. Can Geriatr Soc J Continuing Med Educ. 2014;4(1):21–7.
15. Westra BL, Savik K, Oancea C, Choromanski L, Holmes JH, Bliss DZ. Predicting improvement in urinary and bowel incontinence for home health patients using electronic health record data. J Wound Ostomy Cont Nurs. 2011;38(1):77–87.
16. De Lillo AR, Rose S. Functional bowel disorders in the geriatric patient: constipation, fecal impaction, and fecal incontinence. Am J Gastroenterol. 2000;95(4):901–5.
17. Shah BJ, Chokhavatia S, Rose S. Fecal incontinence in the elderly: FAQ. Am J Gastroenterol. 2012;107(11):1635–46.
18. Petersen RC, Caracciolo B, Brayne C, Gauthier S, Jelic V, Fratiglioni L. Mild cognitive impairment: a concept in evolution. J Intern Med. 2014;275(3):214–28.
19. Wimo A, Jönsson L, Bond J, Prince M, Winblad B, International Alzheimer's Disease. The worldwide economic impact of dementia. Alzheimers Dement. 2010;9(1):1–11.e3.
20. Guthrie DM, Declercq A, Finne-Soveri H, Fries BE, Hirdes JP. The health and well-being of older adults with dual sensory impairment (DSI) in four countries. PLoS One. 2016;11(5):e0155073.
21. Bickley LS. Bates' guide to physical examination and history taking. Philadelphia: Lippincott Williams & Wilkins; 2017.
22. Shah S, Vanclay F, Cooper B. Improving the sensitivity of the Barthel Index for stroke rehabilitation. J Clin Epidemiol. 1989;42(8):703–9.
23. Katz S. Assessing self-maintenance: activities of daily living, mobility, and instrumental activities of daily living. J Am Geriatr Soc. 1983;31(12):721–7.
24. Lawton MP, Brody EM. Assessment of older people: self-maintaining and instrumental activities of daily living. The Gerontologist. 1969;9:179–86.
25. Nasreddine ZS, Phillips NA, Bédirian V, Charbonneau S, Whitehead V, Collin I, et al. The Montreal cognitive assessment, MoCA: a brief screening tool for mild cognitive impairment. J Am Geriatr Soc. 2005;53(4):695–9.
26. Finne-Soveri H, Sorbye LW, Jonsson PV, Carpenter GI, Bernabei R. Increased work-load associated with faecal incontinence among home care patients in 11 European countries. Eur J Pub Health. 2008;18(3):323–8.
27. Gove D, Scerri A, Georges J, van Houten P, Huige N, Hayder-Beichel D, et al. Continence care for people with dementia living at home in Europe: a review of literature with a focus on problems and challenges. J Clin Nurs. 2016;26(3-4):356–65.
28. Mullins J, Bliss DZ, Rolnick S, Henre CA, Jackson J. Barriers to communication with a healthcare provider and health literacy about incontinence among informal caregivers of individuals with dementia. J Wound Ostomy Cont Nurs. 2016;43(5):539–44.
29. Drennan VM, Cole L, Iliffe S. A taboo within a stigma? A qualitative study of managing incontinence with people with dementia living at home. BMC Geriatr. 2011;11:75.
30. Santini S, Andersson G, Lamura G. Impact of incontinence on the quality of life of caregivers of older persons with incontinence: a qualitative study in four European countries. Arch Gerontol Geriatr. 2016;63:92–101.

31. Bliss DZ, Mimura T, Berghmans B, Bharucha A, Chiarioni G, Emmanuel A, et al. Assessment and conservative management of faecal incontinence and quality of life in adults. In: Abrams P, Cardozo L, Wagg A, Wein A, editors. Incontinence. 6th ed. Bristol: International Continence Society; 2017. p. 1993–2085.
32. Registered Nurses Association of Ontario (RNAO). Strategies to support self-management in chronic conditions: collaboration with clients. Toronto: Registered Nurses Association of Ontario; 2010. http://rnao.ca/sites/rnao-ca/files/Strategies_to_Support_Self-Management_in_Chronic_Conditions_-_Collaboration_with_Clients.pdf.
33. Markle-Reid M, Browne G, Gafni A. Nurse-led health promotion interventions improve quality of life in frail older home care clients: lessons learned from three randomized trials in Ontario, Canada. J Eval Clin Pract. 2013;19(1):118–31.
34. Alzheimer's Association. 2014 Alzheimer's disease facts and figures. Alzheimers Dement. 2014;10(2):e47–92.
35. OECD. Pensions at a glance 2015. Paris: OECD Publishing; 2015.
36. Finne-Soveri H, Sørbye L, Jonsson P, Carpenter G, Bernabei R. Increased work-load associated with faecal incontinence among home care patients in 11 European countries. Eur J Pub Health. 2007;18(3):323–8.
37. Varanese S, Birnbaum Z, Rossi R, Di Rocco A. Treatment of advanced Parkinson's disease. Parkinsons Dis. 2010;480260. https://doi.org/10.4061/2010/480260.
38. Smith SM, Soubhi H, Fortin M, Hudon C, O'Dowd T. Managing patients with multimorbidity: systematic review of interventions in primary care and community settings. BMJ. 2012;345:e5205.
39. Bain KT, Holmes HM, Beers MH, Maio V, Handler SM, Pauker SG. Discontinuing medications: a novel approach for revising the prescribing stage of the medication-use process. J Am Geriatr Soc. 2008;56(10):1946–52.
40. Bliss DZ, Norton C. Conservative management of fecal incontinence. Am J Nurs. 2010;110(9):30–8.
41. Surawicz CM, Brandt LJ, Binion DG, Ananthakrishnan AN, Curry SR, Gilligan PH, et al. Guidelines for diagnosis, treatment, and prevention of Clostridium difficile infections. Am J Gastroenterol. 2013;108(4):478–98.
42. Ostaszkiewicz J, Hornby L, Millar L, Ockerby C. The effects of conservative treatment for constipation on symptom severity and quality of life in community-dwelling adults. J Wound Ostomy Cont Nurs. 2010;37(2):193–8.
43. Robbs L, editor. Fecal incontinence: assessment and treatment. Hamilton, ON: McMaster University Press; 2014.
44. Registered Nurses Association of Ontario (RNAO). Prevention of constipation in the older adult population. Toronto: Registered Nurses Association of Ontario; 2011. www.rnao.org/bestpractices/
45. Franklin LE, Spain MP, Edlund BJ. Pharmacological management of chronic constipation in older adults. J Gerontol Nurs. 2012;38(4):9–15.
46. Liu LWC. Chronic constipation: current treatment options. Can J Gastroenterol. 2011;25(Suppl B):22B–8B.
47. Nugent KP. Rectocele pathophysiology and presentation. In Cohen R, Windsor A, editors. Anus: Surgical treatment and pathophysiology. London: Springer; 2013. p.91–6.
48. Hanson L-AM, Schulz JA, Flood CG, Cooley B, Tam F. Vaginal pessaries in managing women with pelvic organ prolapse and urinary incontinence: patient characteristics and factors contributing to success. Int Urogynecol J. 2006;17(2):155–9.
49. McClurg D, Hagen S, Hawkins S, Lowe-Strong A. Abdominal massage for the alleviation of constipation symptoms in people with multiple sclerosis: a randomized controlled feasibility study. Mult Scler J. 2011;17(2):223–33.
50. Doughty D, Jensen LL, editors. Assessment and management of the patient with fecal incontinence and related bowel dysfunction. St. Louis, MO: Mosby Elsevier; 2006.
51. Norton C, editor. Bowel control and managing a misbehaving bowel. Wilmette, IL: The Simon Foundation; 2011.
52. Bliss DZ, Savik K, Jung HJG, Whitebird R, Lowry A, Sheng X. Dietary fiber supplementation for fecal incontinence: a randomized clinical trial. Res Nurs Health. 2014;37(5):367–78.

# Management of Fecal Incontinence in Older Adults in Long-Term Care

<br/>

Lene Elisabeth Blekken, Anne Guttormsen Vinsnes,
Kari Hanne Gjeilo, and Donna Z. Bliss

**Abstract**

Of all the health challenges frail elderly face, fecal incontinence is one of the most dreaded. Lack of knowledge within the field of fecal incontinence is evident. With life expectancy lengthening, the percentage of people who will require care in a nursing home will increase in the years to come. Nursing home patients are the most fragile of the older patients. Among this group, there are often problems connected with defecation, such as constipation, diarrhea, and fecal incontinence. Fecal incontinence is a complex problem. It is therefore necessary to have a broad approach to fecal incontinence, and it is important that nurses have high knowledge and advanced skills when it comes to meeting patients' needs for assessment, care, and treatment. Fecal incontinence can lead to feelings of shame and embarrassment and to a downward spiral of psychological distress, dependency, and poor health. Loose stool, as well as hard stool, can be related to fecal incontinence. Urgency associated with bowel movements is also an important factor. The most important risk factors are functional incapacity, reduced cognitive function, diarrhea, constipation/impaction, stroke, some neurological diseases, diabetes, and comorbidity in general. The level of knowledge among health personnel on the value of good bowel care seems limited. There is at present a relatively limited evidence base from high-quality experimental

L. E. Blekken (✉) · A. G. Vinsnes
Department of Public Health and Nursing, Norwegian University
of Science and Technology (NTNU), Trondheim, Norway
e-mail: lene.blekken@ntnu.no; anne.g.vinsnes@ntnu.no

K. H. Gjeilo
Norwegian University of Science and Technology (NTNU), Trondheim, Norway

St. Olav's Hospital, Trondheim University Hospital, Trondheim, Norway
e-mail: kari.hanne.gjeilo@stolav.no

D. Z. Bliss
University of Minnesota School of Nursing, Minneapolis, MN, USA
e-mail: bliss@umn.edu

© Springer International Publishing AG, part of Springer Nature 2018
D. Z. Bliss (ed.), *Management of Fecal Incontinence for the Advanced Practice Nurse*,
https://doi.org/10.1007/978-3-319-90704-8_8

trials of fecal incontinence, and it remains challenging to provide strong evidence for most interventions. Frail older people require a different care approach addressing the potential role of comorbid disease and current medications, in addition to the functional and cognitive impairment, and should take into account the degree of bother to the person. When appropriate, patient education is important to promote self-management and other coping mechanisms. An environment with physical or social obstacles may impair the ability to maintain continence. This is particularly relevant to individuals who have physical or mental disorders. Good care quality encompasses care personnel to acknowledge the problem of fecal incontinence compassionately. Healthcare personnel should be trained in identification and management of fecal incontinence in nursing home patients.

**Keywords**
Fecal incontinence · Nursing home · Complexity · Dignified care · Comprehensive assessment

## 8.1 Introduction

Of all the health challenges frail elderly face, fecal incontinence is one of the most dreaded; it is a major assault to psychosocial as well as physiologic well-being. Care requires systematic interventions on multiple levels to assure that staff provides individualized, evidence-based care. Clinical improvement efforts aimed at improving care of elders with fecal incontinence must be systematic and evaluated.

## 8.2 Patient Group

With life expectancy lengthening in Western countries, the percentage of people who will require care in a nursing home will increase in the coming decades. As high dependency due to physical or mental impairment is required for admission to nursing homes, most nursing home patients have advanced chronic illnesses and multiple diagnoses, and the vast majority of these individuals are suffering from dementia.

Nursing home patients are the most fragile of older patients. They have multiple diagnoses, are using many different medications, and have a low level of function according to the activities of daily living in general. Hence, nursing home patients are a group of highly dependent older adults. Among this group, there are often problems connected with defecation, such as constipation, diarrhea, and fecal incontinence. It is therefore necessary to have a broad approach to fecal incontinence in nursing homes. It is important that nurses have high knowledge and advanced skills when it comes to meeting patients' needs for assessment, care, and treatment.

Fecal incontinence is prevalent within the group of elderly patients in nursing homes [1–3]. Fecal incontinence among frail elderly is usually a result of many interacting risk factors that include: age-related physical changes, comorbidity, multiple pharmacological treatments, and physical and cognitive reduction [2, 3]. For many of these complexly ill patients, families are an important source of support. Previous research has confirmed that family members continued their involvement and sense of responsibility for care as their elder moved to and remained in a nursing home [4]. Davies and Nolan [5] reported the standards of care which family caregivers regarded as "best care"; however the respondents reported that these expectations were rarely met in full.

## 8.3   Clinical Setting

Future demographic changes portend future pressure to expand nursing home care while maintaining high-care standards with limited resources. Fecal incontinence leads to a high direct and indirect economic burden to the healthcare system and is an important cause of institutionalization of older people [2]. Quality has at least two components that should be addressed: quality of care and quality of life, both of which can be transformed, either positively or negatively by nursing care [4].

Patient care in nursing homes continues to be necessary for those individuals who are no longer able to live at home comfortably or safely. With the shifting demography toward an aging population, nursing homes will continue to be an essential service provided to individuals for the near future. For long-term residents, the nursing home provides a total service, including advanced healthcare, housing, and social care. Nursing home staff are challenged to meet the dual demands of providing a home for long-term residents while managing chronic and acute medical problems. Internationally recognized standards emphasize patient safety, excellence in care, and patient satisfaction in the long-term care of older people. National quality standards for long-term care in several countries include a range of domains relevant to nursing care quality [6]. Also among patients in nursing homes, fecal incontinence is related to feelings of shame and embarrassment [7] and can lead to a downward spiral of psychological distress, dependency, and poor health [2].

## 8.4   Risk Factors for Fecal Incontinence in Nursing Home Patients

### 8.4.1   Age

Age has been confirmed as a risk factor for fecal incontinence in many population-based studies [2]. Normal anorectal physiologic function is complex and relies on several different functions, including anatomic and neurologic factors. A review by

Norton et al. found the results from physiological studies on the aging bowel to vary due to (a) a variety of different techniques used in measuring anorectal function, (b) unclear definition of the normative range of manometric measures for older people, (c) poor matching between cases and controls of clinical factors which may affect gut function (e.g., level of mobility) or inadequate clinical information, and (d) usually small subject numbers. However, studies on healthy older adults report that anorectal function is characterized by a tendency toward an age-related reduction in internal anal sphincter tone (basal pressure) after the age of 70 years in both genders, but to a greater degree in women. There also seems to be a decline in external anal sphincter tone (squeeze pressure) in women after the age of 70 years and in men after the age of 90 years. There seems to be an age-related increase in anorectal sensitivity thresholds and a reduced rectal compliance. However, rectal motility seems to be well preserved [8]. Overall, the physiological data suggest that fecal incontinence should not be considered an inevitable consequence of aging alone [2]. Colonic function in general, and fecal incontinence specifically, appears to be more influenced by factors associated with aging than with aging itself [2].

### 8.4.2  Stool Consistency

Stool consistency is an important factor associated with fecal incontinence. Loose stool [1, 3, 9–11] as well as hard stool [1, 9, 12, 13] can be related to fecal incontinence. Potential reversible causes of loose stool may include excessive laxative use, lactose intolerance, drug-related side effects, and bacterial overgrowth [2]. In the elderly, chronic constipation can lead to fecal impaction. Although a definition of fecal impaction is elusive, it usually refers to the accumulation of hard feces in the rectum and colon that the person cannot evacuate alone [14]. Liquid stools from the proximal colon can bypass the impacted stool, causing overflow incontinence, often mistaken for diarrhea [2]. The research on prevalence and risk factors of impaction is very limited, but indirect data suggest that it is highly prevalent among institutionalized elderly patients [14]. One study investigating prevalence and risk factors for impaction in nursing home patients found a prevalence of 28% with a frequency labeling of impaction as a record of at least two episodes of impaction in the last year and 47% with a frequency labeling of at least one impaction episode within the last year. The same study found a prevalence of 7% based on a rectal examination performed by a physician when the physician described the feces as hard and impacted. They also found that the prevalence of fecal incontinence was 16% among patients without a history of fecal impaction and 28% among those with a history of fecal impaction [14].

### 8.4.3  Urgency

Urgency associated with bowel movements is also an important factor related to fecal incontinence [2]. Many studies do not evaluate urgency as an independent risk factor. However, among the studies that evaluated a sense of urgency associated with bowel movements, urgency is consistently and strongly related to fecal incontinence [2]. Other bowel-related disorders, such as hemorrhoids, posterior vaginal prolapse, irritable bowel syndrome, or complications of prior surgery, can contribute to fecal incontinence in older adults who otherwise would be continent. This might especially become a problem when functional status, mobility, and cognition become impaired. Hence, bowel-related disorders and surgery should be a part of the focused history in older people with fecal incontinence [2].

### 8.4.4  Comorbidities

In patients living in nursing homes, some diseases seem to increase the risk of fecal incontinence. An environment with physical or social obstacles may impair the ability to maintain continence. This is particularly relevant to individuals who have physical or mental disorders. Akpan et al. [9] found that comorbidity in general was associated with fecal incontinence. In male nursing home patients, Aslan et al. found diabetes mellitus to be associated with fecal incontinence, possibly due to impaired rectal sensitivity and sphincter weakness [15]. Neurological diseases associated with fecal incontinence in nursing home patients include neurological disease in general [1], cognitive impairment/dementia [1, 3, 9–12, 16–18], and stroke [12, 15, 17]. However, epidemiological studies suggest that fecal incontinence is associated more with disability-related factors (e.g., locomotion, other functional impairments) than stroke-related factors (e.g., severity, lesion, location) [2]. In addition, poor mobility and an increase in dependency in activities of daily living are shown to be risk factors [3, 9, 17, 18], also after controlling for other variables [1, 3, 11, 12, 15, 19]. In patients living in nursing homes, fecal incontinence most often coexists with urinary incontinence [2].

To conclude, the most important risk factors of fecal incontinence in this group are functional incapacity, reduced cognitive function, diarrhea, constipation/impaction, stroke, some neurological diseases, diabetes, and comorbidity in general [2, 11, 20], making these the most important when assessing patients for risk factors and for targeting management in the individual patient.

### 8.4.5  Functional Fecal Incontinence

Consideration in this group is the concept of *functional fecal incontinence*. Functional fecal incontinence describes fecal incontinence due to mobility problems, toileting self-care or cognitive deficits, or restraints that restrict accessibility to the toilet despite normal bowel sensation and capacity [2]. In a large study of more than 39,000 patients in nursing homes in 27 states in the United States, Bliss et al. observed that 24.6% of patients developed dual incontinence during their nursing home stay. Of these, 35.5% of patients had urinary incontinence only at admission, developing fecal incontinence after admission. Functional limitations in activities of daily living were a significant independent predictor of developing dual incontinence as were older age, having more comorbidities, and worse cognitive function [21].

Since the majority of the patients in long-term care are dependent on care personnel in the prevention and management of fecal incontinence, care personnel need to be aware of the problem and know what the best practice for this group is. The value of good bowel care needs to be emphasized since individualized continence care might be the key in preventing and treating the condition. However, the lack of knowledge among health personnel regarding the value of good bowel care, including appropriate assessment and treatment options, seems limited [20, 22–24]. The use of incontinence pads is the most common management for fecal incontinence in long-term care settings [20, 25, 26]. Harrington et al. found that only 3.7% of nursing home patients with fecal incontinence were offered a bowel training program (diet, fluid, regular schedules) [27].

## 8.5 Evidence Base for Management of Fecal Incontinence in Nursing Home Patients

There is at present a relatively limited evidence base from high-quality experimental trials of fecal incontinence, and it remains challenging to provide strong evidence for most interventions [7]. However, expert consensus is recommending conservative interventions, singly or in combination, for the majority of patients with fecal incontinence as first-line management in the frail patients living in nursing homes. Conservative management is defined as a nonoperative intervention designed to improve fecal incontinence or prevent deterioration. It includes pharmacological treatments [7].

Overall, there are very few trials on treatment of fecal incontinence in the nursing home population. This also includes trials evaluating optimum standards of prescribing in the treatment and prevention of constipation and fecal impaction [2]. Treatment of fecal incontinence in patients living in nursing homes often needs to involve treatment of constipation and fecal impaction as well [2].

Ouslander et al. investigated the effect of prompted voiding on fecal incontinence. They found no significant change in the frequency of incontinent bowel movements, but they did experience a significant increase in number of continent bowel movements and percentages of bowel movements that were continent [28].

Chassagne et al. studied the effect of lactulose alone (group I) compared to lactulose together with daily suppositories and weekly tap water enemas (group II) for reducing fecal incontinence episodes. There were no significant differences between the groups, but the patients in group II achieving complete rectal emptying experienced a significant reduction of fecal incontinence episodes [29].

Schnelle et al. studied the effect of a 3-month multicomponent intervention for improving fecal incontinence and constipation in nursing home patients. The intervention group received toileting assistance and exercise. In addition, to increase nursing home patients' caloric intake, patients were offered a choice of food and fluids several times a day between meals. The intervention was compared to a usual care control group. The intervention group had improvements in bowel movement frequency and the percentage of bowel movements in toilet, but not fewer episodes of fecal incontinence [30].

Goodman et al. tested the effect of a clinical benchmarking tool to improve bowel-related care in patients living in care homes. The study did not demonstrate a significant reduction in bowel-related problems. However, one care home experienced a reduction in episodes of avoidable fecal incontinence [31].

A Cochrane review [32] investigated and compared the effect of biofeedback, pelvic floor exercises, electrical stimulation, and sacral nerve stimulation in adults. The limited number of identified trials, together with methodological weaknesses of many, did not allow for definite conclusions, but there are indications that biofeedback and electrical stimulation may enhance the outcome of treatment compared to electrical stimulation alone or exercises alone. Exercise appears to be less effective than implanted sacral nerve stimulator [32]. Evidence for biofeedback treatment for improving fecal incontinence in older adults with cognitive impairment or physical limitations was not found, but there is no reason why nursing home patients with fecal incontinence may not benefit from biofeedback and exercises if they are able to comply [2].

If associated with loose stools, the antimotility drug, loperamide, may reduce frequency of fecal incontinence (if infection and other causes have been excluded) but should be used with caution in nursing home patients so as not to result in constipation [33].

Overall, it is recognized that in many people, the symptom of fecal incontinence is the result of a complex combination of disordered anatomy and physiology, stool consistency and gut motility, emotional and psychological status, and restricted access to toilet facilities, among other factors [7]. Among patients in nursing homes, the picture is utterly complicated due to functional and cognitive decline making the patients less able to express their needs and more dependent on caregivers in order to adhere to a bowel management program.

There is no reason to suspect why interventions, which have proven efficacy in the community dwelling elderly, should not also be effective in frail older people living in a long-term care setting. Clinicians should, however, take regard of the practicality, potential benefits, and dangers of employing any single intervention in this population.

Effective management to meet the goals of care should be possible for most frail older people [2, 34]. Frail older people require a different approach in addressing the potential role of comorbid disease and current medications, in addition to functional and cognitive impairment. Because risk factors and/or causes of fecal incontinence in this group are multifactorial, a multicomponent assessment and individualized interventions are required in order to treat the condition.

## 8.6   Special Considerations: Physical Examination, Health Assessment, and Symptom Assessment for Older Adults in Nursing Homes

Active case finding for fecal incontinence should be done in all frail older people [2, 34] and even more so in patients in nursing homes due to a higher degree of frailty in general and the high prevalence of severe functional and cognitive impairment in this population. In addition, treatment of fecal incontinence in this group often involves treatment of constipation and fecal impaction as well [2].

In the process of diagnosing and deciding management, a thorough assessment is crucial because of the complexity of interdependent factors associated with fecal incontinence. It is important to capture the holistic picture of the patient. When diagnosing fecal incontinence in frail patients in nursing homes, it is essential to assess what might be the most probable causes in the individual patient. This is an important key in matching the treatment to the patient. The assessment should include:

- Comorbid conditions and medications that could cause or worsen fecal incontinence [2, 34]. In addition to chronic medical conditions in general, the most important comorbid conditions associated with fecal incontinence are neurological diseases, depression, and dementia [2]. A vast number of drugs have direct or indirect effects on the gastrointestinal system, tending to cause constipation, diarrhea, or both in different people [2]. In addition, antianginal and antihypertensive medications may reduce sphincter tone, and ferrous sulfate or antacids may provoke diarrhea [7].
- Functional and cognitive assessment (mobility, transfers, manual dexterity, dressing and undressing ability, ability to toilet) and screening for depression. All in order to assist in diagnosing and to inform individual care need related to bowel management [2, 34].
- Evaluation of age-related reduction in internal and external sphincter function and a digital examination to identify rectal stool impaction causing overflow. In addition, patients who are unaware of the presence of a large fecal bolus in the rectum may have rectal dyschezia and should be considered at risk for recurrent impaction with overflow [2].
- Evaluation of bowel "alarm" symptoms: rectal bleeding, positive blood screening from stool studies, obstructive symptoms, recent onset of constipation or diarrhea, weight loss, and a change in stool form/consistency. These symptoms need more extensive evaluation [34].

In addition to assessing according to the conditions mentioned above, the advanced practice continence nurse must conduct a thorough bowel assessment. See Table 8.1 for an exemplar guideline for bowel assessment.

**Table 8.1**  Exemplar guideline for bowel assessment [35]

*The assessment leads to a determination on onset, cause and type of fecal incontinence, frequency of episodes and any related change in bowel function or stool consistency. In older people the causes are often multiple. The assessment lays the foundation for a nursing diagnosis and choice of interventions*

| | |
|---|---|
| *Frequency of defecation before moving to the nursing home:* <br> ☐ Several times a day <br> ☐ Every day <br> ☐ Between 3 and 6 times a week <br> ☐ Less than 3 times a week <br> ☐ Do not know <br> *Frequency of defecation (the last 7 days)* <br> ☐ Several times a day <br> ☐ Every day <br> ☐ Between 3 and 6 times a week <br> ☐ Less than 3 times a week <br> *Stool color* <br> ☐ Brown black <br> ☐ Brown <br> ☐ Light brown gray <br> *Stool consistency (normally)* <br> ☐ Separate, hard lumps, as nuts <br> ☐ Sausage-like, but lumpy <br> ☐ Like a sausage or a snake, smooth and soft <br> ☐ Fluffy pieces with ragged edges, a mushy stool <br> ☐ Watery, no solid pieces <br> *Pain/discomfort before, during, or after defecation* <br> ☐ Yes <br> ☐ No <br> *Blood in the stool* <br> ☐ Yes <br> ☐ No | *Excessive straining during defecation* <br> ☐ Yes <br> ☐ No <br> *Any changes in the defecation pattern in the last 7 days:* <br> ☐ Yes <br> ☐ No <br> *Frequency of incontinence episodes* <br> ☐ Less than once a month <br> ☐ A few times a month <br> ☐ A few times a week <br> ☐ Every day/night <br> *Does it happen at night (defecation/ incontinence episodes):* <br> ☐ Yes <br> ☐ No <br> *Continent for urine* <br> ☐ Yes <br> ☐ No <br> ☐ The patient has a catheter <br> *If necessary do a rectal examination to evaluate:* <br> ☐ Sore/cracks around the anus <br> ☐ Hemorrhoids <br> ☐ Impaction <br> ☐ Rectal prolapse <br> ☐ Reduced internal/external sphincter tone <br> ☐ Others........................................... |

## 8.7   Fecal Incontinence Management and Expected Outcomes

The extent of the investigation and management should take into account the degree of bother to the frail older person; the goals for care; whether the patient is able to adhere to the intervention due to, e.g., cognitive or functional impairment; and the overall prognosis and life expectancy. As patients living in nursing homes to a large degree are dependent of care personnel to carry out the interventions, you also need to consider what is possible for care personnel to accomplish. In some frail older persons, the only possible outcome may be containment; management with continence products, especially for people with minimal mobility (require assistance of ≥2 people to transfer); advanced dementia (unable to state their name); and/or nocturnal fecal incontinence [34].

Even if very few studies investigating fecal incontinence management in the nursing home population exist, interventions which have proven efficacy in community-dwelling adults or older adults may also be effective in frail older people living in nursing homes [2, 34]. Accordingly, see Chaps. 6 and 7 for these management interventions listed below. Special considerations for older adults in nursing homes are noted.

- Diet modifications
  - In nursing home patients, the risk of malnutrition should be closely monitored when modifying diets.
- Supplementing dietary fiber to improve/firm stool consistency
  - Fiber supplements should be prepared with adequate fluid for safe swallowing; intake of additional fiber should be accompanied with sufficient intake of liquids to prevent constipation.
- Increasing mobility
  - Therapy for increasing mobility may be combined with a plan for establishing a bowel routine or with a toileting plan.
- Medications
  - Evaluate risk of polypharmacy and associated consequences.
- Establishment of regular bowel habits
  - The advanced practice nurse can work with nursing home staff to develop a patient-centered toileting program as needed.
- Taking control and practical coping strategies
  - Strategies should be tailored/modified for a nursing home setting; for example, provide cleansing wipes within stalls where toilets are located rather than expect patients to carry/prepare their own.
- Behavioral therapies
  - Pelvic floor muscle training
    These may be taught individually or in a group which may increase socialization.
  - Biofeedback therapy
  - Neuromodulation including electrical stimulation (ES) therapy
- Devices for fecal incontinence

## 8.7.1 Patient Education

For select cognitively intact older patients with fecal incontinence living in nursing homes, educating them to promote self-management and other coping mechanisms should be undertaken when appropriate. Examples of patient education topics include normal bowel function, reducing the risks of constipation and impaction through dietary and lifestyle measures, and how to take anti-diarrheal medication such as loperamide [2, 7]. Advice about skin care, odor control, and continence aids is also important [2]. For people with cognitive impairment, expert opinion holds that attitude and management methods adopted by care providers are as important as bowel function in maintaining continence [7].

## 8.7.2 Management Compensating for the Consequences of Cognitive Impairment

Expert opinion supports the importance of attempting to establish a regular, predictable pattern of bowel evacuation by patient teaching and adherence to a routine [7]. Because peristaltic contractions of the colon, which are associated with defecation, increase in frequency following awakening from sleep and following meals, the period after breakfast is the best time for scheduled defecation [7]. It is suggested that an effective intervention in managing fecal incontinence in cognitively impaired patients is proximity to the toilet and the ability to recognize it. This might involve removing visual barriers to the toilet in the patients' room; improving signposting both in the patients room and to the publicly available toilets in the units by using bright colors, using pictures, and using the word "toilet" rather than restroom; and placing arrows on the floor that points to the toilet [36]. Also, for some cognitively impaired patients, some kind of prompted toileting program might be beneficial. *Prompted toileting* involves asking on a regular schedule about going to the toilet and giving positive reinforcement when they do. Patients may simply need to be directed to the toilet or reminded of such use at regular intervals. *Scheduled toileting* involves taking the patient to the toilet on a fixed schedule and is recommended as a first approach for persons with cognitive impairment. This might also be efficient in patients who "lack cortical control of the defecation process" but tend to void formed stool following peristaltic movements [36].

## 8.7.3 Management Compensating for the Consequences of Functional Impairment

Ensuring appropriate toilet facilities and convenient access, especially for people with disabilities, is essential [7]. An environment with physical or social obstacles may impair the ability to maintain continence. This is particularly relevant to individuals who have physical or mental disorders. Environmental obstacles include toilet facilities that are physically inaccessible, too few, or distant; they also include clothes that are difficult to manipulate in a hurry, and a variety of other factors which vary with abilities of the individual. The toilet may be too high, leaving the feet dangling, thus making abdominal straining difficult. The toilet may also be too low, making sitting and rising difficult for those with mobility difficulties [7]. Effective bowel evacuation is helped by sitting well-supported, with feet slightly raised upon a step stool if needed to enable appropriate use of abdominal effort, and leaning forward slightly (the squat position). Horizontal grab rails assist pushing up from a seated position, while vertical ones can enable pulling up. For lateral transfer from a wheelchair, both seats need to be at the same height. Where it proves impossible for a person to use the toilet, alternative commodes or chemical toilets are available with appropriate features for individual's needs [7]. If the patient is bed-bound, you can help the patient simulate the squat position by placing the patient in left side-lying position while bending the knees and moving the legs toward the abdomen.

### 8.7.4 Management of Fecal Incontinence Related to Diarrhea, Constipation, and Impaction

As noted above, see Chaps. 6 and 7 for intervention involving diet, fluids, and physical activity. In fecal incontinence related to diarrhea, loperamide may be considered at a low dose to improve stool consistency (if infection and other causes have been excluded) [2, 34]. However, close monitoring for constipation and impaction is needed.

Goodman et al. imply that management of constipation and impaction may lead to improvement in fecal incontinence. This is explained by achieving long-lasting and complete rectal emptying achieved by laxatives, which would reduce the number of episodes of fecal incontinence. On the other hand, it is also suggested that a preoccupation by care personnel on constipation may lead to an overuse of laxatives with a consequence of loose stools and a higher risk of fecal incontinence episodes [36]. However, in patients identified with having constipation/impaction with overflow, effective bowel clearance might be effective in treating fecal incontinence. Complete rectal clearance is required to reduce overflow but may be difficult to achieve in frail patients in nursing homes. Bowel clearance is best achieved by using a combination of laxatives and enemas. After bowel clearance is achieved, the advanced practice nurse should consider maintenance therapy with stimulant or osmotic laxatives. It is very important that type and dosage of laxatives are titrated and individualized, and that the effect is closely monitored in each patient [2]. In addition, suppositories are useful in treating rectal outlet delay and preventing recurrent rectal impaction with regular use [2].

### 8.8 Toward Dignity as a Primary Goal of Continence Care

One of the most important steps to ensure proper diagnosis and management of fecal incontinence in frail patients in nursing homes is for care personnel to compassionately acknowledge the presence of fecal incontinence and initiate assessment and discussion of symptoms. It is a problem that physicians and nurses in nursing homes are not well informed about fecal incontinence. In addition, the stigma, embarrassment, and sensitivity associated with fecal incontinence compel clinicians to give dismissive or blaming responses that may retard patients' care seeking [37].

A lack of awareness or failure to address fecal incontinence by nurses may be part of the reason for the low rate of patient referral by nursing staff to primary care physicians, advanced practice nurses, or continence nurse specialists for further assessment. It may also contribute to the tendency to use containment (e.g. pads only), a passive management strategy, without further evaluation [2]. In addition, both patients and healthcare providers might be influenced by the misperceptions that the condition is part of the natural aging process and therefore "nothing can be done about it" [2]. Nursing home patients with cognitive impairment may be even more dependent on the care personnel to assess for fecal incontinence, explain that it can be managed, and discuss the options of management.

In the guideline shown in Table 8.2, dignity is proposed as an outcome for care. Ostaszkiewicz has developed a framework to guide nurses in how to achieve the goal of dignity in continence care [37]. Dignity is defined as an inherent characteristic of being human; it is subjectively felt as an attribute of the self and is manifest by behaviors that demonstrate respect for self and others [37]. An important concept in understanding dignity is to recognize that what is dignified continence care for one person is not for another person. In order to reach this goal, the most important issues are to:

- Inquire about the persons' (or proxy's) beliefs, goals, and preferences for continence care, and interventions should be based on this information.
- Do the assessment and management within the concept of caring. A central characteristic of caring is empathy. Both caring and empathy are well-known concepts in nursing, but maybe we need to be reminded of the importance of caring by making the effort to really try to understand the other persons' perspective and feelings. Particularly, in nursing home patients, this includes helping the patient adjust to changes in their bodily functions that affect their identity, autonomy, control, and independence.
- Respect personhood in dementia. Most of the patients in nursing homes have some degree of cognitive impairment. It is important to acknowledge that for many care personnel, it is challenging to manage the interpersonal aspects of providing continence care for people who are cognitively impaired because they often have to negotiate consent for care. This is psychologically and physically demanding, especially if other challenging behaviors are concurrently present. In order to respect personhood, you need to develop a culture of care that focuses on the person, not the different symptoms where the person becomes the "wanderer," the "demented," and the "aggressive demented."

**Table 8.2** Example of a guideline on diagnostic assessment and management

| Nursing diagnosis: fecal incontinence/ risk of fecal incontinence | Management to consider |
|---|---|
| *Potential causes/risk factors to consider* <br> • Constipation <br> • Impaction <br> • Chronic diarrhea <br> • Acute diarrhea <br> • Incomplete emptying of bowel <br> • Loss of rectal sphincter control <br> • Impaired reservoir capacity <br> • Prior rectal surgery <br> • Impaired cognition/dementia but with cortical control of the defecation process (e.g., can't remember where the WC is) <br> • Advanced dementia with no control of the defecation process <br> • Stress <br> • Apathy/depression <br> • Toileting self-care deficit <br> • Impaired mobility <br> • Inactivity <br> • Frailty <br> • Upper motor nerve damage <br> • Lower motor nerve damage <br> • Inadequate toileting (privacy, timeliness, position for defecation) <br> • Medication <br> • Laxative abuse/misuse <br> • Environmental factors (e.g., inaccessible bath room) <br> • Insufficient intake of dietary fibers (should be 25–30 g per day) <br> • Insufficient intake of fluids (should be 1500–2000 mL per 24 h) | • Inquire (patient/proxy) about beliefs, goals, and preferences for continence care <br> • Discuss management options and expected result with patient <br> • Teach patient about specific foods that are assistive in promoting bowel regularity <br> • Provide foods that are assistive in promoting bowel regularity <br> • Avoid foods that can cause diarrhea <br> • Implement scheduled/prompted toileting program, as appropriate <br> • Administer bowel record/bowel diary <br> • Implement program for physical activity, as appropriate <br> • Facilitate personal rituals <br> • Ensure proper seating on the toilet/on the bedpan <br> • Offer toileting assistance, as appropriate <br> • Manual removal of stool bulbs from the rectum <br> • Perform rectal examination, as appropriate <br> • Monitor for adequate bowel evacuation <br> • Monitor bowel movements including frequency, consistence, shape, volume, and color, as appropriate <br> • Monitor diet and fluid requirements <br> • Monitor bowel sounds <br> • Monitor for signs and symptoms of diarrhea, constipation, and impaction <br> • Administer laxatives, as appropriate <br> • Monitor for adverse effects of medication administration <br> • Wash perineal area with soap and water and dry it thoroughly after each stool <br> • Provide proper skin creams in the perineal area <br> • Ensure privacy <br> • Keep bed and clothing clean <br> • Manage incontinence pad, as needed <br> • Manage anal plug, as needed |

*Patient outcomes to consider*
• Independent continence (person never been incontinent or continent as result of treatment)
• Controlled continence (continent with an intervention, e.g., behavioral treatment, toileting assistance)
• Contained continence (incontinence that is contained with incontinence products)
• Recognition/use of toilet
• Minimization of leakage/improvement of symptom
• Skin integrity
• Comfort
• Minimization of distress
• Dignity

Refs. [35–37, 44, 45]

## 8.9    Disparities in Care

In studies of nursing homes in the United States, Bliss and colleagues observed racial and ethnic disparities in the management of incontinence (including fecal and dual incontinence) as well as its prevention. For nursing home admissions of Hispanic descent, disparities were found in the time to cure incontinence [38] and in receiving conservative management of incontinence [39]. For Black/African American nursing home patients, there were significant disparities in receiving management of dual incontinence that developed after admission [40], in conservative management of any new incontinence which included behavioral therapies [39], and in the prevention of incontinence [41]. Recommendations for eliminating disparities in incontinence care include developing an organizational culture and model of care committed to equity [42, 43]. This development would include becoming aware of any disparities, implementing interventions for improvement that engage staff at all levels and are based on patient needs, and benchmarking and communicating progress. Achieving equity in nursing home care is consistent with the goal of providing care that maintains patients' dignity.

## 8.10   Communication and Continuity of Care

In addition to the greater emphasis that needs to be placed on systematic and effective management of fecal incontinence in patients in nursing homes, there is also an accompanying need for sound communication between the care personnel [2]. In treating patients with complex health problems within a complex healthcare system, the advanced practice continence nurse needs a decision support system that captures a holistic picture of the patient. At the same time, the decision support system must be able to facilitate an individualized assessment and match an individual's symptoms and characteristics with evidence-based continence care.

Table 8.2 shows an example of a fecal incontinence guideline facilitating individualized assessment and management of fecal incontinence in nursing home patients. Even though this guideline facilitates an individualized assessment of patients in nursing homes, the proposals for management need to be further individualized. For example, the guideline may facilitate the individualized nursing diagnosis: fecal incontinence related to loose stools, possibly due to excessive laxatives, urgency, and reduced mobility. The guideline suggests several interventions related to this diagnosis, e.g., offer toilet assistance as appropriate and administer laxatives as appropriate. What "appropriate" is in the individual patient demands knowledge, clinical reasoning skills among care personnel, and contextually situated decision-making.

## 8.11   Educating Nursing Home Staff

Since healthcare personnel seem to have a low awareness of fecal incontinence and to lack knowledge about assessment strategies and best practice management options, they should receive training in the identification and management of fecal incontinence in nursing home patients. For patients with cognitive impairment, expert opinion suggests that attitude and management methods adopted by care providers are as important as bowel function in maintaining continence. Hence, there seems to be a need to implement a change in practice in order to improve patient care related to fecal incontinence. There are different opinions on how to implement new practice [46]. However, even though the evidence is not fully conclusive, implementation science research suggest that the most effective method for changing the behavior of health-care personnel in long-term care settings involves multifaceted educational efforts such as written materials or toolkits, combined with individual educational visits, small group training, or feedback [47, 48]. Important staff outcomes are increased knowledge, change of attitude toward believing that fecal incontinence is not an inevitable consequence of aging and that it can be treated, confidence, and work satisfaction [36]. Box 8.1 shows an example of a multifaceted educational program as an implementation of change strategy developed and evaluated by Blekken et al. [49, 50].

The effect of the implementation strategy was evaluated by a cluster-randomized trial involving 20 nursing home wards. Primary outcome was frequency of fecal incontinence episodes in patients. Two of the secondary outcomes were change in knowledge among registered nurses and change in documented care for fecal incontinence by health personnel, as registered in the electronic patient record as individualized care plans. The protocol for the study is published [49]. The trial is finished, but analyses are not finalized. Preliminary analyses indicate no significant effect on frequency of fecal incontinence in patients. However, analyses indicate a significant change in knowledge and in documented care. Why this implementation strategy did not work as hypothesized is up for discussion. One potential reason is

---

**Box 8.1: An exemplar educational program with an intervention period of 3 months**

(a) Initial workshop [48] (7 h):
  - 3 h theoretical introduction targeting knowledge, attitudes, and skills
    - Example content:
      Anatomy and physiology of the bowel in general and on the aging bowel
      Risk factors for incontinence in nursing home patients
      Difference between fecal incontinence, diarrhea, and constipation
      Discussion about attitudes, stigma, and shame related to fecal incontinence
      Skills for assessing and managing fecal incontinence
  - 3.5 h cased-based discussions using the fecal incontinence guideline (see Tables 8.1 and 8.2)
(b) Recruitment of a local opinion leader [51] responsible for
  - Motivating and engaging care staff in general between outreach meetings
  - Facilitating adherence to the program together with the care manager
(c) Six 1.5 h educational outreach meetings [48] focusing on
  - Empowering care staff in critical and clinical reasoning on managing fecal incontinence
  - Facilitating nursing home-specific strategies to ensure continuity of care

that an intervention period of 3 months is too short for the entire care staff, within a complex organizational setting, to change their practice for fecal incontinence care and for patients to respond to treatment. Another reason might be the problem of continuity of care. Even though thorough assessments and individualized care plans were developed, these authors do not know whether all of the care staff on all shifts followed the instructions. Third, the interventions focused only on the patients with fecal incontinence. Maybe it would have been wise to also focus on prevention of fecal incontinence in patients still continent. In addition, even though we to some degree focused on attitudes and believe in the educational intervention, the investigators did not focus on the concepts of dignity, empathy, therapeutic communication, and the acknowledgment of stigma and person-centered care. According to the dignity of continence care framework, this might be essential in the process of fostering change of care in nursing homes in addition to educating staff [37].

## 8.12 Person-Centered Care

Goodman et al. have explored the theory and research on the possible effect of person-centered care on management of fecal incontinence [36]. The theory encapsulates the person-centered care approach in that a person's needs, wants, and abilities, specifically in relation to toileting and continence, will prevent and/or reduce reversible fecal incontinence. Although Goodman et al. found extensive literature on person-centered care in nursing homes [36], very little of it provided details about how it should be delivered and about what kind of outcomes that were likely to be achieved. However, it is reasonable to believe that when emotional bonds between caregivers and patients are discouraged by managers, burnout among staff occurs more frequently, leading to absence, higher turnover, and a task-oriented approach resulting in low-quality fecal incontinence care. On the other hand, when interactions and the formation of bonds with patients are valued, staff might develop a person-centered working style and focus on patients as individuals with different needs and preferences [36], leading to individualized strategies to optimize the patient's autonomy and continence [37]. Goodman et al. also refer to a study with promising results investigating the effect of a combination of person-centered care together with a standardized package of care [36]. The mechanism of interest may have been that staff were more likely to promote bowel health when the individual needs of the patient were systematically considered and linked to a standardized checklist. The guideline used by Blekken [35] is an example of a standardized checklist that can be used in an implementation of change processes together with concepts of person-centered care.

## 8.13 Ongoing Management and Reassessment

Optimal fecal incontinence management is usually possible with the approaches described in this chapter. If initial management fails to achieve the desired goals, the next steps are reassessment and treatment of contributing comorbidity and/or functional impairment.

If frail older people have either other significant symptoms (e.g., pain or other bowel "alarm" symptoms as described above) or fecal incontinence symptoms that cannot be classified as urgency or passive leakage or other complicated comorbidities which the primary clinician cannot address, specialist referral should be considered. Referral should also be considered if response to initial management is insufficient. The type of referral will depend on local resources and reason for referral: colorectal surgeons, gastroenterologist, physiotherapists (functional and cognitive impairment), and continence nurse specialist. Referral decision should consider goals of care, patient desire for invasive therapy, and estimated remaining life expectancy.

Box 8.2 presents a case study showing how an educational intervention for nursing home care staff improved their ability to better manage fecal incontinence in one of their patients.

---

**Box 8.2: Case Study**

As part of being involved in an educational intervention in nursing homes, nurses were learning about best practice fecal incontinence care. An essential focus in the intervention was for nurses to learn how to do a thorough and holistic assessment of the patients, including bowel function in general and fecal incontinence in particular. The nurses were coached to use their assessment findings along with risk factors and possible causes of fecal incontinence to guide planned interventions.

In one of the nursing homes, the nurses were assessing the patients and identifying the patients with fecal incontinence. The next step was to discuss possible causes in the individual patients in order to decide how to treat the symptom. In this process, one of the first questions was frequency of fecal incontinence episodes. Carl is a 92-year-old man living in the nursing home. The patient was diagnosed with a moderate cognitive impairment, and he is dependent on care related to functional impairments in activities of daily living. When discussing Carl's situation, the nurses reasoned that the frequency of fecal incontinence was one to two times a week. The nurses kept a bowel diary for 2 weeks and then reviewed it. After further discussion, the nurses realized that the episodes of fecal incontinence only occurred on Saturdays and Sundays. They also realized that Carl on weekdays had normal stool consistency, while on weekends he had loose stools combined with urge. Because of his cognitive impairment and mobility problems, he could not get to the toilet in time. Then they asked themselves why…why does Carl have normal stool consistency on weekdays and loose stools on weekends? What happens in weekends and not on weekdays? After further discussions with other members of the nursing home staff including the dietary aides who assisted Carl with eating, they hypothesized that a possible reason could be the Saturday porridge made of milk and rice. This porridge is only served on Saturday. Carl loves this porridge and eats a large serving every week.

The nurses diagnosed Carl with fecal incontinence related to lactose intolerance. In this case, fecal incontinence was managed by using lactose-free milk in the Saturday porridge. After the change, Carl's fecal incontinence eventually resolved.

# References

1. Chassagne P, Landrin I, Neveu C, Czernichow P, Bouaniche M, Doucet J, et al. Fecal incontinence in the institutionalized elderly: incidence, risk factors, and prognosis. Am J Med. 1999;106(2):185–90.
2. Wagg A, Chen LK, Johnson T II, Kirschner-Hermanns R, Kuchel G, Markland A, et al. Incontinence in frail older persons. In: Abrams P, Cardozo L, Wagg A, Wein A, editors. Incontinence. 6th ed. Bristol: International Continence Society; 2017. p. 1309–441.
3. Saga S, Vinsnes AG, Morkved S, Norton C, Seim A. Prevalence and correlates of fecal incontinence among nursing home residents: a population-based cross-sectional study. BMC Geriatr. 2013;13:87.
4. Vinsnes AG, Nakrem S, Harkless GE, Seim A. Quality of care in Norwegian nursing homes–typology of family perceptions. J Clin Nurs. 2012;21(1–2):243–54.
5. Davies S, Nolan M. 'Making it better': self-perceived roles of family caregivers of older people living in care homes: a qualitative study. Int J Nurs Stud. 2006;43(3):281–91.
6. Nakrem S, Vinsnes AG, Harkless GE, Paulsen B, Seim A. Nursing sensitive quality indicators for nursing home care: international review of literature, policy and practice. Int J Nurs Stud. 2009;46:848–57.
7. Bliss DZ, Mellgren A, Whitehead WE, Chiarioni G, Emmanuel A, Santoro G, et al. Assessment and conservative management of faecal incontinence and quality of life in adults. In: Abrams P, Cardozo L, Khoury S, Wein A, editors. Incontinence. 5th ed. The Netherlands: ICUD-EAU; 2013. p. 1444–85.
8. Norton C, Whitehead W, Bliss DZ, Harari D, Lang J. Conservative and pharmacological management of faecal incontinence in adults. In: Abrams P, Khoury S, Wein A, editors. Incontinence. 4th ed. Paris: International Continence Society; 2009. p. 1321–86.
9. Akpan A, Gosney MA, Barrett J. Factors contributing to fecal incontinence in older people and outcome of routine management in home, hospital and nursing home settings. Clin Interv Aging. 2007;2(1):139–45.
10. Johanson JF, Irizarry F, Doughty A. Risk factors for fecal incontinence in a nursing home population. J Clin Gastroenterol. 1997;24(3):156–60.
11. Blekken LE, Vinsnes AG, Gjeilo KH, Norton C, Mørkved S, Salvesen Ø, et al. Exploring faecal incontinence in nursing home patients: a cross-sectional study of prevalence and associations derived from the Residents Assessment Instrument for Long-Term Care Facilities. J Adv Nurs. 2016;72(7):1579–91.
12. Nelson R, Furner S, Jesudason V. Fecal incontinence in Wisconsin nursing homes: prevalence and associations. Dis Colon Rectum. 1998;41:1226–9.
13. Kinnunen O. Study of constipation in a geriatric hospital, day hospital, old people's home and at home. Aging Clin Exp Res. 1991;3(2):161–70.
14. Rey E, Barcelo M, Cebrián MJJ, Alvarez-Sanchez A, Diaz-Rubio M, Rocha AL. A nationwide study of prevalence and risk factors for fecal impaction in nursing homes. PLoS One. 2014;9(8):e105281.
15. Aslan E, Beji NK, Erkan HA, Yalcin O, Gungor F. The prevalence of and the related factors for urinary and fecal incontinence among older residing in nursing homes. J Clin Nurs. 2009;18(23):3290–8.
16. Nelson RL, Furner SE. Risk factors for the development of fecal and urinary incontinence in Wisconsin nursing home residents. Maturitas. 2005;52:26–31.
17. Brocklehurst J, Dickinson E, Windsor J. Laxatives and faecal incontinence in long-term care. Nurs Stand. 1999;13(52):32–6.
18. Borrie MJ, Davidson HA. Incontinence in institutions: costs and contributing factors. Can Med Assoc J. 1992;147(3):322–8.
19. Wang J, Kane RL, Eberly LE, Virnig BA, Chang L-H. The effects of resident and nursing home characteristics on activities of daily living. J Gerontol A Biomed Sci Med Sci. 2009;64(4):473–80.
20. Saga S. Understanding faecal incontinence in nursing home patients. Doctoral Thesis at Norwegian University of Science and Technology, Trondheim. 2014.
21. Bliss DZ, Gurvich OV, Eberly LE, Harms S. Time to and predictors of dual incontinence in older nursing home admissions. Neurourol Urodyn. 2018;37:229–36.

22. Mangnall J, Taylor P, Thomas S, Watterson L. Continence problems in care homes: auditing assessment and treatment. Nurs Older People. 2006;18(2):20–3.
23. Thekkinkattil DK, Lim M, Finan PJ, Sagar PM, Burke D. Awareness of investigations and treatment of faecal incontinence among the general practitioners: a postal questionnaire survey. Color Dis. 2008;10(3):263–7.
24. Bliss DZ, Mimura T, Berghmans B, Bharucha A, Chiarioni G, Emmanuel A, et al. Assessment and conservative management of faecal incontinence and quality of life in adults. In: Abrams P, Cardozo L, Wagg A, Wein A, editors. Incontinence. 6th ed. Bristol: International Continence Society; 2017. p. 1993–2085.
25. Roe B, Flanagan L, Jack B, Barrett J, Chung A, Shaw C, et al. Systematic review of the management of incontinence and promotion of continence in older people in care homes: descriptive studies with urinary incontinence as primary focus. J Adv Nurs. 2011;67(2):228–50.
26. Rodriguez NA, Sackley CM, Badger FJ. Exploring the facets of continence care: a continence survey of care homes for older people in Birmingham. J Clin Nurs. 2007;16(5):954–62.
27. Harrington C, Carrillo H, Dowdell M, Tang PP, Blank BW. Nursing facilities, staffing, residents and facility deficiencies, 2005 through 2010. San Francisco: University of California; 2011.
28. Ouslander JG. Effects of prompted voiding on fecal continence among nursing home residents. J Am Geriatr Soc. 1996;44(4):424–8.
29. Chassagne P. Does treatment of constipation improve faecal incontinence in institutionalized elderly patients? Age Ageing. 2000;29(2):159–64.
30. Schnelle JF, Leung FW, Rao SS, Beuscher L, Keeler E, Clift JW, et al. A controlled trial of an intervention to improve urinary and fecal incontinence and constipation. J Am Geriatr Soc. 2010;58(8):1504–11.
31. Goodman C, Davies SL, Norton C, Fader M, Morris J, Wells M, et al. Can district nurses and care home staff improve bowel care for older people using a clinical benchmarking tool? Br J Community Nurs. 2013;18(12):580–7.
32. Norton C, Cody JD. Biofeedback and/or sphincter exercises for the treatment of faecal incontinence in adults. Cochrane Database Syst Rev. 2012:1–38.
33. Lauti M, Scott D, Thompson-Fawcett MW. Fibre supplementation in addition to loperamide for faecal incontinence in adults: a randomized trial. Color Dis. 2008;10(6):553–62.
34. Abrams P, Andersson KE, Apostolidis A, Birder L, Bliss DZ, Brubaker L, et al. Recommendations of the International Scientific Committee: evaluation and treatment of urinary incontinence, pelvis organ prolapse, and faecal incontinence. In: Abrams P, Cardozo L, Wagg A, Wein A, editors. Incontinence. 6th ed. Bristol: International Continence Society; 2017. p. 2549–619.
35. Blekken LE. Faecal incontinence, constipation and laxative use: epidemiology and development of an implementation strategy for improving incontinence care in nursing homes. Doctoral Thesis at Norwegian University of Science and Technology, Trondheim. 2016.
36. Goodman C, Norton C, Buswell M, Russell B, Harari D, Harwood R, et al. Managing faecal incontinence in people with advanced dementia resident in care homes (FINCH) study: a realist synthesis of the evidence. Health Technol Assess. 2017;21(42):1–220.
37. Ostaszkiewicz J. Reframing continence care in care-dependence. Geriatr Nurs. 2017;38:520–6.
38. Bliss DZ, Gurvich O, Savik K, Eberly L, Harms S, Wyman JF. Racial and ethnic disparities in time to cure of incontinence present at nursing home admission. J Health Dispar Res Pract. 2014;7(3):96–113.
39. Bliss DZ, Gurvich OV, Savik K, Harms S, Wyman JF, Mueller C, et al., editors. Racial and ethnic disparities in the management of incontinence of nursing home residents. J Wound Ostomy Continence Nurs. 2017;44(3S). https://doi.org/10.1097/WON.0000000000000331.
40. Wyman JF, Bliss D.Z., Gurvich, O., Savik, K., Eberly, L.E., Harms, S., Mueller, C.A., Virnig, B. Racial and ethnic disparities in the time to dual incontinence and its treatment in older adults after nursing home admission. Ann Gerontol Geriatr Res 2017;4(1) 1047: 1–8.
41. Bliss DZ, Gurvich OV, Eberly LE, Savik K, Harms S, Wyman JF, et al. Racial disparities in primary prevention of incontinence among older adults at nursing home admission. Neurourol Urodyn. 2017;36:1124–30.
42. Chin MH, Clarke AR, Nocon RS, Casey AA, Goddu AP, Keesecker NM, et al. A roadmap and best practices for organizations to reduce racial and ethnic disparities in health care. J Gen Intern Med. 2012;27(8):992–1000.

43. Smith DB. Eliminating the disparities in treatment: the link to healing a nation. J Healthc Manag. 2002;47(3):156–60.
44. Herdman T. Nursing diagnoses. Definition and classification (2012–2014). Chichester: Wiley-Blackwell/North America Nursing Diagnosis Associations International; 2012.
45. Butcher HK, Bulechek GM, Dochterman JM, Wagner C. Nursing interventions classification (NIC). 6th ed. St. Louis, MO: Mosby, Inc. Elsevier; 2013.
46. Grol R, Wensing M. Implementation of change in healthcare: a complex problem. Improving patient care. Hoboken, NJ: John Wiley & Sons, Ltd, 2013. p. 1–17.
47. Grol R, Grimshaw J. From best evidence to best practice: effective implementation of change in patients' care. Lancet. 2003;362(9391):1225–30.
48. Grimshaw JM, Eccles MP, Lavis JN, Hill SJ, Squires JE. Knowledge translation of research findings. Implement Sci. 2012;7(1):50.
49. Blekken LE, Vinsnes AG, Gjeilo KH, Mørkved S, Salvesen O, Norton C, et al. Effect of a multifaceted educational program for care staff concerning fecal incontinence in nursing home patients: study protocol of a cluster randomized controlled trial. Trials. 2015;16:69.
50. Blekken LE, Nakrem S, Gjeilo KH, Norton C, Morkved S, Vinsnes AG. Feasibility, acceptability, and adherence of two educational programs for care staff concerning nursing home patients' fecal incontinence: a pilot study preceding a cluster-randomized controlled trial. Implement Sci. 2015;10:72.
51. Flodgren G, Parmelli E, Doumit G, Gattellari M, O'Brien MA, Grimshaw J, et al. Local opinion leaders: effects on professional practice and health care outcomes. Cochrane Database Syst Rev. 2011. https://doi.org/10.1002/14651858.CD000125.pub4

# Management of Fecal Incontinence in Adults with Neurogenic Bowel Dysfunction

9

Tamara Dickinson, Sharon Eustice, and Nikki Cotterill

## Abstract

Neurogenic bowel dysfunction can be classified according to the location of the lesion or disease and can be seen in patients with any central nervous system benign or neoplastic pathology. In the case of spinal cord lesions or disease, the level of the lesion and its complete or incomplete cord damage will determine the type of neurogenic bowel dysfunction. The dysfunction seen in patients with multiple sclerosis is thought to be multifactorial and can be affected by medications, mobility, and comorbidities aside from the disease itself. This chapter explains the management of fecal incontinence in patients with neurogenic bowel dysfunction for the advanced practice continence nurse. It addresses initial conservative strategies that include optimizing stool consistency and scheduled toilet regimes and techniques to assist with stool evacuation. Secondary interventions to be considered including pelvic floor muscle training, biofeedback, anal plugs and transanal irrigation are also discussed. The chapter reviews the important role of quality of life and practicality in management plan for fecal incontinence developed by the advanced practice continence nurse for these patients.

T. Dickinson (✉)
Radiation Oncology, Southwestern Medical Center, Harold C. Simmons Comprehensive Cancer Center, Dallas, TX, USA
e-mail: tamara.dickinson@utsouthwestern.edu

S. Eustice
Cornwall Foundation Trust, Truro Health Park, Infirmary Hill, Truro, Cornwall, UK
e-mail: sharoneustice@nhs.net

N. Cotterill
Bristol Urological Institute (Learning and Research), Southmead Hospital, North Bristol NHS Trust, Bristol, UK
e-mail: Nikki.cotterill@bui.ac.uk

© Springer International Publishing AG, part of Springer Nature 2018
D. Z. Bliss (ed.), *Management of Fecal Incontinence for the Advanced Practice Nurse*,
https://doi.org/10.1007/978-3-319-90704-8_9

**Keywords**
Neurogenic bowel · Spinal cord injury · Multiple sclerosis · Transanal irrigation
Bowel regimen

## 9.1    Introduction

Normal defecation is largely dependent on intact and properly functioning neurologic pathways. Alterations in bowel function can be debilitating. According to Roy, the ability of humans to be ever adapting creates a constant state of becoming an integrated and whole being across the lifespan and health continuum [1]. Patients with neurologic disorders suffer a multitude of shifts in function which can test one's ability to adapt.

## 9.2    How Neurologic Disease Affects Defecatory Dysfunction

Neurogenic bowel dysfunction can be classified according to the location of the lesion or disease. Reflex bowel typically occurs with damage to the brain or spinal cord above the sacral reflex center (S2–S4), while areflexic bowel is usually related to a lesion or damage at or below the conus medullaris [2]. Conditions associated with neurogenic bowel dysfunction include spinal cord injury, multiple sclerosis, spina bifida, cauda equina syndrome, cerebral palsy, stroke, Parkinson's disease, as well as any central nervous system benign or neoplastic pathology. Signs and symptoms of reflex neurogenic bowel dysfunction include a loss of sensation, inability to postpone defecation, altered colonic motility causing erratic bowel function, slow colon transit time, and dyssynergic defecation [2]. Areflexic bowel dysfunction is characterized also by a lack of sensation and inability to postpone defecation; the dysfunction is different in that there is a dysfunctional delivery of stool to the sigmoid and rectum, denervation of the external anal sphincter, and reduced tone of the internal anal sphincter [2]. Constipation in the setting of a slow colon transit time can result in infrequent hard stools along with bloating and abdominal pain. Outlet constipation (or dyssynergic defecation) is often associated with excessive straining and may result in the need for manual evacuation [2].

All neurogenic defecatory dysfunction depends on the location or level of the lesion or injury and in the case of a spinal cord injury, if it is a complete or incomplete injury. Any lesion or injury above the S2–S4 sacral nerves preserves the reflex activity of the anal sphincter and rectum [3]. A spinal cord injury at or below S3 leaves a flaccid anal sphincter and rectum. Spinal cord injuries to the lumbar and sacral regions decrease transit time in the colon, while cervical and thoracic injuries reduce compliance of the colon and often increase transit time [3].

Up to two thirds of patients with multiple sclerosis have bowel symptoms that range from constipation to fecal incontinence [4]. Multiple sclerosis does involve extrinsic autonomic dysfunction, which can cause alterations in lower gastrointestinal motility, sensation, and dyssynergic sphincter activity [4]. Bowel problems can be multifactorial in this patient population and are influenced by medications, mobility, and comorbidities. Research in multiple sclerosis often uses the Expanded Disability Status Scale (EDSS) to classify disability and impairment. It is believed that the amount of disability in these patients is associated with the extent of demyelination of the spinal cord. Preziosi et al. [4] correlated the Neurogenic Bowel Dysfunction (NBD) tool with the Expanded Disability Status Scale (EDSS) suggesting that bowel complaints may be directly related to spinal cord involvement of the disease.

Neurogenic bowel dysfunction likely plays a role in other neurologic conditions and, as in multiple sclerosis, may be multifactorial. Patients with disorders such as dementia, Alzheimer's, Parkinson's, stroke, and cerebral palsy likely have a neurogenic component. Polypharmacy and lack of awareness may also play a role. Clinical assessment is a fundamental component of understanding the category of risk for patients and possible interventions (see Fig. 9.1 and Table 9.1).

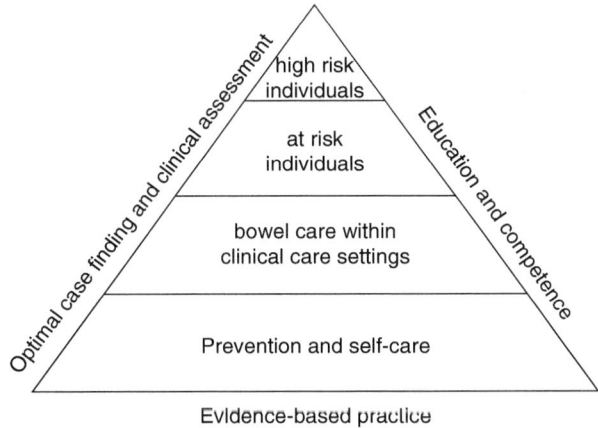

**Fig. 9.1** Categories of bowel care risk. Printed with permission from NHS England Excellence in Continence Care Subgroup—bowel care

**Table 9.1** Examples of and interventions for bowel care by risk group

| Category | Examples | Intervention |
|---|---|---|
| High-risk individuals | Spinal cord injury (those at risk of autonomic dysreflexia; perforation) | Will require combination of oral and rectal interventions to maximize safety and reduce harm |
| At-risk individuals | Neurogenic conditions; children, young people, and adults with learning disability and social communication difficulties; post-surgery; immobility; frailty; critically ill; palliative care | May require combination of oral and rectal interventions to manage bowel dysfunction |
| Bowel care function within clinical care settings | All children, young people, and adults accessing primary, community, and secondary care | Enquiring at first presentation if any bother with bowel function and seek clarification/confirmation with sub-questions if either yes or no response |
| Prevention | Self-care approach to good bowel function | Health promotion via retail, voluntary, and statutory settings |

## 9.3    Special Considerations for Assessment and Patient Education

The assessment phase should include questions regarding their current bowel and bladder regimen/management, pre-neurologic diagnosis bowel function, sensation, and a quality of life evaluation. The ability to use hands and arms, fine motor skills, balance, and mobility as well as toilet accessibility and caregiver support need to be considered when planning for care of the patient with neurogenic bowel dysfunction. Patients need general education about good bowel health and screening procedures such as colonoscopy [5].

## 9.4    Initial Conservative Management

### 9.4.1    Expected Outcomes

In the presence of neurological disease, expected outcomes for bowel care are to avoid fecal incontinence and regulate bowel evacuation. Management of bowel evacuation using conservative strategies can reduce the occurrence of fecal incontinence and is the first line of treatment (see Box 9.1). The two strategies to regulate bowel emptying are optimizing stool consistency and the establishment of a scheduled toileting regime (also known as a bowel care program), for which intense patient education is key to their success [6].

Absorbent products are a useful adjunct to most therapies, lessening a person's concern about potential visible leakage and promoting socialization and public outings [7].

### 9.4.2    Optimizing Stool Consistency

Information and advice is required to establish a regular, healthy, balanced diet to optimize bowel motility and subsequent stool consistency. Dietary and fluid management advice can be tailored to the requirements of the individual. For example, adjusting the fiber intake (of both soluble and insoluble types) to reduce bloating and flatulence improves stool consistency and minimizes soiling. Specific bowel irritants should be considered such as caffeine, alcohol, and artificial additives which can cause looser stools [8]. A review of medication should be undertaken to identify potentially modifiable factors that may affect the bowel. In addition, medications such as stool softeners may be considered [5]. The advanced practice nurse has a key role in patient education to optimize outcomes through manipulation of these modifiable factors.

### 9.4.3    Scheduled Toileting/Bowel Care Regime

Identifying a regular time for emptying the bowel promotes the establishment of an achievable pattern. Advantage should be taken of natural bowel contraction enhancements such as the gastrocolic response (following a warm drink, for example), which can be used to tailor the most optimal elimination time for the individual. Having a bowel movement once a day or on alternate days is advised, but there is no "normal" frequency, which must be considered to achieve a realistic regime. Promoting privacy and good positioning that exploits gravity to achieve bowel emptying is a further area of patient education that can be overlooked, but is key to the establishment of a routine [9]. Medications to enhance bowel movements such as laxatives (stimulant (short-term use) or osmotic preparations), suppositories, and enemas may also be considered in appropriate circumstances. Correct administration should be carefully considered in order to maximize effects. Developing a bowel care program requires understanding of the areflexic or reflex (flaccid) bowel type [10] (see Fig. 9.2).

Specific techniques can also be considered to assist with bowel evacuation when additional efforts to empty the rectal contents may be required. Digital rectal stimulation involves inserting a gloved, lubricated finger into the anal canal using a circular motion, to cause a reflex contraction of the colon and rectum. Manual stool evacuation is performed to physically remove stool from the rectum with a gloved finger. Using the heel or palm of the hand on the abdomen to massage the bowel contents through the colon toward the rectum can be useful for some patients with multiple sclerosis or spinal cord injury [8]. In a similar manner, a Valsalva maneuver to provide additional pressure to move the bowel contents along the colon can be considered. Appropriate assessment and caution is advised for the above strategies to avoid trauma to the anal region and responses such as autonomic dysreflexia [11].

It is noted that the above strategies require significant "buy-in" from the patient, a willingness to embrace the techniques, and in some cases, assistance to conduct

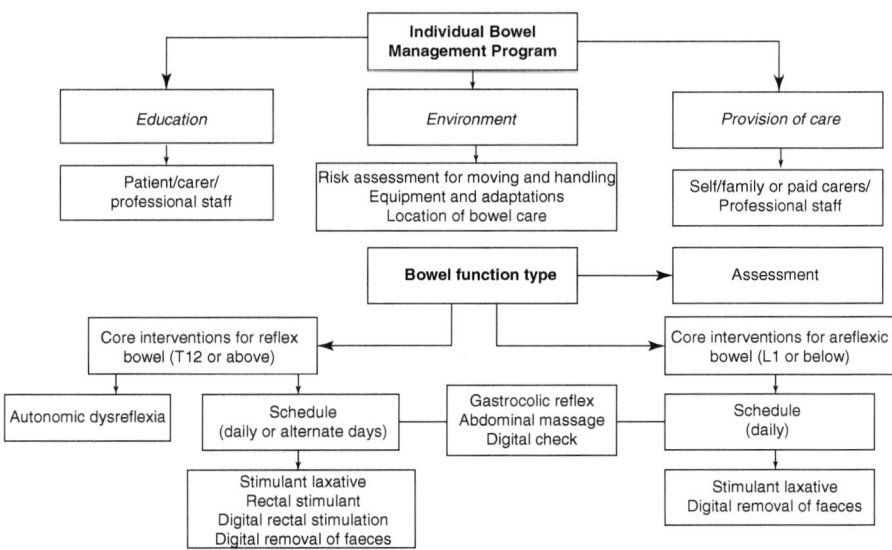

**Fig. 9.2**  Example of a bowel care program for patients with neurogenic fecal incontinence

the advice. The advanced practice nurse has a role in establishing the acceptability to the patient and/or caregivers of these strategies in addition to assisting or educating them regarding the technical aspects. The feasibility of such modifications must therefore be considered from the patient's perspective and also with consideration of their the bowel function prior to the neurological disease, if relevant, to set realistic targets. Personal circumstances and financial implications must not be overlooked as barriers to the achievement of potentially successful interventions.

## 9.5    Specific Conservative and Behavioral Interventions

When maintaining fecal continence remains problematic despite the implementation of effective strategies to maximize stool consistency and evacuation habits, further intervention can be considered. Techniques to train the pelvic floor muscles and evaluate the anal sphincter, which are integral to maintaining continence, are described.

### 9.5.1    Pelvic Floor Muscle Training

Originally developed for the management of urinary incontinence, the integrity of the pelvic floor to the entire continence mechanism has been recognized, and benefits for fecal incontinence have also been proposed [12, 13]. A program of repetitive contraction and relaxation of the pelvic floor, including the external anal sphincter and puborectalis muscle, is prescribed in order to promote increased strength in the region. Programs may include biofeedback to assist the patient to perform the training correctly [14]. There is no standardized program for pelvic floor muscle training, but there is recognition that endurance and strength training are required to provide optimal continence improvements. One example protocol can be found in a study by Hung et al. [15]. Fifty-one patients after surgery for colorectal cancer (and not patients with fecal incontinence of neurogenic causes) were instructed to perform four sessions of pelvic floor muscle exercises every day with 20 contractions per session. Quality of life related to fecal incontinence improved, especially in the first 6 months, albeit the effects on fecal incontinence symptoms were not measured. Studies of the effects of pelvic floor muscle training with or without biofeedback for fecal incontinence often include patients with fecal incontinence of various etiologies. Studies of its effectiveness specifically in patients with neurogenic involvement are needed.

### 9.5.2    Neuromodulation/Electrostimulation/Magnetic
          Stimulation/Biofeedback

The above methods provide stimulation to the muscles or nerves that control the bowel through electrodes, needles, or magnetic fields (see Chap. 6). The aim of these techniques is to passively stimulate, assist in correct identification, and modify nerve activity in order to achieve improved coordination and ability of the components to control continence. These methods can be utilized in combination with biofeedback to convey information about this usually unconscious process, in order to be able to impose more voluntary control when required. Sensory training can also be incorporated to improve sensation of rectal filling.

### 9.5.3  Anal Plug/Anal Insert/Vaginal Bowel Device

When additional security is required to limit fecal incontinence, an anal plug or insert that are inserted into the rectum provides a physical barrier to reduce the chance of an incontinence episode [7] (see Chap. 6). Plug retention has proven a problem for some, but in limited studies, benefits have been reported [9]. Another option for women is a vaginal bowel device that presses the rectum closed from the vaginal side using a balloon that is inserted then inflated in the rectum (see Chap. 6).

## 9.6  Secondary Management and Expected Outcomes

Where conservative measures fail to result in sufficient management of fecal incontinence, surgical options are available. Outcomes vary however, and the emphasis should be on exhausting all conservative strategies before considering surgery, and appropriate assessment is essential to maximize results. The advanced practice nurse has a role in counseling patients regarding the available options, in partnership with their medical team, and to ensuring patients arrive at an informed decision regarding their further treatment.

## 9.7  Transanal Irrigation

The advancement of transanal irrigation over the last few years has brought significant opportunity for symptom management to patients with neurogenic and non-neurogenic bowel disorders. Symptom management has witnessed the research and knowledge pool on transanal irrigation gathering pace [5]. That said, there continues to be a lack of robust clinical evidence despite transanal irrigation systems populating the market. Uncontrolled studies provide the vast majority of evidence, except for one multicenter randomized controlled trial [16]. This study, based on 87 patients with neurogenic bowel dysfunction, offers compelling evidence of a positive transanal irrigation effect when compared to standard bowel care. Transanal irrigation systems are securing a position in clinical care when standard bowel care has reached its potential and the patient continues to suffer with symptoms. Symptoms from chronic constipation, obstructive defecation disorders, and/or fecal incontinence have been found to be managed safely and successfully with transanal irrigation [17]. Such has been the success of this intervention, that the market has a variety of products available, therefore increasing choice.

### 9.7.1 What Does Transanal Irrigation Involve?

The principle of transanal irrigation is to flush out the rectum and lower colon of stool using tepid tap water. Water is instilled via a catheter or cone, which is inserted into the rectum. Some catheters are self-retaining with balloon inflations, attached via tubing to a water bag. It is not yet completely understood if it is the mechanical effect of the washout or stimulation of a colonic mass movement that leads to gravity-led expulsion of the water bringing the stool along with it once the catheter or cone is removed [18, 19]. Transanal irrigation systems provide patient instructions and should be followed carefully to maximize effect and safety. In particular, the risks of rectal perforation need to be explained and discussed, even though the risk is low [20, 21]. Unfortunately, evidence is lacking on which system works best and for whom. In particular, the effectiveness and impact of low or high volumes of irrigating fluid is not yet known [22]. Therefore, until more evidence becomes available, selecting the best product for the patient depends on clinical experience and judgment of the advanced practice nurse and specific clinical and lifestyle needs of the patient [23] (see Figs. 9.3 and 9.4).

### 9.7.2 When Should Transanal Irrigation Be Considered?

When standard conservative measures have been exhausted, which tend to be classified as first-line options (e.g., lifestyle measures, pharmacotherapy, biofeedback, suppositories, digital removal of feces, and stimulation), transanal irrigation is generally positioned as second-line management [17, 24] and mostly recommended for constipation and/or fecal incontinence. Alternatively, the International Consultation

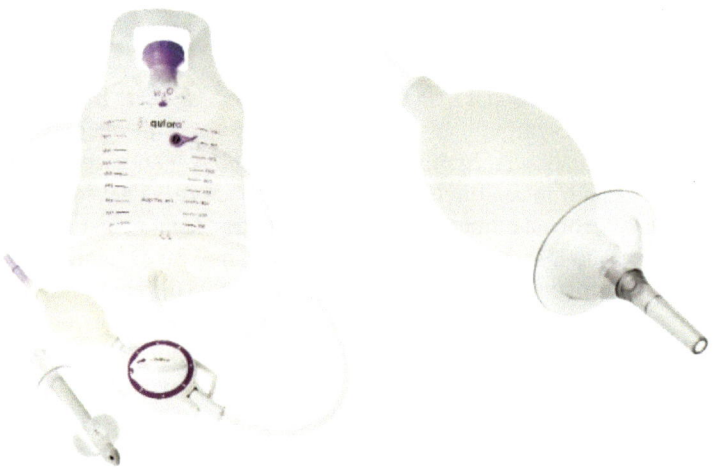

**Fig. 9.3** Qufora IrriSedo Balloon (left side). Qufora IrriSedo Mini (right side). Reproduced with permission from MacGregor Healthcare Ltd

**Fig. 9.4** Peristeen® anal irrigation system. Reproduced with permission from Coloplast Ltd

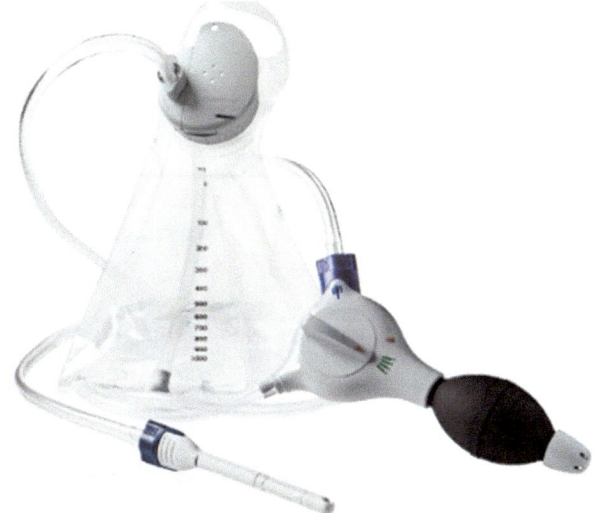

on Incontinence (ICI) committee proffers a useful decision-making tool, whereby transanal irrigation is positioned at both initial and specialist management of fecal incontinence [14]. Once transanal irrigation is chosen following careful patient selection, the consultation with the patient should not be rushed, ensuring enough time for questions. High-quality preparation and teaching of transanal irrigation will increase success of the procedure and reduce anxiety. It has been suggested that the attention to teaching and less technical issues experienced at an early stage is likely to increase sustainability of transanal irrigation [25].

Lowering the risk of fecal incontinence is often high priority for patients, and use of transanal irrigation is a key consideration to reduce this risk [26]. In their survey study of 143 participants with neurogenic bowel dysfunction, Nafees et al. [26] identified that the main attributes for choosing transanal irrigation were reducing the risk of fecal incontinence, the frequency of use (every other day as opposed to daily), and reducing urinary tract infections.

Reestablishing bowel control is a key aim of transanal irrigation and can maximize quality of life [27]. Once the patient commences transanal irrigation, timely follow-up and review is critical. Undoubtedly, new questions and concerns will emerge which will need to be addressed in a timely manner. Follow-up assessment may identify practical problems or a need to adjust irrigating fluid volume or combine transanal irrigation with laxatives [19].

### 9.7.3   Effectiveness of Transanal Irrigation

Transanal irrigation has become a popular option for patients and healthcare professionals alike, especially for those experiencing spinal cord injury or multiple sclerosis [28–30]. Indeed, the impact of transanal irrigation on improving quality of life is

**Box 9.1 Summary of Interventions for Patients with Neurogenic Causes of Fecal Incontinence**
*Initial conservative interventions*

- Lifestyle variations
- Food and fluid intake
- Laxative use
- Optimizing stool consistency
- Scheduled toileting/bowel care program
- Absorbent products for containment

*Secondary conservative interventions*

- To promote emptying of the rectum
    - Suppositories, mini-enemas, enemas
    - Digital stimulation
    - Digital removal of feces
    - Transanal irrigation
- Mechanical barriers to fecal leakage
    - Anal plug, insert, or vaginal bowel device
- Behavioral therapy or neuromodulation
    - Pelvic floor muscle training, biofeedback, electrical stimulation, etc.

*Surgical interventions*

- Sacral nerve stimulation (SNS)
- Sphincter repair
- Antegrade continence enema
- Artificial anal/bowel sphincter
- Colostomy formation

gaining momentum in the literature and is now becoming grounded in clinical pathways.

While quality of life is fortunately central to patient experience, the issue of compliance is something to consider as more knowledge is gained. Compliance was investigated in a retrospective study of 108 patients using transanal irrigation for constipation or fecal incontinence, only 43% continued to use irrigation after 1 year [25]. Of the 108 patients, 38% had a neurogenic bowel. Those that continued beyond a year tended to use it for fecal incontinence. Reasons for stopping transanal irrigation were technical issues, lack of efficacy, and constraints on time. Likewise, Juul and Christensen [31] identified similar findings in their study of 507 patients who were invited to use transanal irrigation. At 12 months follow-up, only 43% continued using irrigation [31]. What is not yet clear within the literature are the specific criteria that can predict those who are most likely to benefit from transanal irrigation in the longer term.

Over £14.8 million was spent on rectal irrigation systems between June and August 2016 across England and Wales [32]. Further investigation into cost-effectiveness of transanal irrigation offers confidence that this transanal irrigation intervention is beneficial for users when compared to standard bowel care [33].

## 9.8    Surgical Treatment

Fecal continence relies on a complex interplay between neural and muscular control. Even with extensive efforts to optimize lifestyle and dietary factors, incompetent muscular and neural function can diminish the potential for success and may require more intensive intervention including surgery [5]. Surgical options for patients with neurological disease are very similar for those without, the main aim being to improve deficits or to provide a manageable alternative where this is not possible (see Box 9.1). The main surgical procedures are detailed in Chap. 12 and include:

- Anatomical surgeries—anal sphincter repair and artificial anal sphincter
- Neural procedures—sacral nerve stimulation
- Alternative solutions—colostomy formation, antegrade continence enema (ACE)

The antegrade continence enema (ACE) is not detailed elsewhere in this book and thus is explained here. The ACE is a procedure to create a continent colonic stoma. It uses the principles of antegrade colonic washout through a catheterizable channel to enable the bowel to be emptied at a convenient time and exert more control over bowel activity [34]. This procedure, now performed laparoscopically, has been used more commonly among children, but success has also been reported among adult neurogenic patients. The main complication associated with ACE is the possibility of stoma stenosis.

## 9.9    Quality of Life Considerations

Quality of life is a significant consideration with regard to all of the above treatment interventions where the impact of the interventions themselves must not be overlooked. The evaluation of quality of life outcomes is recommended to evaluate patient perceived benefits or disadvantages. Along with the assessment of incontinence symptom outcomes, evaluation of quality of life is necessary to understand improvements or deterioration from the patient's perspective [35]. The advanced practice nurse has a particular role in ensuring quality of life impact is considered for each patient in terms of their presenting symptoms and potential consequences of treatment. Education and the provision of advice to enable patients to make balanced decisions regarding their care is a vital component to the advanced practice nurse specialist role.

Practical considerations regarding treatment intervention should also not be overlooked. Factors such as manual dexterity, comorbidity, caregiver availability, and toilet facilities are all intrinsic to the feasibility of treatment options. Careful discussion with patients regarding their treatment options and the resulting considerations must be given sufficient time in order to make fully informed decisions.

The latest review by the sixth International Consultation on Incontinence and International Continence Society provides updated algorithms to guide assessment and conservative and specialized management for patients with neurogenic fecal incontinence [14]. The algorithms provide a practical resource for the advanced practice continence nurse.

### 9.9.1  When to Refer

Primary care providers should refer these patients for specialist care. Most patients with neurogenic bowel dysfunction will require a tertiary multidisciplinary approach for much of their care. If patients do not respond to initial management referrals to colorectal surgery, physical medicine or urogynecology may be warranted for further investigations (such as manometry, ultrasound, MRI, and EMG) and more complex management.

Boxes 9.2 and 9.3 present case studies illustrating common problems of patients who have fecal incontinence due to neurological causes and their management by an advanced practice nurse.

---

**Box 9.2 Case Study 1: Sarah**

Sarah was an active mother of teenagers when it was discovered that the cause of her lower extremity weakness was a benign spinal cord tumor in the sacral region. She underwent a resection of the tumor and "recovered" with only bowel and bladder sequelae. She was unable to empty her bladder or evacuate her bowels on her own. Intermittent catheterization was initiated and she found this process simple. Her bowel management was more challenging. Her neurosurgeon had maximized her doses of stool softeners so she would not become constipated.

When Sarah saw an advanced practice continence specialist nurse, she revealed that her stools were so soft that they were the consistency of peanut butter. She was unable to manually remove her stools and was unable to pass them on her own due to the level of her lesion.

The advanced practice continence specialist nurse discontinued her stool softeners, and as a result, Sarah's stools became a manageable consistency for manual evacuation.

**Box 9.3 Case Study 2: Ben**

Ben is 34 years old and sustained a T5 spinal cord injury in his early 20s following a motor cycle accident. He underwent intensive rehabilitation in a spinal injury unit. Ben's bladder care was managed with a suprapubic catheter (his preference as opposed to intermittent self-catheterization). With multidisciplinary team support, Ben was settled into an adapted single-story dwelling along with equipment to enable his independence.

Because of the risk of autonomic dysreflexia, Ben was taught how to recognize the signs and symptoms of this condition and was provided with medication to use as required. Oversight of his progress from the rehabilitation team was scheduled every few months.

Ben was receiving bowel care three times weekly from the local nursing team. He used a bisacodyl suppository, along with digital removal of feces and digital stimulation. The success of this program varied, influenced by his lifestyle choices. The team needed to visit twice on the bowel care days. Ben did not like sitting on the toilet, but it was agreed that he would work toward this. However, Ben had been putting on weight due to his preference for takeaway foods and beer intake; thus, he struggled to transfer easily.

Ben was keen to explore transanal irrigation and had done his own online research and spoken with friends who were using it. Following discussions with Ben, his preference for independence with bowel care was his key aim. He recognized that for this to succeed his contribution to adjusting his lifestyle choices was paramount.

An advanced practice nurse on the rehab team assisted Ben in obtaining the needed supplies and educated him about transanal irrigation. He was satisfied with the positive bowel results of this therapy. His success motivated him to work on reducing weight and eating a more nutritious diet. The advanced practice nurse scheduled a follow-up appointment with Ben in 1 month.

# References

1. Roy C, Whetsell MV, Frederickson K. The Roy adaptation model and research. Nurs Sci Q. 2009;22(3):209–11.
2. Gardiner A, Wallace E. Identifying patient problems and devising care pathways with the neurogenic bowel dysfunction score. Gastrointestinal Nurs. 2014;12(Suppl 2):S17–23.
3. Solomons J, Woodward S. Digital removal of faeces in the bowel management of patients with spinal cord injury: a review. Br J Neurosci Nurs. 2013;9(5). https://doi.org/10.12968/bjnn.2013.9.5.216.
4. Preziosi G, Raptis DA, Raeburn A, Thiruppathy K, Panicker J, Emmanuel A. Gut dysfunction in patients with multiple sclerosis and the role of spinal cord involvement in the disease. Eur J Gastroenterol Hepatol. 2013;25(9):1044–50.
5. Apostolidis A, Drake D, Emmanuel A, Gajewski J, Hamid R, Heesakkers J, et al. Neurologic urinary and faecal incontinence. In: Abrams P, Cardozo L, Wagg A, Wein A, editors. Incontinence. 6th ed. Bristol, UK: International Continence Society; 2017. p. 1093–308.

6. Cotterill N, Madersbacher H, Wyndaele JJ, Apostolidis A, Drake M, Gajewski J, et al. Neurogenic bowel dysfunction: Clinical management recommendations of the neurologic incontinence committee. Presented at the proceedings of the 5th International Consultation on Incontinence. Paris, FR, 2013.
7. Beeckman D, Cottenden A, Fader M, Buckley B, Kitson-Reynolds E, Moore K, et al. Management using continence products. In: Abrams P, Cardozo L, Wagg A, Wein A, editors. Incontinence. 6th ed. Bristol, UK: International Continence Society; 2017. p. 2303–426.
8. Emmanuel A. Managing neurogenic bowel dysfunction. Clin Rehabil. 2010;24(6):483–8.
9. Krassioukov A, Eng JJ, Claxton G, Sakakibara BM, Shum S. Neurogenic bowel management after spinal cord injury: a systematic review of the evidence. Spinal Cord. 2010;48(10):718–33.
10. Coggrave M, Ash D, Adcock C. Guidelines for management of neurogenic bowel dysfunction in individuals with central neurological conditions. Multidisciplinary Association of Spinal Cord Injury Professionals. 2012.
11. Wyndaele JJ, Kovindha A, Madersbacher H, Radziszewski P, Ruffion A, Schurch B, et al. Neurologic urinary and fecal incontinence. In: Abrams P, Cardozo L, Khoury S, Wein A, editors. Incontinence. 4th ed. Plymouth: Health Publication Ltd; 2009. p. 793–960.
12. Bliss DZ, Mimura T, Berghmans B, Bharucha A, Chiaroni G, Emmanuel A, et al. Assessment and conservative management of faecal incontinence and quality of life in adults. In: Abrams P, Cardozo L, Wagg A, Wein A, editors. Incontinence. 6th ed. Bristol, UK: International Continence Society; 2017. p. 1993–2086.
13. Dumoulin C, Adewuyi T, Booth J, Bradley C, Burgio K, Hagen S, et al. Adult conservative management. In: Abrams P, Cardozo L, Wagg A, Wein A, editors. Incontinence. 6th ed. Bristol, UK: International Continence Society; 2017. p. 1443–628.
14. Apostolidis A, Drake D, Emmanuel A, Gajewski J, Hamid R, Heesakkers J, et al. Algorithms for faecal incontinence in neurological patients. In: Abrams P, Cardozo L, Wagg A, Wein A, editors. Incontinence. 6th ed. Bristol, UK: International Continence Society; 2017. p. 2597–600.
15. Hung SL, Lin YH, Yang HY, Kao CC, Tung HY, Wei LH. Pelvic floor muscle exercise for fecal incontinence quality of life after coloanal anastomosis. J Clin Nurs. 2016;25(17-18):2658–68.
16. Christensen P, Bazzocchi G, Coggrave M, Abel R, Hultling C, Krogh K, et al. A randomized, controlled trial of transanal irrigation versus conservative bowel management in spinal cord-injured patients. Gastroenterology. 2006;131(3):738–47.
17. Benezech A, Bouvier M, Vitton V. Faecal incontinence: current knowledges and perspectives. World J Gastrointest Pathophysiol. 2016;7(1):59–71.
18. Bazzocchi G, Giuberti R. Irrigation, lavage, colonic hydrotherapy: from beauty center to clinic? Tech Coloproctol. 2017;21(1):1–4.
19. Christensen P, Krogh K, Buntzen S, Payandeh F, Laurberg S. Long-term outcome and safety of transanal irrigation for constipation and fecal incontinence. Dis Colon Rectum. 2009;52(2):286–92.
20. Memon S, Bissett IP. Rectal perforation following transanal irrigation. ANZ J Surg. 2016;86(5):412–3.
21. Christensen P, Krogh K, Perrouin-Verbe B, Leder D, Bazzocchi G, Petersen Jakobsen B, et al. Global audit on bowel perforations related to transanal irrigation. Tech Coloproctol. 2016;20(2):109–15.
22. Emmett C, Close H, Mason J, Taheri S, Stevens N, Eldridge S, et al. Low-volume versus high-volume initiated trans-anal irrigation therapy in adults with chronic constipation: study protocol for a randomised controlled trial. Trials. 2017;18(1):151. http://europepmc.org/articles/PMC5374566?pdf=render. doi.org/10.1186/s13063-017-1882-y
23. Emmanuel AV, Krogh K, Bazzocchi G, Leroi AM, Bremers A, Leder D, et al. Consensus review of best practice of transanal irrigation in adults. Spinal Cord. 2013;51(10):732–8.
24. The National Institute for Health and Care Excellence (NICE). Faecal incontinence in adults: Management 2007. Available from: https://www.nice.org.uk/guidance/cg49.
25. Bildstein C, Melchior C, Gourcerol G, Boueyre E, Bridoux V, Vérin E, et al. Predictive factors for compliance with transanal irrigation for the treatment of defecation disorders. World J Gastroenterol. 2017;23(11):2029–36.

26. Nafees B, Lloyd AJ, Ballinger RS, Emmanuel A. Managing neurogenic bowel dysfunction: what do patients prefer? A discrete choice experiment of patient preferences for transanal irrigation and standard bowel management. Patient Prefer Adherence. 2016;10:195–204. Available from: http://europepmc.org/articles/PMC4764299?pdf=render.
27. Emmanuel A. Review of the efficacy and safety of transanal irrigation for neurogenic bowel dysfunction. Spinal Cord. 2010;48(9):664–73.
28. Passananti V, Wilton A, Preziosi G, Storrie JB, Emmanuel A. Long-term efficacy and safety of transanal irrigation in multiple sclerosis. Neurogastroenterol Motil. 2016;28(9):1349–55.
29. Fourtassi M, Charvier K, Hajjioui A, Have L, Rode G. Transanal irrigations in the management of bowel dysfunction and disordered defecation after spinal cord injury. Ann Phys Rehabil Med. 2011;54:e309.
30. Lloyd K. How transanal irrigation changed my life. Gastrointestinal Nurs. 2014;12(Sup2):S4–6.
31. Juul T, Christensen P. Prospective evaluation of transanal irrigation for fecal incontinence and constipation. Tech Coloproctol. 2017;21(5):363–71.
32. PrescQIPP. Rectal irrigation. 2017. Available from: https://prescqipp.info/rectal-irrigation/send/348-rectal-irrigation-drop-list/3294-bulletin-171-rectal-irrigation-drop-list-briefing.
33. Emmanuel A, Kumar G, Christensen P, Mealing S, Størling ZM, Andersen F, et al. Long-term cost-effectiveness of transanal irrigation in patients with neurogenic bowel dysfunction. PLoS One. 2016;11(8):e0159394. Available from: http://europepmc.org/abstract/MED/27557052.
34. Malouf A. Surgical treatment of faecal incontinence. In: Norton C, Chelvanayagam S, editors. Bowel continence nursing. 1st ed. Buckinghamshire: Beaconsfield Publishers Lts; 2004. p. 150–64.
35. Castro-Diaz D, Robinson D, Bosch R, Costantini E, Cotterill N, Espuna-Pons M, et al. Patient-reported outcome assessment. In: Abrams P, Cardozo L, Wagg A, Wein A, editors. Incontinence. 6th ed. Bristol, UK: International Continence Society; 2017. p. 541–670.

# Management of Fecal Incontinence in Acutely Ill and Critically Ill Hospitalized Adults

# 10

Marcia Carr and Kathleen F. Hunter

**Abstract**

The focus of this chapter is to explain the management of fecal incontinence in adult patients who are admitted to an acute care hospital who have either chronic (pre-existing) or transient (reversible, short-term) fecal incontinence. Effective management can minimize or eliminate adverse patient outcomes such as skin breakdown, infections, and patient discomfort from fecal leakage. Included in the care approaches will be containment/collection products that are currently used for fecal incontinence in acute care and critical care. This chapter will also describe efforts toward prevention of fecal incontinence in this population.

**Keywords**

Hospital · Acute · Critical care · Management · Strategies

M. Carr (✉)
Medicine, Geriatric Medicine, Geriatric Psychiatry, Nurse Continence Advisor, Fraser Health, Delta, BC, Canada

Adjunct Professor, University of British Columbia, School of Nursing, Vancouver, BC, Canada

Adjunct Professor, University of Victoria, School of Nursing, Victoria, BC, Canada

Gerontology Research Department, Adjunct Professor, Simon Fraser University, Burnaby, BC, Canada

Clinical Assistant, McMaster University, School of Nursing, Hamilton, ON, Canada

Guest Professor, Fujian Medical University, Fuzhou, China

K. F. Hunter
Faculty of Nursing, University of Alberta, Edmonton, AB, Canada

Glenrose Hospital Continence Clinic, Edmonton, AB, Canada
e-mail: kathleen.hunter@ualberta.ca

© Springer International Publishing AG, part of Springer Nature 2018
D. Z. Bliss (ed.), *Management of Fecal Incontinence for the Advanced Practice Nurse*,
https://doi.org/10.1007/978-3-319-90704-8_10

## 10.1 Introduction

Although the epidemiology of fecal incontinence, including information about hospitalized and critical care patients, is addressed in Chap. 4, it is noteworthy to emphasize that Akpan et al. [1] reported that loose stools, which exacerbate fecal incontinence, were more prevalent in hospitalized older adults with fecal incontinence than those in rehabilitation, nursing home, or home settings. These authors also reported that functional disability, which also influences the development of fecal incontinence, was more prevalent in the hospitalized group. Barriers to assessment and management of fecal incontinence in the acute care setting include poor understanding and recognition of geriatric syndromes [2], lack of assessment of fecal incontinence by generalist nurses and physicians [2, 3], lack of adoption of standardized assessment and protocols on admission and throughout the patients' stay in hospital in the acute care setting [4], and practitioner omission or patient declining a focused physical examination including digital rectal exam [1, 3]. Additionally, patients in critical care are at a high risk for fecal incontinence with most experiencing at least one episode [5, 6].

The devastating impact of fecal incontinence on an already compromised patient group can add stress to patients, families, and caregivers when there is a loss of voluntary bowel control. One anecdotal report provided to her nurse on a surgical unit was from a 92-year-old patient who was postoperative from a right hip arthroplasty. She lived in an assisted living residence, however, was incontinent for bowel movements in the hospital. She felt so humiliated and embarrassed that she could not get to the toilet in time; she said "I would rather have suffered the hip pain for the rest of my life than to have pooped my pants and have to be cleaned up by you. I would rather die than have to live with having no control over my bowels now." This patient can be returned to her fecal continence status through proactive care management. More detailed case studies presented later in this chapter will illustrate different scenarios on how to better manage and prevent fecal incontinence.

In acute and critically ill patients, the potential clinical concerns associated with fecal incontinence, especially due to diarrhea, include loss of fluid and electrolytes, infection control issues, alterations in skin integrity (e.g., incontinence dermatitis), and increased hygiene needs [7]. Older patients in acute care, especially those with some degree of disability, often lack privacy when defecating and may not be able to clean themselves after a fecal incontinence episode, even when they are aware they have had a bowel accident [8]. Whether the fecal incontinence is pre-existing or newly developed, patients, families, and care providers may start questioning the patient's future abilities to regain either a total continent or acceptable continent state again. Fecal incontinence is one of the most common reasons for moving the elderly to nursing homes [9].

The care and management of hospitalized patients with fecal incontinence can be complex and challenging. The health-care providers' assessment, diagnosis, and treatment approaches can make the difference between episodic fecal incontinence or ongoing fecal incontinence. Studies have found that there is a lack of adequate knowledge by the care staff, especially in critical care, of normal bowel function and the multiple factors that contribute to fecal incontinence [2, 10]. In a large multi-country survey of nursing staff, physicians, and other health-care providers in intensive care units in Germany, Italy, Spain, and the United Kingdom (UK), Bayón García and colleagues [4] found that critical care nurses and physicians had limited (low to moderate) self-rated awareness of the clinical risks of acute fecal incontinence. Reducing the risk of cross contamination (61% of physicians, 42% of nurses) and protection of skin integrity (30% of physician, 42% of nurses) were identified as the most important clinical objectives for fecal incontinence management. Seventy-three percent (73%) of respondents reported using a fecal management system to contain feces to reduce these risks, although only half of the settings had protocols to guide their use. Differences were also seen in the perception of burden of fecal incontinence on nursing staff. Physicians estimated the number of nursing staff needed to manage a fecal incontinence episode as two, while nurses reported three nursing staff were needed, although only 7% of both groups rated the amount of time to manage fecal incontinence as a challenge. Lack of dignity and perceived impact on quality of life were also rated low in terms of challenges (6% of physicians, 10% of nurses), which may reflect the focus on management of other life-threatening challenges in the inpatient setting.

Reactive, rather than proactive, interventions that would prevent hospital-acquired adverse events such as urinary tract infections, incontinence dermatitis, other skin breakdown, and wound infections have been found in a number of research studies [10]. In the UK, a national audit of adherence to the guidance from The National Institute for Health and Care Excellence (NICE) for fecal incontinence that included the hospital setting showed lower rates of assessment of bowel history in patients 65 years and older compared to those less than 65, little documentation of focused examination (digital rectal examination, neurological, cognition, functional ability) and identification of factors contributing to fecal incontinence in either group, and few patients with a documented treatment plan for fecal incontinence [3]. The report notes that impact of fecal incontinence on quality of life was particularly poorly documented in the hospital setting.

It is essential that all care providers identify etiologies and factors that are either producing or contributing to the pre-existing or new-onset fecal incontinence, and advanced practice nurses have a key role to play in leading change in the hospital setting. It is important that the practitioner adopts a conceptual model from which to categorize fecal incontinence. This will assist in determining how etiologies, underlying causes, and contributing factors to fecal incontinence can be organized for assessment and management strategies to be applied. Bliss et al. [11] categorize the etiologies of fecal incontinence as shown in Table 10.1.

Rao [12] categorizes fecal incontinence more concisely as an interruption or disruption in the structure and/or function of the anorectal unit. Structural changes will affect the anal sphincter, rectum, pudendal nerve, puborectalis muscle, and central and autonomic nervous system. Examples of possible causes are obstetrical injury, trauma, excessive straining, hemorrhoid surgery, neuropathies, stroke, and radiation scarring. Examples of functional changes could be caused from adverse drug responses, impaction, diarrhea, and dementia.

**Table 10.1** Etiologies of fecal incontinence

| Category etiology | Examples |
|---|---|
| Neuro-sensory-motor dysfunction of the anal sphincter or pelvic floor | • Obstetrical injury to the perineum that extends to the anus and/or rectum<br>• Anorectal trauma<br>• Neurological insult—spinal cord injury, stroke, acquired brain injury<br>• Neurodegenerative disease—multiple sclerosis, amyotrophic lateral sclerosis, Parkinson's disease, Alzheimer's dementia<br>• Rectocele, rectal/anal prolapse—oozing of stool<br>• Diabetes mellitus |
| Abnormal colonic transit | • Dumping syndrome—tube feeding (too rapid)<br>• Gastric bypass surgery<br>• Adverse effects of medications, foods, fluids—lactose intolerance<br>• Over- or underuse of appropriate bowel management medications<br>• Knowledge deficit of normal individual defecation pattern |
| Loose or liquid stool | • Infection—*Clostridium difficile*, food-borne pathogenic bacteria (botulism, salmonella), viruses (norovirus), and gastroenteritis<br>• Ova/parasites<br>• Gastrointestinal surgery—bowel resection, reversal of an ostomy<br>• Hepatic detoxification—osmotic cleansing (e.g., encephalopathy requiring large doses of lactulose) |
| Decreased intestinal capacity with overflow | • Bowel obstruction from tumor or fecal impaction leading to bypassing<br>• Anticholinergic medications (action or side effect)—causing constipation and fecal bypassing |
| Idiopathy—a disease or condition that arises spontaneously or for which the cause is unknown | • Inflammation—inflammatory bowel syndrome (diarrhea or constipation forms) and inflammatory bowel disease (Crohn's, ulcerative colitis, diverticulitis) |
| Functional limitations in mobility and cognitive ability also contribute substantially to the risk of fecal incontinence | • Functional mobility impairment<br> – Inability to independently respond to defecation urge in a timely way to get to the toilet or on the toilet<br> – Requires assistive device to defecate<br> – Inability to remove clothing when getting to the toilet<br> – Immobility<br>• Psychiatric disorders (e.g., depression, anxiety) |

Any leakage of feces is considered fecal incontinence. The current ICI 6 publication has defined three subtypes of passive, urge, and functional fecal incontinence. Identifying the subtype of fecal incontinence facilitates the advanced practice nurse's ability to develop the management plan and determine effectiveness of the approaches.

As detailed in Chap. 5, determining how to manage fecal incontinence starts with assessing the patient's usual baseline bowel movement, frequency and pattern, stool form or consistency, level of defecation control, presence of complicating factors such as hemorrhoids or pain on defecation, and use of any containment or collection devices. The above assessment is optimally conducted at the patient's initial arrival into the hospital whether through the emergency department or direct admission to the hospital unit. Using the same documentation forms throughout the patient's stay, no matter where they may be transferred during their hospital stay, is imperative. Uniform documentation facilitates the ability to evaluate the effectiveness of management and patient outcomes related to fecal incontinence. Initiating early management interventions that prevent constipation, diarrhea, and ultimately fecal incontinence with related skin breakdown or infections is considered the best care practice for all patients.

One approach that has been developed and mandated by the British Columbia, Ministry of Health (2012), is the 48/6 structured protocol. The protocol includes patient-centered questions that target six common issues (cognition, pain, malnutrition, medications, functional mobility, bowel/bladder incontinence). The patient or family complete the prescreening questionnaire that is based on the patient's status 2 weeks prior to coming to the hospital. This becomes the baseline on which care planning will be developed. Examples of questions are:

In the past 2 weeks before coming to the hospital,

- Did you have full control over your bowel elimination?
- Have you ever had a problem getting to the toilet in time to empty your bowels?
- Have you ever had an accident when you soiled your clothing with stool?
- Do you have any problems with your bowels?
- What is your usual pattern and type of bowel movements? (Bristol stool chart)
- When was the last time that you had a bowel movement? What was it like? (Bristol stool chart)

Based upon a "yes" response to any of the questions, the care provider completes a more in-depth assessment. Then a care plan must be completed within 48 h that proactively manages the identified bowel elimination issues. Once transferred to an admitted patient location, the mandate requires consistent evaluation of effectiveness of the care plan which includes ongoing assessments, documentation, and auditing of the patient's bowel status.

This type of "forcing function" for care providers to always address bowel care enables proactive and preventive actions to ensure improved patient outcomes. Since all British Columbia Health Authorities are required to audit and report to the Ministry, the completion rates and outcomes of the 48/6 program, which demonstrate compliance, support accountability and the importance of diligent care.

## 10.2    Initial Interventions for Management

The initiation of a bowel care plan from the first assessment enables timely and proactive interventions and positive patient outcomes. Chapter 5 describes what should be assessed when making a differential diagnosis of fecal incontinence. The components of a general bowel assessment are provided in the assessment chapter. A separate bowel record for monitoring bowel movements is needed in order to better identify patterns, issues, and effectiveness of interventions. When this information is not easily accessible and tracked, the importance for proactive bowel management care is lowered. The hospitalized patient's daily bowel monitoring form should include the admission date, date/time/amount of last bowel movement prior to admission, any bowel-related medical problems (e.g., irritable/inflammatory bowel syndromes/diseases, chronic constipation or diarrhea, bowel continence status), and patient's self-reported usual bowel movement pattern (e.g., every day after breakfast, every 3 days). Using a feces consistency chart to specify type of stool (see Chap. 5) enables standardization for accuracy of description of the actual stool being eliminated. Furthermore, the bowel record should contain the date and time of the bowel movement, the type and amount eliminated (e.g., small (less than 120 mL), medium (greater than 120 mL and less than or equal to 240 mL), large (greater than 240 mL and less than or equal to 480 mL), or x-large (greater than 480 mL)), any interventions that were done, and effectiveness of the interventions.

Often physicians or nurse practitioners will order "bowel protocol" as part of their general hospital admission orders. This may vary as to what the order actually includes or excludes and what the practitioner assumes this order will do. Therefore, a standardized evidence-based bowel protocol that is incorporated into all physician/nurse practitioner's admission orders enables both timely interventions and consistency of interventions that can facilitate accurate evaluation of effectiveness or noneffectiveness throughout the patient's hospitalization. A standardized protocol enables the nurses to be consistent in "when, how, and what" to use for bowel care.

The following is an example protocol for general medical patients that the nurse can initiate should the patient become constipated or have diarrhea. The nurse can follow up with the ordering physician/nurse practitioner for further treatment orders if needed.

1. An admission bowel protocol order is written by a physician or nurse practitioner as a "when needed" (prn) order and includes preventive interventions to do prior to initiating medications for bowel movements (e.g., referral to registered dietitian for food and fluid intake changes; increase in water-based fluid intake, and ambulate patient following meals).
2. A patient-centered criteria that would trigger the initiation of the medication-based part of the protocol (e.g., patient straining to have bowel movement with no results/hard stool; no bowel movement in past 2 days).
3. The medication-based part of the protocol.
   (a) Specific medications to be used if constipation is present with and without impaction

- Constipation is a contributing factor to fecal incontinence, as straining during defecation can weaken the pelvic floor muscles and sphincters resulting in involuntary stool leakage. Furthermore, if the constipation progresses to the point of stool impaction, bypassing of liquid feces around the hard stool results.
- With impaction: osmotic and stimulant laxative orally along with suppository OR enema.
- Without impaction: osmotic and/or stimulant laxative.

(b) Specific medications if diarrhea is present and bypassing or infection has been ruled out
- Bulking agent or antidiarrheal

(c) Specific medications if patient has non-cancer opioid-induced constipation
- Osmotic and stimulant laxative
- Chloride channel activator [13]

Patients in critical care units present with higher risks for developing infections and skin damage (i.e., dermatitis or pressure injury) if they are fecally incontinent [14, 15] due to immobility from medically induced sedation and/or presenting medical conditions. Therefore, the patient frequently becomes transiently incontinent. The patient's dependency on the care staff increases the need to proactively assess and manage bowel function. The consequences of a lack of management are added physical, psychological, and financial burdens with harmful outcomes.

A critical care bowel management assessment tool to manage fecal incontinence is a care imperative for this patient population, especially when they have a bowel management system in place. Proprietary bowel management systems consisting of an intrarectal catheter with a retention balloon can cause complications that include damage to the rectal mucosa with necrosis and fistula formation, bleeding, temporary anal atony, and excess leakage of stool around the catheter [16].

## 10.3   Management Options for Patients with Fecal Incontinence in Acute and Critical Care

The management options presented will focus on the most challenging fecal incontinence experienced by adult patients in acute and critical care. Diarrhea is the most common symptom associated with fecal incontinence in transient fecal incontinence in acute and critically ill patients [17]. Since diarrhea overwhelms all the patient's continence-preserving mechanisms because it alters stool consistency and transit times and challenges the efficacy of the sphincter mechanisms [6], the advanced practice continence nurse should first determine what the underlying cause is as this will help to select the right management approach. There is a paucity of good, independent (i.e., non-manufacturer written) evidence about the efficacy of products or devices for managing fecal incontinence in acute and critical care. Use is often determined by clinician or patient preference and/or cost. Table 10.2 summarizes the various categories and types of products.

**Table 10.2** Products and devices for managing fecal incontinence in acutely or critically ill hospitalized patients

| Approach type | Products used |
|---|---|
| External containment/collection | • Absorbent incontinence pads (wearable, surface protective)<br>• External fecal collector |
| Indwelling tube for collection | • Rectal catheter with retention balloon |
| Indwelling tube for collection and irrigation | • Fecal management and irrigation systems |
| Pharmacological treatment | • Bulking agents<br>• Antidiarrheal medications<br>• Antimicrobials if diagnosed causation is infectious agent |
| Specific for recurrent, resistant *Clostridium difficile* | • Fecal transplant through fecal irrigation system |

The care goals for any of the products or devices used to manage fecal incontinence in hospitalized patients are:

1. Effectively contain/collect liquid/semi-formed stool, control odor, and, for body-worn absorptive products, are leak proof
2. Prevent infectious organisms (e.g., *Clostridium difficile*) from spreading
3. Ensure preservation of intact perineal and adjacent skin
4. Patient acceptability and comfort (insertion, removal, and for body-worn absorptive products, wearability)
5. Offer ability to measure accurate patient output when required
6. Maintain patency of drainage without obstruction (e.g., for catheter or pouch devices)
7. Staff is able to safely and easily use
8. Products are cost-effective and save care time
9. Made of latex-free materials

Selection of any product should have these goals in mind in order to achieve the best outcomes for the patient.

## 10.4 External Containment/Collection

### 10.4.1 Absorbent Products

#### 10.4.1.1 Body-Worn Products
There are two different types of absorbent products, body-worn/wearable and surface protection. Body-worn absorbent products include various types of pads that are held in place with a panty or belt, pull-up underwear that is all-in-one with pad and stretch panty, and full brief pad (also referred to as adult diaper). The surface

protection pad is a specifically designed absorbent pad that is placed onto the chair or low-pressure mattress. The main purpose of absorbent products is to contain the leaked feces. The liquid portion of feces will be absorbed into the core of the pad; however, any solid material will remain on the pad surface which can soil and irritate the adjacent skin and perineal openings (e.g., urethra and vagina). The perineal and adjacent body areas to where the pad has covered or stool leaked must be thoroughly cleansed quickly after the diarrheal episode because of the caustic effects on the skin.

Despite great improvements in product quality, odor remains an ongoing patient issue. Additionally, skin barrier/protective creams and ointments that transfer from the patient and adhere to the surface of the pad will reduce absorption of any fluids and, therefore, will reduce protection of the skin. For this aforementioned reason, barriers should be applied sparingly so that they do not transfer onto the absorbent surface. This may require more frequent reapplication of the skin barrier.

### 10.4.1.2   Surface Protector

If the patient is on any type of low-pressure mattress or surface, wearable pads cannot be used to contain the stool. Low-pressure mattresses or seating cushions are designed to offload pressure to prevent skin breakdown. There is a specific surface protection pad that is placed under the patient directly onto the chair or mattress directly. The reason for these specially designed pads is that they do not affect the efficacy of low-pressure surfaces but are highly absorbent of fluids (e.g., urine or liquid stool). They have the same limitations as the wearable products that require timely changing and skin care and provide limited protection against skin irritation of more formed stool.

### 10.4.2  External Fecal Collector/Perianal Pouch

Another option for external containment of frequent liquid stools is a fecal collector (also called a perianal pouch) (see Fig. 10.1). This product is comprised of a pouch and ring-shaped adhesive wafer that is cut to fit to cover the anus. The pouch is connected to a bedside drainage bag that collects the liquid stool. The skin must be free of any skin care products, completely dry, and intact before application. It is imperative that the device be applied in a timely manner after diarrhea develops in order to keep the damaging effects of liquid stool away from sensitive skin areas at high risk for breakdown. Since it is completely external, it is a noninvasive closed collection unit that facilitates infection control of loose liquid stool and has no limit to how long it can be worn to manage diarrhea. It does not have the same risks as internal devices that can impact the internal continence mechanisms and rectal mucosa because they must be inserted past the anal sphincter into the rectal vault [18].

**Fig. 10.1** A fecal collector or perianal pouch (Reprinted with permission from the European Association of Urology and the International Consultation on Incontinence)

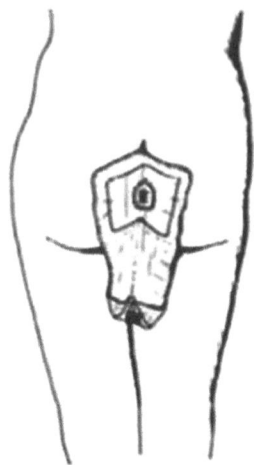

The external fecal collector does meet the care goals. One advantage of the external fecal collector is that as the diarrhea resolves, it can still collect more formed stool and will not become blocked as can internal catheters. Furthermore, it is a Class I medical device (very minimal potential for harm [19]), so that lack of safety of use is not an issue unless the patient has an allergy to the adhesive.

Fecal collectors do have a number of disadvantages. Patients that are ambulatory, agitated, and obese (weight between buttocks negate stool flow) or have movements that would dislodge the device or obstruct fecal flow (e.g., sliding up/down in bed, sitting) are not good candidates for external fecal collectors. It is essential that there is close monitoring to ensure intact placement and functioning of the device as any stool leakage defeats the rationale for diverting the liquid feces away from the skin. A fecal collector cannot be used on denuded skin, moist skin, or skin that has product (e.g., emollients, protectors) as the adhesive will not adhere securely enough to maintain operational function of the device. If leakage happens because the device has pulled away, the skin is then directly exposed to the irritating effects of liquid stool resulting in skin breakdown. Staff applying the device must be specifically educated and competency validated on correct application, troubleshooting, removal, and monitoring. When external fecal collectors fail, it often is due to unsuccessful adhesive adherence or patient movements that dislodge or obstruct the devices' functionality. Any procedures that require accessing the rectum once the device is in place (e.g., rectal medications, examinations) cannot be done unless the device is removed and a new one reapplied. Application and maintenance tips that may assist the staff to ensure placement and adherence of the external fecal collector are listed in Box 10.1.

Some manufacturers have a helpful user guide on their website that assists when deciding to use this product and for applying it on the patient.

---

**Box 10.1 Application Steps and Maintenance Tips for a Fecal Collector/ Perianal Pouch**

1. Assess the patient's abilities and readiness to cooperate with the application. Preferable to apply as close to the last time defecation of liquid stool occurred.
2. Gather all supplies needed before starting to apply the device because once started you will need to work quickly and efficiently. Supplies include a external fecal collector (and close the drainage port), ostomy stoma powder (to apply over any denuded skin if needed), nonalcohol skin sealant, and any absorbent pads that are to be placed between the buttocks to keep area dry, tube connector, and bedside drainage bag.
3. May need to cut the adhesive opening into an oval shape that will fit over the anus. Make sure that there is adequate adhesive area to apply to the skin and cut edges are smooth. If not, then it is unlikely that this device will work for the patient.
4. Position the patient on the side with top leg bent and supported with a pillow to ensure perianal viewing exposure.
5. Have two staff work as a team. One who ensures that the patient's position and perianal area remain clearly visible and DRY for the person applying the device. Clip away (do NOT shave) any hair where the ring will be placed.
6. Cleanse with non-moisturizing soap and water. Be sure to rinse well and dry thoroughly. At this point, a small absorbent pad may be placed over area to absorb any residual moisture.
7. If there is any denuded skin, assess the area where the adhesive will be placed is intact. Surrounding denuded skin, apply stoma powder.
8. As long as the skin is completely intact, apply nonalcohol skin sealant where the adhesive ring will be placed.
9. Remove adhesive protector paper from ring and fold ring in half.
10. Firmly expose anus, and apply the ring opening over the anal opening evenly without creating any wrinkles on the adhesive surface. Firmly press around the ring adhesive area.
11. Hook up to bedside drainage bag depending on the volume of liquid stool being eliminated and over what time period.
12. For cognitively intact patients, reinforce not sitting or lying directly on pouch and monitor periodically.

## 10.5    Indwelling Tubes for Collection

There are a variety of indwelling tube devices that will collect liquid stool. Selection requires clear criteria for use that is determined by assessment of an individual patient's need. As with any indwelling tube system that is anchored through the use of an inflatable balloon, there must be intact anatomical structures through which the tube is inserted and where the balloon will be inflated without causing circulatory obstruction or prevent liquid stool from leaking out. Invasive devices should be used judiciously because of their limitations, contraindications, precautions, and unanswered questions about long-term effects [18].

### 10.5.1  Rectal Catheter with Retention Balloon

A rectal catheter with an inflatable balloon is an older technology to collect only liquid stool through an indwelling secured tube attached to an external drainage bag. It does meet the requirements of diverting the liquid stool away from the perianal skin and prevents infectious contamination through closed system collection. However, it does not control odor, can leak around the catheter, and can obstruct elimination especially when stool becomes more formed. There are two styles—one balloon and two balloons. The fact that the majority of rectal catheters contain latex and the balloon volume can inflate to an exceptional size (750–1000 cc), there is a high potential to cause ischemic pressure to the rectal wall, become an actual obstruction, or create internal open lesions or perforation [20, 21]. The balloon requires scheduled deflation and reinflation in order to try to prevent the aforementioned adverse effects. The literature and expert opinion does not support the use of this type of rectal catheter with balloon as a safe option because of their potential to cause anorectal necrosis [21].

### 10.6    Fecal/Bowel Management Systems

Fecal or bowel management systems are closed-system catheters that are made of non-latex (silicone) material inserted through the anus into the rectum and secured with a low-pressure inflatable balloon that is filled with water to collect liquid feces. They drain feces into an external collection bag by gravity. These catheter systems are medical devices that are primarily used for hospitalized critically ill patients who are bedbound and have liquid/loose stools. They aim to prevent liquid stool from making contact with the skin and the spread of infectious stool. This catheter system has a lumen for irrigating the rectum and intentionally keeping stools liquid for better flow through the catheter and to instill medications [22, 23].

Each manufacturer provides specific indications, contraindications, use instructions, complication alerts, and recommendations for their product. Additionally, a physician or nurse practitioner order is required before inserting any of these indwelling devices. Nurses are typically the clinicians who insert, maintain, and remove these devices. Each brand of fecal/bowel catheter system has its own design for ease of insertion and prevention of discomfort on insertion. Each brand has its own way of controlling odor and collection bag usage instructions, i.e., whether they are single-use or empty/clean/reconnect.

Device-specific education, knowledge, and skill competency is a requirement for any staff that will be using this type of device. It is important that a digital rectal exam be done first to assess whether the liquid stool may be caused from bypassing impacted feces. Any impacted feces must be cleared before using this type of device. The retention balloon is designed to be low pressure, reducing the risk of anorectal trauma. Maintenance of the device involves close monitoring and documentation in the nursing notes. Maintenance includes checking catheter patency and leakage on a regular schedule, irrigating the catheter to maintain patency as needed, and inspecting the perianal skin for any breakdown. The amount of cuff inflation,the position of the catheter, and the ongoing need for its use should also be documented. Box 10.2 lists important steps for insertion and management of one of these systems.

Fecal or bowel management systems are contraindicated in patients who have had recent lower large bowel or rectal surgery, rectal or anal injury, stricture or stenosis, mucosal impairment, rectal/anal tumor, or severe hemorrhoids are not candidates for these devices. Possible disadvantages are incurred overall costs that include staff education to use and validation of knowledge/skill competency, expense for the device, and system maintenance equipment. Developing a checklist of contraindications for using a fecal/bowel management system can assist the advanced practice

---

**Box 10.2 Key Steps for Insertion and Maintenance of a Fecal/Bowel Management System**

1. Properly position the patient so the rectum can be well visualized (typically on the left side) during insertion.
2. Lubricate the balloon end of the catheter for ease and comfort of insertion.
3. After inserting the catheter, inflate the balloon per manufacturer's instructions and never over-inflating it.
4. Position the external part of the catheter so as to avoid kinks and obstructions; regularly check the catheter for patency.
5. Avoid tugging on the catheter to prevent damage to the anal sphincter and internal mucosa from the inflated balloon.
6. Maintain the drainage bag below the patient to facilitate flow of feces by gravity.
7. Use the correct port/lumen for irrigating the rectum or instilling medications.
8. Regularly assess the skin around the catheter for seepage/leakage of feces and skin damage and treating skin damage as needed (see Chap. 13).
9. Monitor the patient to avoid tugging or removal of the catheter.
10. Deflate the balloon completely prior to catheter removal.

**Table 10.3** Example of a checklist of contraindications for using a fecal/bowel management system

| If one or more of the following are present, do not start FMS until MRP consulted | | |
| --- | --- | --- |
| Contraindications | Yes | No |
| Lower large bowel/rectal surgery within last year | | |
| Rectal/anal injury or trauma | | |
| Severe rectal/anal stricture or stenosis | | |
| Suspected or confirmed rectal mucosa impairment (i.e., severe/ischemic proctitis, mucosal ulcerations) | | |
| Confirmed rectal/anal tumor | | |
| Severe hemorrhoids | | |
| Fecal impaction | | |
| Neutropenia—consult MRP | | |
| Date Inserted: _____ | Nurse's Signature: _____ | |
| Date for removal: _____ (29 days from insertion (record on nursing record) | | |
| Date removed: _____ Reason: _____ Signature: _____ | | |

*FMS* fecal management system; *MRP* most responsible physician

continence nurse in deciding whether to order one for a patient. An example of a checklist used at a Canadian hospital is in Table 10.3.

Peart and Richardson [24] reported on a quality improvement program that had a critical care bowel management assessment tool, adapted from Edwards [25], and that standardized bowel assessment and management. The focus is on decreasing skin damage and pressure ulcers and appropriate use of proprietary bowel management systems in critical care. The authors were in advanced practice nursing roles. The tool leads nurses through a process that includes ruling out fecal overflow associated with constipation, assessment of skin integrity, current continence/mobility, and results in a risk rating. Low-risk patients are placed on a skin care protocol and reassessed every 12 h. High-risk patients are considered for a bowel management system based on stool form/consistency. Those with loose or watery stool are potential candidates for the system. Figure 10.2 shows an example, from the Fraser Health authority in British Columbia, Canada, of an algorithm that uses consistency of stool to assist the advanced practice nurse in deciding whether to insert and use a fecal/bowel collection device (with or without irrigation) to manage the fecal incontinence.

Fecal/bowel management systems are advantageous because they meet all the care goals. Additionally, if the patient should expel the device or it is accidentally pulled out, the risk of rectal trauma is minimized, and the catheter can be reinserted. The devices can remain in place for up to 29 consecutive days without being changed. However, as with any device, there is always the risk and the potential to

**Decision Making Tool for Insertion and Use of Fecal/Bowel Management System**

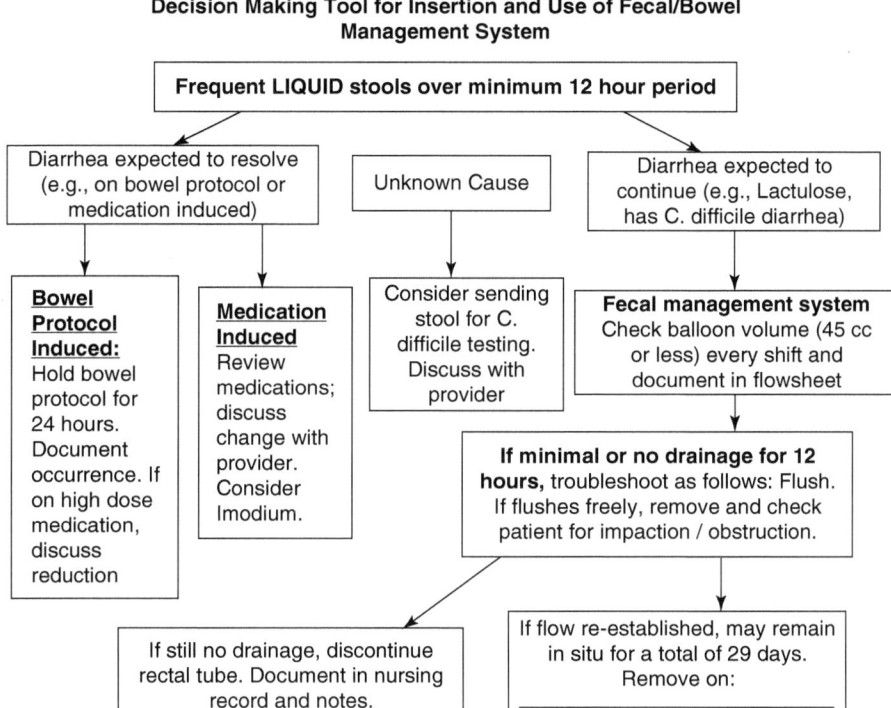

**Fig. 10.2** Decision-making algorithm for insertion and use of a fecal/bowel management system (© 2015 Fraser Health Authority (FHA) Criteria for Use of Fecal Management Systems Critical Care. FHA authorizes use/reproduction/modification of this publication for non-commercial healthcare/educational purposes only. All other rights reserved. FHA disclaims all liability for use by third parties. Final judgment about the propriety of any clinical practice rests with the health care provider)

cause adverse events (e.g., bleeding, rectal erosion, fistula formation). Meticulous, strict, and timed monitoring and documentation is required to decrease adverse events from occurring.

## 10.7   Pharmacologic Treatment

As with any drug therapy, it is essential to target either the causative organism or disease or have a clear pharmacological goal with a measurable outcome. For example, if the causative organism is *Clostridium difficile*, then appropriate antimicrobial therapy (e.g., oral flagyl or vancomycin) would be the expected physician/nurse practitioner's order. However, if the presenting symptom is too fast intestinal transit time with the need to reduce intestinal peristalsis, slowing transit time, an antidiarrheal medication (e.g., loperamide) may be ordered. When transit time is slowed, it will also decrease elimination urgency and frequency to enable the anal sphincter to respond more adequately. The caution is not to overdose or overuse antidiarrheal medications as they can lead to constipation, megacolon, and central nervous system side effects. Bulking agents (e.g., psyllium) may be used to help firm the stool so that it is not as liquid. Adding more insoluble and soluble fiber to the diet may also act as a bulking agent. Collaborating with the registered dietitian on diet modifications is recommended. Irrigations through the fecal/bowel management system may also ensure patency for drainage.

When the treatment goal is to have the patient's stool be either liquid or semi-formed in order to be able to use a fecal/bowel management system, the pharmacological approach may include a combination of a cathartic stimulant (e.g., senna-based like Senokot, bisacodyl) and osmotic laxative (e.g., lactulose, PEG 3350). Patients that are receiving opioids need a proactive management plan that prevents constipation and possible impaction. Since a number of patients in acute care and critical care are prescribed opioids for pain management, they are more susceptible to opioid-induced constipation. Methylnaltrexone (available as Relistor[R]) is a subcutaneous injectable drug that is used specifically for opioid-induced constipation without decreasing the effects of the opioid itself. When given alongside opioid therapy, it is designed to displace the opioid from binding to peripheral receptors in the gut, decreasing the opioid's constipating effects and inducing laxation. Its use in patients who have acute pain as seen in the acute, critically ill, or palliative care when opioid therapy is needed has been highly beneficial for symptom management.

Tube feeding often may cause diarrhea due to various reasons such as the most common one known as "dumping syndrome" (too fast a transit through the bowel). It is important to work with the registered dietitian to manage the feedings and achieve the required nutritional intake. Identifying a tube-feeding formula that is better tolerated or possibly slowing down the rate of administration should be tried before considering any antidiarrheal medications.

## 10.8    Prevention of Fecal Incontinence

Nurses are pivotal to preventing the development of transient fecal incontinence while patients are in acute or critical care. Furthermore, nursing care has a direct impact for those patients who came to the hospital with chronic fecal incontinence. Increased illness burden, for example, from skin breakdown, infections, and psychological stress can be directly correlated with fecal incontinence. Therefore, preventive care interventions are as much of a priority as managing fecal incontinence for this vulnerable population. The advanced practice continence nurse promotes prevention of fecal incontinence (see Box 10.3).

The primary nurse for the patient should ensure the implementation of a continence care plan that includes assessment and interventions from the occupational therapist, physiotherapist, pharmacist, and registered dietitian.

**Box 10.3 Interventions for Prevention of Fecal Incontinence in Acutely or Critically Ill Hospitalized Patients**

- Monitor fluid intake to ensure adequate hydration to prevent constipation.
- Mobilize and/or ambulate patients at least two to three times a day to stimulate bowel peristalsis.
- Monitor food intake paying attention to fiber intake to ensure a regular pattern of elimination of a formed stool. Referral to a registered dietitian as needed. Possible addition of a fruit-based laxative (30 mL) daily. If the patient's glomerular filtration rate (an indication of kidney function) is less than 30 mL/min, fruit-based laxative is contraindicated.
- Provide privacy when patient is toileting. An odor-reducing deodorizer can be used if noxious odor is present.
- Ensure correct positioning of patient on the toilet or commode (thighs at 30° to buttocks). This may require a foot stool that the patient plants their feet on. Commodes placed over the toilet are of particular concern because they are high and often result with the patient's feet dangling rather than being supported.
- Protect vulnerable perianal skin from urine and stool. This includes impeccable perineal cleansing, timely changing of collection/containment products, and application of appropriate skin protectants (see Chap. 13).
- Routinely ask the patient after breakfast whether they need to toilet. This timing takes advantage of the gastrocolic reflex after meals.
- Complete and review the bowel record every shift in order to detect early if a problem is arising.

## 10.9   Special Consideration: Morbidly Obese Patients with Fecal Incontinence

There have been an increasing number of patients who are morbidly obese presenting to acute and critical care units in hospital. The challenges are greater in managing fecal incontinence as it is more difficult to toilet, mobilize, and care for them due to their obesity. However, it is important to have appropriate equipment and supplies specifically designed to assist with their care. The bariatric equipment available includes beds, chairs, low-pressure surfaces (mattresses, cushions), commodes, wheelchairs, and patient transfer lifts. Wearable containment products (e.g., pads with panties, pull-ups, full briefs) all come in bariatric sizes. The other collection and containment products can be used for a bariatric patient but may need extension tubing added to facilitate drainage.

## 10.10  Expected Patient Outcomes for Fecal Incontinence in Acute Care and Critical Care

The expected patient outcome for transient and/or chronic fecal incontinence is that at discharge, the patient's bowel function returns to their usual baseline. Patient teaching on good bowel hygiene practices would include adequate intake of non-caffeinated fluids, intake of adequate soluble and non-soluble fiber, and walking or exercising after a meal to engage the gastrocolic reflex. Additionally, emphasizing that when the urge to defecate is felt, it is important to respond in a timely manner as delaying may result in fecal incontinence. Proper positioning on the toilet with the upper legs at a 30-degree angle to the buttocks and feet flat on the floor enables the external anal sphincter to relax. A small foot stool under the feet may be needed to achieve this angle (See Fig. 6.1 in Chap. 6). Additionally trying to set a daily routine ensures adequate time to completely evacuate. The use of laxatives or suppositories should be used with caution and a discussion with their primary care provider or a nurse continence advisor is advised.

For patients that have an ongoing problem with fecal incontinence at discharge, a referral to a nurse continence specialist, continence service in the community, or advanced practice nurse either in the hospital or community is recommended. These nurses and/or services have additional evidence-based knowledge and skills to assess, diagnose, and conservatively treat fecal incontinence [26]. Furthermore, they are able to determine when other health-care providers may be helpful for the patient to be seen by or, if in an advanced practice role that includes prescribing and ordering of lab and diagnostic imaging tests, may undertake further investigation or referral [27].

## 10.11  Summary

Fecal incontinence in acute and critical care patients is often a complex and challenging problem for the patient and their caregivers. Nurses in all positions of care, from the generalist direct care bedside nurse, continence specialty nurse, to the advanced practice continence nurse, have a major role to play in preventing the development of fecal incontinence and associated skin breakdown and infections. However, when fecal incontinence is present, it is imperative that nurses are knowledgeable and have the requisite skills to develop and carry out an appropriate fecal incontinence management care plan. Furthermore, the direct bedside care nurses are the 24/7 professionals who have the most consistent contact with the patient and thus observe what is needed, provide the appropriate intervention, evaluate the effectiveness of the interventions, and implement a change in the approach. Continence specialty nurses and advanced practice continence nurses may recommend or order the plan of care, provide consultation, and monitor the patient's response. These nurses also educate the general nursing staff and facilitate system changes that enable improvements to the care for patients with fecal incontinence. This may include selecting and evaluating products and devices for the management of fecal incontinence, development of best practice clinical guidelines for fecal incontinence, and development of protocols and documentation requirements and records for fecal management systems.

Ultimately, the goal for patients with either transient or chronic fecal incontinence in acute and critical is to prevent what is preventable, reverse what is reversible, and better manage what is not changeable.

Case studies illustrating common examples of the occurrence of fecal incontinence in hospitalized patients are presented in Boxes 10.4, 10.5, and 10.6. Each case study highlights the management of the patient by an advanced practice nurse.

---

**Box 10.4 Case 1: Hospitalized Older Adult with Acute** *Clostridium difficile-*
**Associated Diarrhea**

Millie (as she prefers to be called) is an 82-year-old, married female that lives with her 84-year-old husband, Fred, in their own two-story house in a suburban area outside of a major city. Both have been active and independent and enjoying active vacations. They have an upcoming Caribbean cruise in 1 month and are concerned that Mille will not be able to go.

She was admitted 2 days ago to the local community hospital with a urinary tract infection, dehydration from nausea with vomiting, and exacerbation of her heart failure. She has a delirium and has been restless, disorientated, and pulling out her IV and indwelling catheter. It was decided to discontinue the IV and catheter for they were contributing to her discomfort and thus her challenging behaviors. She now is on oral antibiotics, furosemide, and monitored intake and output. Additionally, her gait and balance are unsteady that she requires assistance for all ambulation. Fred has been very attentive and helps as much as he can. He keeps saying that "this is not my gentle Millie."

Prior to admission, she was continent of stool but did have stress urinary incontinence which she managed with pull-ups just in case she did not make it in time to a toilet when they were out. However, Fred reports that she always preferred getting herself to a toilet rather than wet the pull-up. She has occasional constipation and only once developed diarrhea while on vacation in another country. She always managed to make it to a toilet as she was determined not to have an "accident" and embarrass herself.

Yesterday Millie had six, liquid and explosive stools that required care as she could not get to the toilet on her own or in time. She was transferred to an isolation room, as the culture was positive for *Clostridium difficile* (*C. difficile*). She was started immediately on metronidazole. So far, today she has had five, very liquid stools, and her anal area is quite red but still intact. She cries out saying "Stop! It hurts" each time she is being cleansed after a stool. Millie stays in bed most of the time as she sleeps between diarrhea episodes. It is taking two care providers (nurse and health-care aide) to clean Millie and change her bed linens and absorbent products. She is wearing a full incontinence brief (with adhesive tab fasteners) to contain the stool. The pull-up type of external containment is no longer appropriate because of her poor balance and inability to lift herself up to pull the product up. A zinc-based skin protectant is being used to try to prevent her perianal region from breaking down. Fred is quite distressed by how Millie has declined so rapidly and fears she may be dying. He has asked that he be allowed to stay with her as much as possible.

### Care Plan

*The advanced practice continence nurse would order the following interventions/treatments for the generalist bedside nurse to follow:*

- Teach husband about *C. difficile* infection and how to use isolation techniques whenever he is in the room.
- The advanced practice nurse will reassure husband that Millie should return to fecal continence after *C. difficile* infection is resolved and that her symptoms are not indications that she is dying.
- Apply zinc-based, antihistamine protective cream to anal area and surrounding skin with every cleansing.
  - This cream may not only protect the perianal skin from the caustic effects of the diarrhea, but the topical antihistamine may also help to relieve the pain. However, since the barrier cream may block the absorption of liquid into the containment product, there is increase potential for leakage and thus spread of *C. difficile* organisms or spores.
- Since Millie is primarily in bed or in a chair resting, assess whether an external fecal collection pouch would be a better choice.
- The skin is reddened but still intact. She is not moving around much, so the likelihood that the closed system, external fecal collection pouch will remain secured and prevent spread of infectious stool is good. The pouch should be connected to a drainage bag to accurately measure fecal output in order to assess need for hydration. Use of a fecal collection pouch will decrease the perianal pain she feels from cleansing.
- Give 650 mg acetaminophen every 6 h regularly for pain.
  - The analgesic given on a regular basis rather than as needed will assist with keeping her proactively comfortable.
- Record changes in stool frequency and form/consistency to evaluate effectiveness of antimicrobial treatment.
- Discharge referral to continence clinic to see a nurse continence advisor to assess and conservatively manage her stress urinary incontinence.

### Outcome

The external fecal collection pouch attached to a bedside drainage bag was applied successfully. Her husband, Fred, reassured Millie throughout the application. Millie became much more comfortable and settled without the frequent need to change her absorbent brief and the pain from cleaning her skin. She no longer needed the acetaminophen for pain. The perianal skin decreased in redness and remained intact.

After seeing how Millie became more comfortable, Fred expressed his gratefulness for her care and his renewed hope that Millie would be her "old self" again once she got over all her acute illnesses. Millie's *C. difficile* infection, fecal incontinence, and urinary tract infection resolved and concurrently so did her delirium. No other patients on the unit became infected with *C. difficile* during Millie's stay due to closed containment and disposal of the infected stool and infection precautions followed by the nursing staff. Millie agreed that seeing a nurse continence advisor for her stress urinary incontinence would be prudent as she just thought it was a normal part of aging.

**Box 10.5 Case 2: Hospitalized Surgical Patient After Reversal of an Ostomy**
Malcolm is a 25-year-old male, who was diagnosed with ulcerative colitis and initially treated with a colostomy due to the extent of the acute lesions. Malcolm has had his colostomy for about 1 year now. He has been anxious to have the ostomy reversed because he is to be married in 3 months and does not want to have the embarrassment of the ongoing care of the ostomy especially on his honeymoon. His fiancée, Debbie, seems very supportive but quite anxious as she has limited knowledge of Malcolm's chronic disease and the lifelong implications. She said to the nurse that Malcolm does everything himself so she has little to do with it. However, she says that she has a very weak stomach and that if she became needed to help, she would have problems with that.

Malcolm is now 2 days postoperative reversal of the ostomy. His postoperative recovery has been excellent, especially because he was in good physical and mental health. He is eating and drinking a regular diet, ambulating independently, and well managed for pain with regular acetaminophen. Although he knew that he might experience some fecal incontinence, he was nevertheless devastated when it happened today for the third time. He has been having semiformed stools throughout the day. He states that once he feels the urge that he has less than a few minutes to get to a toilet, he loses stool. He is wearing a medium-sized continence pad held in place by his underwear. Malcolm states that all this is so embarrassing for him, especially when he knows he has gone into the pad and it smells. He is to be discharged tomorrow and feeling quite fearful and anxious that his fecal incontinence will continue. He is afraid to tell Debbie, as he knows how squeamish she is about the whole situation.

**Care Plan**

*The advanced practice nurse would order the following:*

- Referral to registered dietician for high fiber diet change and counseling.
- Referral to pharmacist for medication counseling reuse of bulking medications.
- Referral to physiotherapist to reinforce pre-op teaching of pelvic floor exercises and urge suppression.
- Referral to social worker for counseling on the impact on their relationship.
- Discuss with fiancée and Malcolm about contacting Crohn's and Colitis Society for ongoing education and support groups.
- Referral to the pelvic floor physiotherapist in the community at discharge to further treat the pelvic floor muscles.
- Referral to community continence clinic for nurse continence advisor for follow-up on Malcolm's bowel status, teaching both fiancée and Malcolm management strategies.

---

**Box 10.6 Case 3: Intubated Unconscious Patient in Cardiac Critical Care Unit**

Jennie is a 45-year-old lawyer who was admitted yesterday to the critical care unit. She has had a "terrible cold" for the last 3 weeks with a progressive productive cough, chills, fever, and fatigue. She has been self-treating with over-the-counter medications as she has had a critical case that she has been working night and day to prepare for a court hearing in a few days.

Jennie collapsed at work and was transported to emergency via ambulance. Her diagnosis is septic pneumonia. She is intubated and unconscious, becoming restless when in pain and when needing different positioning especially for incontinence. She has two IVs and an indwelling urinary catheter and is on a pressure release mattress. She had soft, mush-like stools today, which contaminated the catheter. Her perianal skin is reddened and so far, the skin is intact. Her elimination is managed with a disposable bed protector pad specifically designed for low-pressure surfaces.

**Care Plan**

*The advanced practice continence nurse would order the following interventions/treatments for the generalist bedside nurse to follow:*

- Use the critical care algorithm to determine whether a fecal management system should be started for Jennie.
- Assess whether there is an ongoing need for the catheter.
- Ensure no containment product is placed on patient while she is on a pressure release mattress. Place collection disposable pad in place on mattress.

# References

1. Akpan A, Gosney MA, Barrett J. Factors contributing to fecal incontinence in older people and outcome of routine management in home, hospital and nursing home settings. Clin Interv Aging. 2007;2(1):139–45.
2. Nair B, O'Dea J, Lim L, Thakkinstian A. Prevalence of geriatric 'syndromes' in a tertiary hospital. Australas J Ageing. 2000;19(2):81–4.
3. Harari D, Husk J, Lowe D, Wagg A. National audit of continence care: Adherence to National Institute for Health and Clinical Excellence (NICE) guidance in older versus younger adults with faecal incontinence. Age Ageing. 2014;43(6):785–93.
4. Bayón García C, Binks R, De Luca E, Dierkes C, Franci A, Gallart E, et al. Prevalence, management and clinical challenges associated with acute faecal incontinence in the ICU and critical care settings: the FIRST cross-sectional descriptive survey. Intensive Crit Care Nurs. 2012;28(4):242–50.
5. Dobb GJ. Diarrhoea in the critically ill. Intensive Care Med. 1986;12(3):113–5.
6. Beitz JM. Fecal incontinence in acutely and critically ill patients: options in management. Ostomy Wound Manage. 2006;52(12):56–8. 60, 62–66.
7. Rees J, Sharpe A. The use of bowel management systems in the high-dependency setting. Br J Nurs. 2009;18(Sup3):S19–24.
8. Akpan A, Gosney MA, Barrett J. Privacy for defecation and fecal incontinence in older adults. J Wound Ostomy Cont Nurs. 2006;33(5):536–40.
9. International Foundation for Functional Gastrointestinal Disorders. Available from www.iffgd.org.
10. National Institute of Health and Care Excellence (NICE). Fecal incontinence: the management of fecal incontinence in adults 2007. Available from https://www.nice.org.uk/guidance/cg49.
11. Bliss DZ, Norton CA, Miller J, Krissovich M. Directions for future nursing research on fecal incontinence. Nurs Res. 2004;53(6 Suppl):S15–21.
12. Rao SSC. Pathophysiology of adult fecal incontinence. Gastroenterology. 2004;126:S14–22.
13. Nelson AD, Camilleri M. Opioid-induced constipation: advances and clinical guidance. Ther Adv Chronic Dis. 2016;7(2):121–34.
14. Wishin J, Gallagher TJ, McCann E. Emerging options for the management of fecal incontinence in hospitalized patients. J Wound Ostomy Cont Nurs. 2008;35(1):104–10.
15. Bianchi J, Segovia-Gomez T. The dangers of faecal incontinence in the at-risk patient. Wounds Int. 2012;3(3):15–21.
16. Whiteley I, Sinclair G, Lyons AM, Riccardi R. A retrospective review of outcomes using a fecal management system in acute care patients. Ostomy Wound Manage. 2014;60(12):37–43.
17. Bliss DZ, Johnson S, Savik K, Clabots CR, Gerding DN. Fecal incontinence in hospitalized patients who are acutely ill. Nurs Res. 2000;49(2):101–8.
18. Nelson JA, Daniels AU, Dodds WJ. Rectal balloons: complications, causes, and recommendations. Invest Radiol. 1979;14(1):48–59.
19. United States Food and Drug Administration. Center for devices and radiographical health: device classes 2006. Available from www.fda.gov/cdrh/devadvice/3132.html.
20. Bosley C. Three methods of stool management for patients with diarrhea. Ostomy Wound Manage. 1994;40(1):52.
21. Doughty DB, Jensen LL, editors. Assessment and management of the patient with fecal incontinence. 3rd ed. St. Louis, MO: Mosby Elsevier; 2006.
22. Keshava A, Renwick A, Stewart P, Pilley A. A nonsurgical means of fecal diversion: the Zassi Bowel Management System. Dis Colon Rectum. 2007;50(7):1017–22.
23. Powers J, Bliss DZ. Product options for faecal incontinence management in acute care. J World Council Enterostomal Therapy. 2012;32(1):20–3.
24. Peart J, Richardson A. Developing a critical care bowel management assessment tool to manage faecal incontinence. Nurs Crit Care. 2015;20(1):34–40.

25. Edwards J. Development of a bowel management assessment tool. Poster presented at Wounds UK Conference, UK. 2011.
26. Paterson J, Ostaszkiewicz J, Suyasa IGPD, Skelly J, Bellefeuille L. Development and validation of the role profile of the nurse continence specialist: a project of the International Continence Society. J Wound Ostomy Cont Nurs. 2016;43(6):641–7.
27. Hunter KF. ICS update in continence care: the role of the nurse continence specialist in continence services. Urology News. 2016;20(6):46–8.

# Management of Fecal/Anal Incontinence During Pregnancy and Postpartum

# 11

Christina Hegan and Marlene Corton

**Abstract**

This chapter discusses the potential pathophysiology of anal and/or fecal incontinence during pregnancy and the postpartum period and prevalence of such incontinence, appropriate assessment, and various treatment options. This chapter explains risk factors associated with fecal incontinence in first and subsequent pregnancies and the postpartum, including risks associated with obstetrical anal sphincter injuries, pudendal nerve injury, and chronic fourth-degree lacerations. Quality of life and impact on psychosocial factors, including sexual function, are also discussed. Case studies are provided to emphasize the role of the advanced practice nurse in assessment and treatment of fecal incontinence within this special population.

**Keywords**

Fecal incontinence · Anal incontinence · Pregnancy · Postpartum · Obstetrical anal sphincter injuries

## 11.1 Introduction

Anal incontinence is defined as the involuntary loss of gas, feces, and/or mucus [1]. Fecal incontinence is defined as the involuntary loss of feces only [1]. Anal and/or fecal incontinence is a life-altering condition sometimes associated with onset during pregnancy [2] or the postpartum period [3]. Fecal incontinence is twice as likely

C. Hegan (✉) · M. Corton
Division of Female Pelvic Medicine and Reconstructive Surgery, University of Texas
Southwestern Medical Center, Urogynecology Clinic, Dallas, TX, USA
e-mail: Christy.hicks@utsouthwestern.edu; Marlene.corton@utsouthwestern.edu

among parous women as nonparous women [2] but may occur with new onset during a first pregnancy. Van Brummen et al. (2006) conducted a prospective cohort study of 487 nulliparous women reporting a 42.3% rate of new-onset anal incontinence and 3.9% rate of new-onset fecal incontinence in first pregnancies [4]. Various theories regarding pathophysiology have been proposed. Among parous women, the most common cause theorized is previous overt or occult anal sphincter injury associated with third- or fourth-degree laceration during vaginal childbirth [3]. Anal and/or fecal incontinence can greatly impact quality of life [5, 6]. Identification and effective treatment are important in order to prevent psychological, emotional, and/or physical impact on patient lives [7].

## 11.2    Etiology of Anal and Fecal Incontinence in Pregnancy

There is very little data regarding fecal incontinence first reported during pregnancy, especially in regard to first pregnancies. Factors that may affect fecal incontinence include stool volume, consistency, transit, rectal distensibility, anal sphincter function, anorectal sensation, and reflexes [8]. During pregnancy, hormonal changes may play an important role in physiological changes of the colon, anus, rectum, and pelvic floor musculature [2]. One theory for fecal incontinence during pregnancy suggests that the hormone relaxin secreted during the first trimester may contribute to fecal incontinence in pregnancy through depolymerization of collagen bonds [9]. Loosening of collagen ligaments may have direct effect on the perineal body and rectovaginal septum [9]. The hormone progesterone may influence fecal continence during pregnancy through ligament laxity, which may stretch the pubic symphysis and potentially contribute to pelvic floor muscle dysfunction and, subsequently, defecatory dysfunction, pelvic organ prolapse, perineal descent, and difficult defecation [8]. Furthermore, progesterone may play a role in smooth muscle relaxation of the anal sphincters [8]. Androgen, estrogen, and progesterone receptors can be found within the anal epithelium below the dentate line, potentially effecting anal sphincter function [8].

   Another factor that may influence fecal continence during pregnancy is the increase in abdominal pressure as a result of increasing uterine size and volume [9]. The enlarged uterus may press against the large intestine [9] and pelvic floor musculature, resulting in dysfunction [8]. Anal canal elongation may contribute to another mechanism of anal continence during pregnancy through increasing flow resistance [10]. Flow resistance may occur when the anal canal elongates, but anal canal volume remains constant, potentially impeding flow of stool [10]. The anal mucosa accounts for a third of the anal volume, calculated by the sum of inner and outer areas of the internal anal sphincter and external anal sphincter, increasing in volume during the last half of pregnancy [10]. The anus elongates, increasing anal volume by 20% during this phase, and returns to its normal state postpartum [10]. The puborectalis muscle, which is one of the levator ani muscles, also provides support to the anorectal junction, possibly acting as another mechanism of continence [11].

## 11.3 Prevalence and Risk Factors for Anal and Fecal Incontinence in Pregnancy

Reported prevalence rates of fecal incontinence in pregnancy vary but have been reported to be between 3% and 9% by the end of the first trimester and around 3% at 36 weeks of gestation [2]. One cross-sectional study of 228 pregnant women reported rates of prevalence as high as 10% during pregnancy [9]. It is reported that anal incontinence may be most prevalent in the third trimester of pregnancy [12], with prevalence rates as high as 65% in pregnancy [13], with up to a 42.3% incidence in first-time pregnancies [4]. Risk factors for fecal incontinence in pregnancy include advanced maternal age, body mass index, excessive weight gain during pregnancy, strenuous physical activity, and cigarette smoking (see Box 11.1) [14]. Risk factors for anal incontinence during pregnancy include maternal age, excessive weight gain during pregnancy, obesity, and unemployment status [15]. Obesity may play a role through increased abdominal pressure on an already weakened pelvic floor and, consequently, may impair healing and/or deteriorate anal sphincter repairs [16]. Therefore, one might consider that with more women waiting to have children until later in life and the increasing rates of obesity in our society, anal and fecal incontinence rates among pregnant women are likely to increase. With limited information available regarding anal and fecal incontinence in pregnancy, more research is needed for further understanding of the etiologies of anal and fecal incontinence during the antepartum period.

## 11.4 Etiology of Anal and Fecal Incontinence in Postpartum Women

Among postpartum women, a more common explanation for anal and fecal incontinence is overt and occult anal sphincter tears and/or injury [3]. Risk factors for fecal incontinence in the postpartum period include tears involving the external anal sphincter and/or internal anal sphincter, operative vaginal deliveries, median

**Box 11.1: Risk Factors for Fecal Incontinence in Pregnancy**
- Advanced maternal age
- Body mass index
- Excessive weight gain in pregnancy
- Strenuous physical activity
- Cigarette smoking

In subsequent pregnancies:

- History of transient fecal incontinence in first pregnancy
- History of occult sphincter tear in first pregnancy

episiotomies, and multiple vaginal deliveries [3]. Data suggests that anal sphincter tears contribute to 45% of anal incontinence cases in postpartum women [17].

## 11.4.1 Obstetrical Anal Sphincter Injuries

Third- and fourth-degree lacerations (see Fig. 11.1), often referred to as obstetrical anal sphincter injuries, may greatly influence the probability of developing fecal incontinence in the postpartum period [3]. Third-degree obstetric lacerations may disrupt the external anal sphincter, either partially or completely [3, 18]. They may also extend to the internal anal sphincter [18]. The World Health Organization (WHO) classifies third-degree obstetric lacerations by percentage of damage to the external anal sphincter and presence of internal anal sphincter involvement [18]. Partial external anal sphincter disruption of less than 50% thickness is classified as a 3a third-degree obstetric laceration [18]. Classification 3b involves damage of over 50% thickness to the external anal sphincter [18]. Classification 3c includes disruption that extends into the internal anal sphincter [18]. Fourth-degree obstetric lacerations disrupt the external anal sphincter, the internal anal sphincter, and anorectal mucosa [3, 18]. While both third- and fourth-degree lacerations may contribute to an increased risk for fecal incontinence, it has been hypothesized that fourth-degree lacerations may carry an increased risk compared to third-degree lacerations due to muscle contracture forces during the healing process [19]. In third- and fourth-degree lacerations that involve greater than 50% of the external anal sphincter (3b or 3c), theories suggest that the constant resting tone of the internal and external anal sphincters may contribute to further separation of the external anal sphincter during healing [19]. Whereas, it is hypothesized that in lacerations of less than 50% (3a), muscle

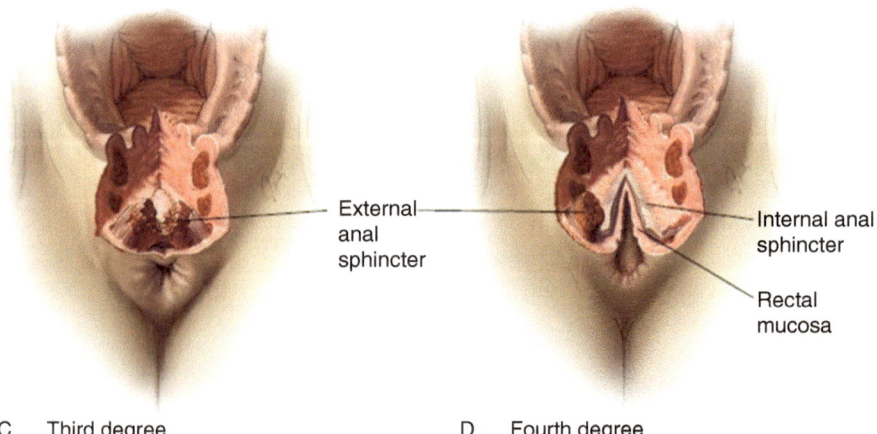

C     Third degree                          D     Fourth degree

**Fig. 11.1** Third- and fourth-degree obstetrical anal sphincter injuries (Reprinted with permission from Dr. Shayzreen Roshanravan and Dr. Marlene Corton)

contractions usually aid in healing of the obstetrical anal sphincter injuries [19]. This is important to consider given that the anal sphincter muscles are unique, maintaining a constant state of contraction [11]. The internal anal sphincter contributes up to 85% of anal canal resting pressure, while the external anal sphincter contributes approximately 15% [11]. The external anal sphincter contributes to continence by voluntarily contracting muscle, similar to a Kegel contraction, when one feels the desire to defecate or when continence is threated [11]. It is also proposed that the internal anal sphincter may be damaged independently of the external anal sphincter as a consequence of shearing forces from the descent of the infant head during vaginal childbirth [5]. Because the internal anal sphincter contributes up to 85% of anal canal resting pressure [11], isolated internal anal sphincter injury may lead to flatus incontinence [20]. Denervation injury may also occur [11].

Magnetic resonance imaging studies have demonstrated higher prevalence of levator ani muscle damage in women suffering from anal sphincter tears, suggesting that the combination of sphincter tear and levator ani damage may contribute to an increased risk for fecal incontinence [21]. One retrospective analysis by Sultan et al. (1994) reported the incidence of fecal incontinence and fecal urgency to be as high as half of the women requiring surgical repair of postdelivery tears involving the external anal sphincter and/or internal anal sphincter [22]. Tin et al. (2010) reported that roughly one to two thirds of women with third-degree lacerations may develop fecal incontinence [6]. However, data on prevalence of fecal incontinence after third-degree obstetric laceration was limited based on small population sample size and was not reproducible in the recent Behavioral Therapy of Obstetric Sphincter Tears (BOOST) study conducted by the Pelvic Floor Disorders Network [19]. In the BOOST study, incidence of fecal incontinence in 343 women after anal sphincter injury repair was reported as 7%, 4%, and 9% at 6 weeks, 12 weeks, and 24 weeks, respectively [19]. The BOOST study, which started as a clinical trial, was converted to an observational cohort study due to the lack of reported fecal incontinence after third- or fourth-degree obstetrical anal sphincter injuries [19]. Suspected causes for previously reported high rates of fecal incontinence in other studies include potential nerve injury, inadequate surgical repair, and/or partial dehiscence of surgical repair due to faulty healing from competing muscle contraction forces on the anal sphincter complex [3].

## 11.4.2 Chronic Fourth-Degree Lacerations/Cloacal-Like Deformities

If left unrecognized or if breakdown occurs, third- or fourth-degree lacerations may result in chronic fourth-degree lacerations, also known as cloacal-like deformities (see Fig. 11.2) [23]. Cloacal-like deformities occur in 0.3% of deliveries complicated by third- or fourth-degree obstetric laceration [23]. Cloacal-like deformities occur when there is complete disruption of the perineal body with a wide-angle anterior anal sphincter defect and loss of the rectovaginal septum, allowing for potential flow of flatus and stool from the rectum to the vagina [23]. The primary

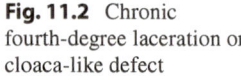

**Fig. 11.2** Chronic
fourth-degree laceration or
cloaca-like defect

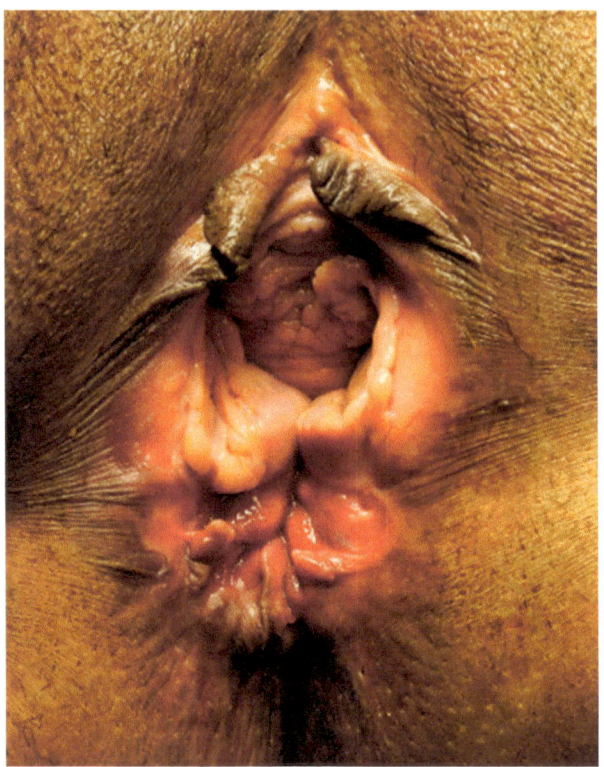

symptom of a cloacal-like defect is fecal incontinence with the possible complaint
of stool also passing from the vagina [23]. There may be complete loss of continence of stool [23]. Additional complaints include skin irritations, sexual dysfunction, and emotional, psychological, and social distress [23].

### 11.4.3 Risk Factors for Obstetrical Anal Sphincter Injuries

Midline episiotomies are known risk factors for third- or fourth-degree lacerations
[3]. Mediolateral episiotomies, conversely, do not carry increased risk of anal
sphincter injury and, thus, are preferred by some practitioners when an episiotomy
is clinically indicated [3].

Assisted operative vaginal delivery with the use of forceps or vacuum may also
increase the risk for anal sphincter tear [3]. However, forceps use has been shown to
double the risk for fecal incontinence in comparison to vacuum-assisted deliveries
[24]. It has been suggested that cesarean delivery may be somewhat protective in
prevention of postpartum fecal incontinence [3]. However, studies have demonstrated this is not always the case, as emergency cesarean deliveries performed in
the second stage of labor cannot protect against the already influenced neurophysiological damage to the pelvic floor [3]. In addition, a retrospective cohort study by

Nygaard et al. (1997) showed that anal incontinence rates among middle age women do not differ significantly based on mode of previous delivery(ies) [25]. In this study, fecal incontinence rates were shown to be the same 30 years postpartum, regardless of vaginal delivery with or without obstetric anal sphincter injury or cesarean delivery [25].

Anal sphincter disruption is not the only cause of anal incontinence [13]. Other anatomical and/or physiological processes likely contribute given the similar rates of anal incontinence found comparatively in both nulliparous and primiparous women [13]. In some cases, anal incontinence may improve and even cease after delivery, suggesting pregnancy may hold a more important role in the development of anal incontinence [26].

## 11.4.4  Rectovaginal and Anovaginal Fistula

Although rare, one must also assess any women who presents with postpartum fecal incontinence for potential rectovaginal or anovaginal fistula (see Fig. 11.3) [3]. This is not common in developed countries but often present due to prolonged labor causing pressure necrosis, breakdown of third- or fourth-degree laceration repairs, or infected

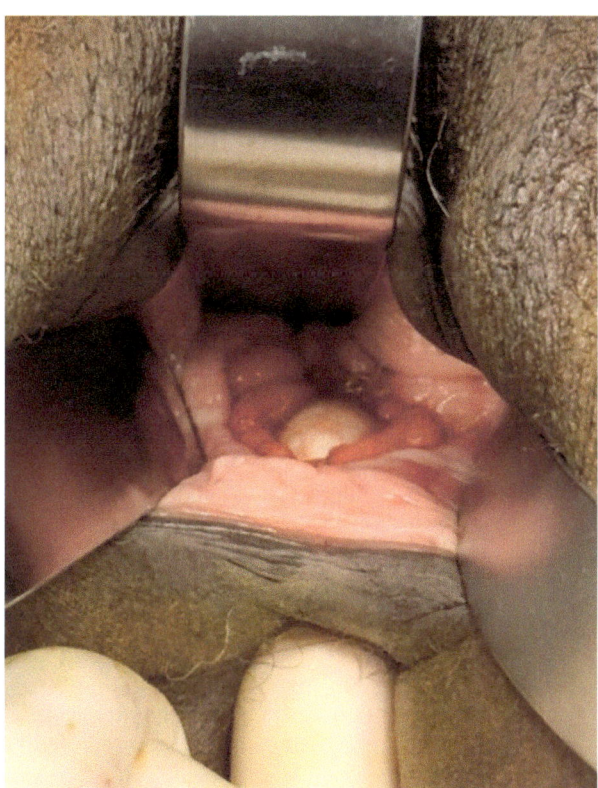

**Fig. 11.3** Rectovaginal fistula

episiotomy sites [3]. When considering differential diagnoses, women with rectovaginal fistula usually present with complaints of fecal stool or drainage per vagina and/or chronic or recurrent vaginitis, while women with anal incontinence usually present with complaints of fecal urgency with or without accidental bowel losses and/or loss of stool or flatus from the anus without awareness [27].

### 11.4.5  Pudendal Nerve Injury

Pudendal nerve injury sustained during pregnancy or the vaginal birth process may also play a role in the development of postpartum fecal incontinence [18]. Mechanical damage to the anal sphincter during the second stage of labor may result in compression or stretching injuries to the pudendal nerve, resulting in neuropathy [18]. In a study of 71 women, it has been reported that the pubococcygeus and anal sphincter sustained denervation injury in up to 42%–80% of vaginal deliveries with progressive nerve damage based on findings from electrophysiological tests conducted 2–3 days after delivery [28]. However, in most of the same women, nerve damage resolved within 2 months postpartum and did not relate to symptoms of fecal incontinence [28]. It has also been suggested that pudendal nerve injury during childbirth may lead to functional asymmetry of anal sphincter innervation, which is associated with the development of fecal incontinence, as well [29].

### 11.4.6  Other Risk Factors for Postpartum Anal and Fecal Incontinence

Other risk factors that may influence fecal incontinence in the postpartum period include high body mass index, prolonged pushing in the second stage of labor, smoking cigarettes [30], fetal macrosomia [31], and constipation [32]. Epidural analgesia may also contribute to increased risk due to the risk of prolonged labor [33] and risk of need for operative delivery in these circumstances [34]. However, there is some controversy to this, as epidural analgesia may also relax the pelvic floor and avert pelvic floor trauma and potential lacerations [34]. Women with a narrow subpubic arch may also be more prone to postpartum anal incontinence due to prolonged labor, but these women have not been found to have higher incidences of anal sphincter damage by vaginal or operative delivery than women with wide angle subpubic arches [35].

### 11.5  Etiology of Fecal Incontinence in Subsequent Pregnancies

Among subsequent deliveries, there is controversial evidence regarding recurrence of anal sphincter damage [31]. It has been reported that up to 35% of primiparous vaginal deliveries are associated with occult sphincter injuries [36]. In a study of

107 women by Corton et al. (2013), endoanal sonography detected anal sphincter defects in 12% of primiparous women [37]. The same study estimated a total of 17.8% of vaginally delivered primiparous women sustained anal sphincter injury as detected by both clinical diagnosis and sonography [37]. In another prospective study of 20,111 consecutive vaginal deliveries, only 5% of women who suffered third-degree laceration during their first delivery sustained additional anal sphincter injury [38]. Other studies have suggested a five- to sevenfold increase in risk for recurrent anal sphincter disruption and increased risk with prior third- or fourth-degree laceration involving high birthweight infants [39, 40]. In women who suffered transient fecal incontinence and/or occult sphincter tear with their first child, there is an increased risk for fecal incontinence after subsequent vaginal deliveries [5, 41]. Other risk factors for sustaining further anal sphincter damage in subsequent delivery include operative vaginal deliveries and episiotomy [31].

## 11.6   Prevalence and Risk Factors for Anal and Fecal Incontinence in Postpartum Women and Subsequent Pregnancies

In an observational cohort study of 8,774 surveys of postpartum women, there was a reported 29% incidence of fecal incontinence with nearly half of these women reporting incontinence of stool and 38% reporting incontinence of flatus only [30]. Nearly half of women reporting fecal incontinence stated that they started experiencing fecal incontinence after their first delivery, and more than 25% of these women began to experience fecal incontinence within the first 6 months postpartum [30]. In another observational cohort study of 343 women, the incidence of postpartum fecal incontinence among primiparous women who sustained obstetrical anal sphincter injuries was reported to be 7% at 6 weeks postpartum, 4% at 12 weeks postpartum, and 9% at 24 weeks postpartum, while anal incontinence was reported to be 24% at 24 weeks postpartum [19].

Roughly two thirds of women with flatus incontinence after vaginal delivery will have resolution of symptoms by 12 months postpartum [5]. In a prospective 5-year cohort study of 349 nulliparous women, data suggests that if anal incontinence persists at or after 9 months postpartum, it will most likely persist and worsen with time [41]. In primiparous women with obstetrical anal sphincter injuries and fecal incontinence persisting at 9 months postpartum, approximately 50% were reported to have persistent symptoms 5 years later [41]. Twenty-five percent of women without clinically diagnosed anal sphincter injury reported anal incontinence at 9 months postpartum with 32% having persisting symptoms at 5 years postpartum [41]. This rate increased to 34% in women with subsequent deliveries [41]. This indicates that a woman with a sphincter tear has an eightfold increased risk for developing anal incontinence at 5 years postpartum if she had anal incontinence at 9 months postpartum [41]. Most studies regarding subsequent deliveries indicate that additional childbirth incidences increase the risk for developing anal incontinence [41]. In this prospective 5-year cohort study, anal incontinence symptoms were noted to increase

**Box 11.2: Summary of Main Points to Consider in Clinical Decision-Making and Patient Education**
- If a woman sustains an obstetrical anal sphincter injury with first delivery, she has a 7% chance of fecal incontinence within the first 6 weeks postpartum, a 4% chance at 12 weeks, and a 9% chance at 24 weeks [19].
- In primiparous women who sustained obstetrical anal sphincter injuries and report anal incontinence at 9 months postpartum, there is a 50% chance that their anal incontinence symptoms will persist or worsen within 5 years postpartum [41]. However, anal incontinence has not been shown to persist at the same rate 30 years postpartum [25].
- If a primiparous woman sustained an obstetrical anal sphincter injury with first delivery, she has a 4–8% higher rate of another obstetrical anal sphincter injury with subsequent vaginal birth [18].
- If a woman sustained an obstetrical anal sphincter injury with first delivery with or without anal incontinence postpartum, a cesarean delivery may be recommended with subsequent pregnancy [5].
- Main risk factors for obstetrical anal sphincter injuries in primiparous women are midline episiotomies, assisted operative vaginal delivery, high body mass index, prolonged pushing during the second stage of labor, smoking cigarettes, fetal macrosomia, constipation, connective tissue disease, and Asian, Indian, and Filipino race [3, 5, 30–32].

from 3% to 10% with a second vaginal delivery without anal sphincter disruption [41]. Subsequent anal sphincter tear rates have been reported to be 4%–8% [18]. See Box 11.2 for further considerations in clinical decision-making and patient education.

## 11.7   History and Physical: Special Considerations

In assessment of fecal continence among pregnant and postpartum women, one must take into special consideration any comorbidities or acute conditions that may affect continence by taking a careful history and physical. One of the most common bowel disorders, irritable bowel syndrome, may have an impact on fecal incontinence in postpartum women [42]. In general, women with irritable bowel syndrome may have irregular bowel consistency and defecation frequency [42]. These erratic fluctuations may cause alterations in continence [42]. One prospective observational study assessed 208 women prior to delivery and during the postpartum period, as well as an additional 104 primigravid women postpartum only. It was found that in the first 6 weeks postpartum, irritable bowel syndrome symptoms may be exacerbated and subsequently contribute to an increased risk for postpartum fecal incontinence in women who deliver via vaginal delivery [42]. In contrast, women who delivered via cesarean delivery were not reported to have higher rates of fecal incontinence [42]. Irritable bowel syndrome symptoms were not associated with any increased risk for obstetrical anal sphincter injuries [42]. In these circumstances, it is also imperative to rule out inflammatory bowel disease and colorectal cancer [27, 43]. Colorectal cancer may often present with new-onset bowel changes, fluctuating between constipation and diarrhea or presenting with narrow ribbonlike stools [43]. In patients with inflammatory bowel disease, such as ulcerative colitis and Crohn's disease, rectal compliance may be poor, and some patients may experience chronic diarrhea [27]. These patients are at a higher risk for developing fecal incontinence [27]. If there is any suspicion for potential inflammatory bowel disease or colorectal cancer pathology, referral to a gastroenterologist is warranted [43].

In regard to acute conditions, the most severe of differential diagnoses must include cauda equina syndrome [44]. Lower back pain is common among pregnant women and is generally attributable to hormonal changes and increasing stress on the lumbosacral spine from a gravid uterus [44]. However, lumbar disk herniation is considered an obstetric emergency [44]. Cauda equina syndrome involves lumbar disk herniation that may present with bilateral sciatica-type pain, bilateral leg weakness, and diminished sensation over the buttocks, perineum, and inner thighs, as well as loss of continence, both urinary and fecal [43, 44]. If not treated immediately, it may progress to permanent neurological sequelae [43]. Symptoms warranting an advanced evaluation include severe back and/or leg pain in pregnancy [44]. Assessment should include rectal examination to determine anorectal sensation and magnetic resonance imaging (MRI) of the lumbosacral spine [44]. Minor lumbar disk herniation that does not lead to cauda equina syndrome may be managed conservatively [44]. Massive disk herniation that leads to cauda equina syndrome in pregnancy is generally considered a surgical emergency [44].

Bothersome lumbar disk herniation only occurs in about 1/10,000 pregnancies, and only a few cases have been reported to progress to cauda equina syndrome [44]. In a presented case study, anal sphincter dysfunction resolved after surgical intervention, but anorectal sensation was diminished for an additional 6 months [44]. The assessment and identification of cauda equina syndrome in pregnancy are imperative in order to provide emergency care and avoid potential permanent motor loss and permanent urinary and fecal incontinence or dysfunction [44].

## 11.8 Assessment of Anal and Fecal Incontinence in Pregnancy and Postpartum

It is an expert opinion that one should consider careful baseline assessment of anorectal symptoms during pregnancy. With up to 29% of women experiencing fecal incontinence postpartum, and surveys indicating fecal incontinence occurring at 6 months postpartum [30] and 9 months postpartum [41], postpartum assessment of pregnancy sequelae must continue past the standard 6–8 weeks postpartum checkup [30]. Assessment may include physical examination to detect fecal smearing, obstetrical scarring, perineal descent, hemorrhoids, anal warts, rectal prolapse, and/ or the classic dovetail sign (see Fig. 11.4) seen with anterior disruption or separation

**Fig. 11.4** Dovetail sign: anterior separation of the external anal sphincter

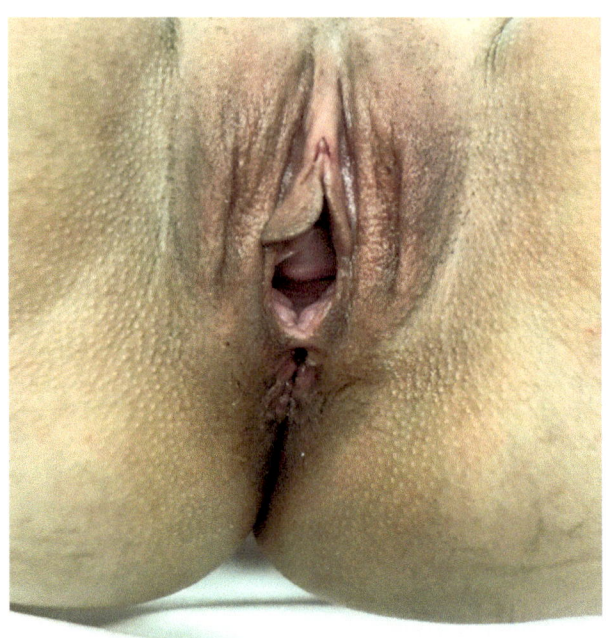

of the external anal sphincter [27]. Examination should also include assessment of the pudendal nerve by checking for the presence of an anal wink in response to light stimulus, such as with a cotton swab, on the perianal area [27]. Digital anorectal examination allows for evaluation of palpable anorectal masses and/or fecal impaction [27]. In addition, the tone and contraction of the anal sphincters can be assessed [27]. Valsalva maneuvers can aid in detection of perineal descent, pelvic organ prolapse, and/or rectal prolapse [27]. In women who endorse accidental bowel losses, additional evaluation should include validated condition-specific questionnaires [33]. If warranted by the initial history and physical examination, some women may undergo anal endosonography, colonoscopy and/or barium enema [27], MR defecography, anorectal manometry [33], electromyography, or pudendal nerve motor latency testing [27]. Anorectal manometry, electromyography, and pudendal nerve motor latency testing may not be indicated for clinical assessment but are utilized more in the setting of clinical research.

## 11.9    Assessment for Anal Sphincter Injury

Evaluation with the use of endoanal or transperineal sonography may aid in detection of occult anal sphincter tears postpartum [45]. If a sphincter defect is suspected on postpartum physical examination and noted by endoanal or transperineal sonography, an anal sphincteroplasty can be considered [45]. With up to 35% of primiparous women [36, 46] and 44% of multiparous women [46] having anal sphincter defects, anal endosonography provides a useful tool in assessment and diagnosis of occult sphincter injuries [46]. Based on a multicenter prospective cohort study of

251 primiparous women by the Pelvic Floor Disorders Network, those with evidence of occult defects have greater risk of having fecal incontinence compared to primiparous women with no sonographic evidence of anal sphincter gaps or disruption [47].

Anal endosonography may be done at 6 weeks postpartum to assess for anal sphincter tears among any woman who has delivered vaginally [46]. Transperineal and transvaginal ultrasound may also be utilized to assess for sphincter disruption with minimal discomfort compared to anal endosonography [48]. Surgical intervention may or may not be necessary depending on the presence of anal sphincter gaps [47] and the relationship between ultrasound findings and anorectal symptoms [49]. However, anal sphincteroplasty is not a simple or benign procedure. It carries risk of further sphincter damage and risk of pudendal neuropathy [27]. Emphasis should always be placed on aggressive behavioral measures and supervised pelvic floor exercises with or without biofeedback [27].

Perhaps more important than sonographic evaluation is routine intrapartum anorectal examination in the setting of a second-degree laceration or any extensive perineal laceration [37]. In a prospective observational study of 107 women who underwent postpartum endoanal sonography with no clinical evidence of obstetrical anal sphincter injuries at the time of delivery, 12.1% of women demonstrated anal sphincter defect compared with 6.5% diagnosed by clinical observation [37]. A significant number of anal sphincter defects were associated with second-degree perineal tears [37]. This indicates that second-degree tears should warrant further evaluation by rectal examination in order to prevent misdiagnosis of potential anal sphincter defects [37]. A thorough intrapartum evaluation of the anorectum can be performed by inserting the gloved index finger of the non-dominant hand to distend the rectum and by placing the index and middle fingers of the dominant hand intravaginally to separate the borders of the laceration in order to visualize the deepest layer of tissue involved [37]. Appropriate lighting and irrigation should be used during this process.

Expert opinion suggests that all women should be screened for anal incontinence at every postpartum visit. Screening may present opportunities for early behavioral and nonsurgical interventions. Expert opinion also recommends that if anal incontinence is present immediately postpartum, one should reassess anal incontinence symptoms at 3 months postpartum, 6 months postpartum, 9 months postpartum, and 12 months postpartum. Given that anal incontinence may not initially present until many years postpartum [18], it is also recommended to assess all women for anal incontinence at least annually.

## 11.10 Conservative Management and Expected Outcomes

### 11.10.1 Pelvic Floor Therapy, Biofeedback, and Electrical Stimulation

It is often recommended to strengthen the pelvic floor musculature during pregnancy in order to prevent postpartum urinary and fecal incontinence [50]. Biofeedback has been utilized to provide computer-guided feedback from rectal balloons to increase patient perception of rectal contents, assist in coordinated sphincter contraction and relaxation as appropriate, and improve anal sphincter strength [51, 52]. One systematic review did not support the use of pelvic floor therapy during the antepartum or postpartum period up to 3 months postpartum to prevent anal or fecal incontinence [50]. Conversely, a recent retrospective quantitative study by Mathe et al. (2016) showed that starting early postpartum pelvic floor therapy may aid in reduction of both anal and fecal incontinence with statistically significant findings [53]. Mathe et al. (2016) suggests beginning pelvic floor therapy within the first month postpartum. [53]. While this study shows promise for reduction in anal and fecal incontinence with early intervention, the study does have multiple weaknesses, including low level of evidence, potential treatment bias, and potential placebo effect [53]. Further research is needed.

Combination therapy consisting of pelvic floor physical therapy with biofeedback with or without anorectal electrical stimulation may aid to increase muscle and sphincter tone in prevention of stool loss [31]. One systematic review from 2013 reviewed 13 randomized control trials that evaluated biofeedback and electrical stimulation for the treatment of fecal incontinence [54]. Twelve trials evaluated biofeedback as treatment alone or in combination with electrical stimulation, while seven trials evaluated effectiveness of electrical stimulation alone [54]. Of these trials, only three were rated of high quality and one rated of moderate quality of evidence [54]. Three out of seven electrical stimulation trials were of average strength evidence, with only two reaching therapeutic windows [54]. However, the systematic review concluded that there was enough statistically significant evidence to advocate the use of biofeedback with concurrent electrical stimulation for the treatment of fecal incontinence with medium frequency amplitude electrical stimulation being the most effective modality [54]. Results indicate that the use of both together is superior to the use of a singular modality [54].

While these combination therapies have been evaluated in women with anal incontinence remote from delivery, further research is needed in regard to combination therapies specific to pregnancy and postpartum. In addition, electrical stimulation is contraindicated in pregnancy and up to 6 weeks postpartum. After 6 weeks postpartum, one may consider electrical stimulation if vaginal bleeding has resolved and episiotomy or obstetric tears have completely healed. Lactation is not listed as a contraindication to electrical stimulation in the manufacturer's packaging.

## 11.10.2 Perineal Stretching and Massage

The use of antenatal perineal stretching and massage has been suggested to lessen the incidence of obstetrical anal sphincter injuries and subsequently lessen the risk for associated anal and fecal incontinence [55]. Findings from a prospective observational study suggested decreased rates of clinically diagnosed sphincter tears and occult sphincter injuries in women over 30 years of age who engaged in antenatal perineal massage starting at 34 weeks gestation [55]. However, these findings were not statistically significant [55]. In addition, intrapartum stretching of the perineal body was found to be unrelated to obstetric tears in another large prospective observational study [56]. Thus, further research is needed.

### 11.10.3 Dietary Modifications

Conservative treatment with dietary modifications, as well as certain medications, may aid with postpartum fecal incontinence symptoms in women with infrequent fecal incontinence [31]. First-line treatment for fecal incontinence is the use of fiber to produce bulkier stools [57]. It is recommended to slowly taper the amount of fiber intake into the diet in an effort to avoid abdominal bloating symptoms [57]. This may be done with a bowel recipe, such as one cup applesauce, one cup of oat bran or unprocessed wheat bran, and ¼ cup of prune juice, tapering up by one to two tablespoons/day each week until desired stool consistency and regularity are achieved [58]. Psyllium has also been shown to have significant effects on reduction of fecal incontinence episodes compared to other fiber supplements [57]. However, in women with decreased rectal compliance, such as those with history of radiation and prior surgery, stool bulking agents may exacerbate symptoms of fecal incontinence [57].

A low residue diet has also been suggested in order to avoid loose stools, which are often associated with fecal frequency and accidental bowel losses in women with fecal incontinence [31]. Avoidance of foods and beverages containing fructose, lactose, artificial sweeteners, caffeine, carbonation, and alcohol should be avoided, as these may aggravate symptoms by increasing stool frequency and/or by making the stool consistency loose [57]. In addition, cured and smoked meats and spicy, fatty, and greasy foods may all contribute to looser stool consistency and increase rates of fecal incontinence [57].

### 11.10.4 Medication Management

Women with severe constipation may experience overflow fecal incontinence [57]. In women with constipation, stool softeners may be helpful [32]. Conversely, constipating medications may be used to reduce fecal incontinence episodes, especially in women with loose stool and diarrhea [5]. One small double-blind crossover study of 30 people compared loperamide hydrochloride (Imodium), codeine phosphate, and diphenoxylate hydrochloride (Lomotil) for the treatment of chronic diarrhea, which is commonly associated with fecal urgency and fecal incontinence [59]. Diphenoxylate was not found to be as effective as loperamide or codeine phosphate [59]. Both codeine phosphate and loperamide were superior in decreasing stool frequency and fecal urgency that some subjects associated with fecal incontinence [59]. Additionally, side effects were most significant for subjects taking diphenoxylate and least significant for subjects taking loperamide [59]. First-line medication should be loperamide due to minimal side effects when compared with codeine phosphate [5] or diphenoxylate [59] and due to its safety during pregnancy [60]. In addition, loperamide increases anal sphincter tone and rectal compliance [61]. Although codeine phosphate is a good second alternative [5], there may be potential risk to a fetus with use in pregnancy [5, 60]. Both medications work to decrease gut transit time and bulk the stool [5]. For some patients, loperamide can cause bothersome constipation [5]. If this occurs, one may consider loperamide syrup, which carries less side effects [5]. Another factor to consider in medication selection is lactation. Codeine phosphate is contraindicated in breastfeeding, while loperamide is considered safe [60]. A third-line alternative medication to consider would be amitriptyline, which aids in decreased bowel frequency and fecal incontinence [5]. Suggested starting dosage of amitriptyline is 20 mg PO QHS [5]. However, 25% of patients may experience side effects of this medication [5]. It is considered safe in lactation but carries potential risk to a fetus when used in pregnancy [60]. Additionally, glycerin suppositories and enemas may be used to evacuate the rectum in order to avoid fecal incontinence, but these may pose risk to a fetus in pregnancy and lactation [31, 60].

## 11.10.5 Products

There are many products on the market to help manage fecal incontinence, such as fecal pads used to prevent underwear soiling, silicone inserts and anal plug devices that seal the rectum to prevent accidental bowel leakage, and other bowel control devices with pump inflated balloons to prevent fecal leakage. Please refer to Chap. 6 regarding more information on these products.

## 11.11 Intrapartum Interventions

Other interventions that have been recommended include the use of vacuum assistance vs. forceps, when needed, and the use of mediolateral episiotomy instead of midline episiotomy, when needed, to prevent risk of trauma to the anal sphincter [62]. However, while mediolateral episiotomy has been shown to decrease the risk of anal sphincter tears, it has not been shown to decrease anal or fecal incontinence rates [48].

### 11.11.1 Mode of Delivery

It is sometimes recommended that women with history of previous third- or fourth-degree laceration with or without persistent fecal incontinence, abnormal manometry, and/or endoanal sonography results should be given the option to deliver by cesarean delivery [18]. Vaginal births after cesarean delivery have also been associated with increased risk of subsequent anal incontinence [63]. However, in women with subsequent vaginal delivery and history of previous obstetrical anal sphincter injuries, repeat vaginal delivery does not necessarily mean sustained damage to the anal sphincter or decreased quality of life [64]. Among women with previous third-degree tears with no fecal incontinence or minimal fecal incontinence, 70% may have subsequent vaginal deliveries with minimal impact on fecal incontinence [65]. Recurrence of obstetrical anal sphincter injuries may occur in up to 8% of second vaginal deliveries [18]. It is important to weigh the risks and benefits of cesarean delivery versus the risk of recurrence of obstetrical anal sphincter injuries, resulting in potential pudendal neuropathy changes and/or need for secondary anal sphincter repair, which is usually not as successful as primary repair [66].

## 11.12 Perineal Clinic

Perineal clinics that care for women who sustained obstetrical anal sphincter injuries are increasingly being implemented throughout the USA [6]. They provide the best setting for education, preventative strategies, and management of anal incontinence in women who sustained obstetrical anal sphincter injuries [6]. These specialty clinics can also provide counseling on future mode of delivery [6].

## 11.13 Percutaneous and Sacral Neuromodulation

Failure of conservative treatment may lead to consideration of either percutaneous or sacral nerve stimulation [31]. Sacral nerve stimulation uses electrical sacral nerve stimulation via an implanted stimulator device to help aid in improvement of fecal incontinence symptoms [31]. It has been reported to improve patient quality of life in 80% of patients treated for fecal incontinence [31].

There is limited evidence regarding the use of sacral neuromodulation for fecal incontinence during pregnancy [67, 68]. Only one case report currently involves the use of continuous sacral neuromodulation throughout the full term of pregnancy for the treatment of fecal incontinence [67]. The patient's fecal incontinence returned postpartum due to lead breakage and displacement, presumably disrupted by vaginal delivery [67]. The patient regained continence after successful postpartum lead replacement [67]. Sacral neuromodulation has been reported for the treatment of symptoms other than fecal incontinence in pregnancy [68]. One systematic review investigated eight cases of sacral neuromodulation throughout a full-term pregnancy [68]. Of these eight cases, two infants were born with congenital anomalies, one with a motor tic and one with a pilonidal sinus [68]. Both infants born with congenital anomalies were from the same mother [68]. It is unknown whether or not the sacral nerve stimulator had a role in the resulting congenital anomalies of the infants [68]. Due to the limited data available regarding modulation in pregnancy, future research is needed [11, 68]. However, one might consider that this treatment would be reserved for severe and refractory cases of fecal incontinence in pregnancy due to the need for anesthesia. It is suggested that sacral neuromodulation in pregnancy be individualized based on the potential benefits vs. risks [68].

Regardless of these few case studies mentioned, it is important to note that the manufacturer does not recommend use during pregnancy. Currently, sacral neuro-modulation is contraindicated in pregnancy.

If women with sacral neuromodulation devices in place opt to keep the device throughout pregnancy, regardless of if the device is turned on or off, cesarean delivery may be considered due to the risk for potential sacral electrode breakage or displacement [67]. However, Mahran et al. (2017) suggest that mode of delivery does not affect postpartum results, as similar incidences have occurred in women with elective cesarean deliveries [68]. This suggests that pregnancy may lead to electrode displacement due to the increasing maternal habitus and accompanying abdominal pressure, regardless of delivery mode [68].

In postpartum women, sacral nerve stimulation may be a very successful option for the treatment of fecal incontinence [5]. Results have shown improvement in symptomatic fecal incontinence in women with both intact and disrupted anal sphincters, both with external anal sphincter and/or internal anal sphincter disruptions [5]. This procedure, unlike an anal sphincteroplasty, carries low or no risk of further sphincter damage [5].

While often used in countries outside the United States (USA), posterior tibial nerve stimulation (PTNS) is not currently approved by the US Food and Drug Administration for the treatment of fecal incontinence in the USA. Studies abroad show mixed results regarding the use of PTNS for the treatment of fecal incontinence [11]. Further research is needed. Some may opt to consider this treatment as an off-label use.

## 11.14  Surgical Intervention

In women with obstetrical anal sphincter injuries, surgical treatment with primary sphincter repair is often preferred in prevention of long-term fecal incontinence [31]. However, there is always the risk for repair failure and/or continued anal and/or fecal incontinence. In a study of 47 primiparous women who delivered vaginally, anal incontinence symptoms persisted in 11% after anal sphincter repair [69]. In another prospective study of 154 women who sustained third-degree lacerations and had subsequent primary anal sphincter repair at the time of delivery, up to 50% of subjects complained of fecal incontinence at 3 months postpartum [49]. Up to 44% of women demonstrate continued internal anal sphincter defect on ultrasound evaluation at short term and further follow-ups after primary sphincter repair [5]. In a telephone interview survey of 71 patients who previously underwent overlapping anal sphincteroplasty, 49 patients were contacted regarding fecal incontinence symptoms [70]. Over 60% of patients contacted reported fecal incontinence at 47–141 months postoperatively [70].

Failed repair may occur due to inappropriate surgical techniques, hematoma formation, wound infections, fecal impaction, and/or missed secondary injury [5]. Risk for long-term sphincter repair failure is currently unknown, but potential theories include sphincter denervation, muscular fibrosis, and muscular atrophy from the aging process [5]. When sphincter damage has been missed or primary repair has failed, it is suggested to wait at least 3 months before considering a secondary repair [5]. Conservative management should be used for the first year after obstetrical anal sphincter injuries, unless incontinence symptoms are severe or large sphincter defect is present [69]. Gracilis muscle transposition and artificial sphincter repairs are only recommended as a last resort due to significant morbidity [69]. In addition, diversion may be considered as a last option but may improve quality of life in select women [69].

In women with fecal incontinence and cloacal-like defects, an anal sphinctero-plasty combined with perineal reconstruction is indicated [23]. Surgical intervention includes separation of the rectum from the vagina, longitudinal reconstruction of the anorectal canal and vagina, anterior overlapping sphincteroplasty, and transverse reconstruction of the perineal body [23] (see Chap. 12). Outcomes have demonstrated improved functionality [23].

## 11.15  Quality of Life

Anal and fecal incontinence can greatly alter a woman's emotional well-being and quality of life [5, 6]. Anxiety, depression, and/or fear of further pregnancy and delivery may all ensue [5]. It is reported that over 25% of women who develop anal incontinence in the postpartum period continue to experience decreased quality of life at 2 years postpartum [71]. Women with more severe fecal incontinence affecting activities of daily living are more likely to report anal incontinence to their healthcare provider, but overall, rates of reporting anal incontinence are low [5, 71]. Only 10% of symptomatic women will actually report anal incontinence, making it all the more important for healthcare providers to routinely screen for these symptoms [5]. Most women fear embarrassment and, therefore, will not report symptoms or seek care [15]. Others assume there are no treatment options, they don't know who to talk to, and/or they don't think their healthcare provider would be interested in treating their fecal incontinence [72].

In addition to fecal incontinence symptoms, other life stressors that may affect quality of life include the need for incontinence products and potential side effects of constipating medications, such as loperamide, which may lead to inconvenience in a new mother's life [5]. Fecal urgency may also contribute to social isolation as women feel the need to stay home near a toilet [5].

Additionally, anal incontinence may impact sexual function postpartum [73]. It has been reported that roughly 81%–87% of women engage in sexual intercourse within 12 weeks postpartum [73]. However, only 40% of women who sustained an obstetrical anal sphincter injury are reported to resume sexual intercourse within 12 weeks postpartum [73]. History of obstetrical anal sphincter injuries and report of worsening anal incontinence within 2 weeks postpartum are strong predictive factors for not resuming sexual intercourse by 12 weeks postpartum [73]. Furthermore, anal incontinence continues to be severe in those prolonging return to intercourse after they have resumed sexual activity [73]. In women who have had anal sphincteroplasty and continue to have fecal incontinence with solid stools, sexual function has been reported to remain poor [73]. Further research is needed on the implications of anal and fecal incontinence on sexual function [73].

It is plausible that body image perception may impact sexual function [7]. While the topic of body image during pregnancy and postpartum has not been investigated thoroughly, there has been some research to suggest a correlation between poor postpartum body image and depression associated with fecal incontinence [7]. Poor body image may consequently affect physical activity, sexual function, and ultimately decreased quality of life [7]. Further research is needed regarding body image perception related to fecal incontinence in pregnancy and the postpartum, and the implication of poor body image perception during pregnancy and the postpartum period.

While there is considerable research to assess the influence of anal and fecal incontinence on a woman's quality of life throughout pregnancy and the postpartum period, there is little research to support appropriate interventions at this time. It is important to assess and identify symptoms in order to expedite treatment and care [72]. In addressing complaints of incontinence, body image perception, sexual dysfunction, and quality of life may improve greatly [7, 72, 73].

## 11.16  Follow-Up Care

Routine pregnancy follow-up is once every 4 weeks and then weekly after 36 weeks of gestation, unless other complications require more frequent visitation. Evaluation of anal and/or fecal incontinence throughout pregnancy should be conducted at routine visit intervals. Recommended postpartum follow-up is within 6 weeks of delivery, unless other complications indicate earlier attention. If fecal incontinence is identified in the immediate postpartum period and pelvic floor therapy is recommended, weekly or every other week visits with a physical therapist may be required for up to 12 weeks. It may be necessary to continue follow-up with a provider at least at 3-month intervals to assess for and treat anal and fecal incontinence symptoms, if present. Three-month follow-up is considered appropriate for any behavioral modifications and/or treatment. One may consider follow-up at 1 month for medication management of newly prescribed medications for anal and/or fecal incontinence. After 3-month intervals for 1 year, one should provide at least annual evaluation of anal and fecal incontinence symptoms.

## 11.17  Team Approach to Care

Given that most pregnant and postpartum women are followed by an obstetrician, gynecologist, or advanced practice nurse in the field of women's health or midwifery, first evaluation is usually within the OB-GYN setting. This provides an opportunity for screening, further evaluation, if warranted, and early conservative interventions. If there is no concern for inflammatory bowel disease or colorectal cancer, many cases of fecal incontinence may be managed conservatively by a nurse practitioner or other advanced practice providers. However, if patients do not

**Table 11.1** Interventions for anal and/or fecal incontinence in pregnancy and postpartum

*Antepartum*

- Dietary modifications
- Physical therapy with biofeedback (no electrical stimulation)
- Over-the-counter products
- Medications
  - Stool bulking agents with fiber supplementation
  - Loperamide
- Previous third- or fourth-degree laceration, history of or current persistent fecal incontinence, abnormal manometry, and/or abnormal endoanal ultrasonography?
  - Use appropriate careful counseling regarding mode of delivery:
    Consider vaginal delivery and with postdelivery plan with physical therapy
    Consider Cesarean delivery

*Intrapartum*

- Vacuum assistance (if operative delivery is clinically indicated)
- Avoid forceps
- Mediolateral episiotomy (if operative delivery is clinically indicated)
- Avoid midline episiotomy (especially if operative assisted vaginal delivery is anticipated)

*Postpartum*

- Dietary modifications
- Physical therapy with biofeedback
- Electrical stimulation
- Over-the-counter products
- Medication Management
  - Stool bulking agent with fiber supplementation
  - Loperamide
- Sacral neuromodulation
- Surgical intervention with anal sphincteroplasty

respond to treatment within 3–4 months, referral to a specialist is warranted. In the event of new-onset fecal incontinence, women may need initial evaluation by a specialist in the area. They may benefit from endoanal ultrasound or endoscopic evaluation. If physical therapy, biofeedback, and/or electrical stimulation are desired as treatment options, a physical therapist and/or advanced practice provider may provide these services. In the setting of fecal incontinence with suspected anal sphincter injury, referral to a specialist is also warranted, as these women may benefit from anal sphincteroplasty or sacral neuromodulation (see Table 11.1).

## 11.18 Multidisciplinary Interventions

One may also consider referral to a dietician and/or nutritionist for evaluation and management of potential dietary contributions to fecal incontinence. In the event that anal and/or fecal incontinence persists despite conservative treatment options, referral to gastroenterology and/or a urogynecologist or colorectal surgeon may be considered to evaluate for other etiologies. Colonoscopy may be considered if there is a significant change in bowel habits, bloody stool, abdominal pain, or weight loss. Fecal incontinence without awareness is a predominant symptom that warrants additional neurologic evaluation.

## 11.19  Innovations

Another new device, currently in clinical trials, is a vaginal bowel control system, Eclipse™, which consists of a balloon that is inserted into the vagina and an inflation pump [57]. Once inflated, the balloon prevents fecal incontinence by pressing the vaginal wall into the rectal space and occluding the rectum [57]. One trial, the LIFE study, has demonstrated the device to provide significant improvement in quality of life and reduction in fecal incontinence episodes [57]. The device is currently being evaluated in another multicenter clinical trial, LIBERATE, for safety, durability, and effectiveness after 3 and 12 months of use [57]. Please see Chap. 6 for more information.

### Conclusion

There are many proposed theories regarding the etiology of anal and fecal incontinence during pregnancy and the postpartum period [3]. In the postpartum period, the most accepted theory is occurrence secondary to obstetrical anal sphincter injuries, either overt or clinically diagnosed and occult, or sonographically diagnosed in those with fecal incontinence [3]. Early identification and treatment may help to improve quality of life for women suffering from anal and/or fecal incontinence. Box 11.3 lists key points to consider. Conservative measures should also be used in initial management if there is no suspicion for inflammatory bowel disease or colorectal cancer. Various treatment options have been suggested, including physical therapy with or without biofeedback and/or electrical stimulation, dietary modifications, medication management, and intrapartum modifications, such as the use of vacuum assistance versus forceps, when clinically indicated, and use of mediolateral episiotomy versus midline episiotomy, when clinically indicated. Other treatments include postpartum surveillance and management in specialized perineal clinics and sacral neuromodulation. For women with fecal incontinence and clinical or sonographic evidence of anal sphincter defect, anal sphincteroplasty continues to be a common treatment option. The choice of treatment should be decided and agreed upon between patient and provider and also take into account the safety of treatment options during the antepartum period and in consideration of potential lactation.

**Box 11.3: Key Points**
- Fecal incontinence or anal incontinence that is first noted in the postpartum period may be related to overt or occult anal sphincter injury [3].
- A thorough history and targeted physical examination can help elucidate etiology [27].
- If there is no apparent evidence of obstetrical anal sphincter injuries on examination or targeted testing, consider and rule out inflammatory bowel disease and colorectal cancer [27, 43].
- Women who sustain obstetrical anal sphincter injuries and/or develop fecal incontinence postpartum should be referred to a perineal clinic where multidisciplinary care can be implemented [6].
- Mode of future delivery post-obstetrical anal sphincter injuries with or without fecal incontinence should be thoroughly discussed by an obstetric care provider and a urogynecologist or other specialists with knowledge of the available data, who can provide risks and benefits to alternatives.
- Referral to a neurologist should be considered if new-onset fecal incontinence is noted during pregnancy, especially in nulliparous women.

Box 11.4 describes a case study about fecal incontinence associated with a cloacal-like defect and a rectovaginal fistula, requiring surgical intervention and highlights the role of the advanced practice nurse in management of such incontinence.

**Box 11.4: Case Study 1**
Mrs. Jones is a 30-year-old female, gravida 1, para 1, referred by her obstetrician to a urogynecology office specializing in female pelvic medicine and reconstructive surgery (FPMRS) for potential anal sphincter repair. She had a spontaneous vaginal delivery about 3 months ago with subsequent episiotomy with extension into the rectum. She presented with complaints of fecal incontinence since this event, as well as fecal urgency and difficulty cleaning after defecation, using up to two rolls of toilet paper sometimes.

The advanced practice nurse conducted a thorough detailed health history through collection of questionnaires and verbal review and questioning. A Modified Manchester Health Questionnaire was administered. Upon review of Modified Manchester Health Questionnaire, the patient demonstrated that her bowel problem "always" affects her life, limits her physical activities, limits her social life, "often" affects her relationship with her spouse and family life, "always" makes her anxious, depressed, and makes her feel bad about herself. Additionally, she indicated that even though she had resumed sexual intercourse by 10 weeks postpartum, she would sometimes have flatus incontinence during sexual activity and that her flatus and fecal symptoms interfered with her desire to have intercourse with her partner.

Original physical examination was conducted by the advanced practice nurse and followed by physical examination by a medical doctor/surgeon in the field of female pelvic medicine and reconstructive surgery. Physical examination revealed a genital hiatus of 2 cm with no perineal body. Only vaginal wall was noted between the vaginal and anal opening. On rectal examination, an anterior anal divet was felt and tender to palpation. A small amount of blood was noted in what appeared to be a pinpoint defect in the distal midline vagina, just above the hymen. No prolapse was visualized.

Diagnosis of cloacal-like defect and anovaginal fistula was made. Patient was subsequently scheduled for an endoanal sonography to visualize extent of anal sphincter muscle defect. She elected for surgical intervention with anal sphincteroplasty and perineal reconstruction. Expectations and complications were discussed, including risk for breakdown, infection, and dyspareunia. The patient desires to proceed with surgery.

Postoperatively, the advanced practice nurse may assist in the inspection of the surgical site prior to discharge, assessing for any sign of infection. Usually, the surgeon will also desire to inspect the surgical site prior to patient discharge, as well.

The advance practice nurse preparing a patient for postoperative discharge educates the patient regarding the following:

- The procedure that was performed and expectations of recovery.
- Signs and symptoms of potential infection or breakdown of the surgical site, including fever, redness, and increased pain from day to day.
- Perineal care with a peri-bottle to clean perineum and educate on the importance of keeping the perineum dry. Pads may be worn for perineal hygiene.
- Avoidance of constipation by slowly advancing the diet, adding bulking agents with fiber into the diet, and avoiding narcotics, if possible. Additionally, education regarding stool softeners may assist in soft stool transit after procedure. One may consider a low residue diet, as well.

The advanced practice nurse will reassess another Modified Manchester Health Questionnaire at 6–8 weeks post-op, when the patient is able to resume normal activity and assess for fecal symptoms, as well as impact on quality of life and sexual function. In any case, the aim is to treat the underlying cause of the fecal and flatus incontinence in hope of improving quality of life, self-perception of body image, and sexual function.

Box 11.5 describes a case study about fecal incontinence associated with loose stools, which presented several years after child birthing. The case study addresses the role of the advanced practice nurse in management of fecal incontinence several years postpartum in the presence of an anterior anal sphincter defect.

**Box 11.5: Case Study 2**
Mrs. Smith is a gravida 4, para 4, 60-year-old female, status post-vaginal hysterectomy with bladder prolapse repair. She presented to clinic with original complaint of bladder prolapse. Upon presentation, she also reported anal incontinence with liquid stool about once a week. She reported that she takes loperamide, one to two tablets as needed to help with liquid stools. Other complaints included dyspareunia secondary to vaginal dryness and mixed urinary incontinence with predominant stress urinary incontinence. Medical history is significant for breast cancer with history of radiation and oral tamoxifen therapy. She also has history of rheumatoid arthritis, diverticulitis, and hypertension. Family history is significant for mother with ovarian cancer.

Pelvic examination was conducted by the advanced practice nurse and physician. Examination revealed a positive cough stress test with vaginal vault prolapse involving stage 1 apical, stage 2 posterior wall, and stage 3 anterior wall prolapse. She leaked urine with both Valsalva and cough maneuvers with prolapse reduced. Pelvic floor muscles were non-tender on examination. The patient underwent urodynamic testing by the advanced practice continence nurse, which demonstrated low-volume stress urinary incontinence with intrinsic sphincter deficiency. The patient proceeded to have robotic-assisted laparoscopic sacral colpopexy with laparoscopic bilateral salpingo-oophorectomy, retropubic exploration with removal of two prolene sutures, retropubic midurethral sling with mesh, and cystourethroscopy with bladder wall biopsy, which resulted negative for malignancy.

Her postoperative course was complicated by an emergency department (ED) visit with 23-h observation for nausea, vomiting, decreased oral intake, and concern for constipation versus ileus versus obstruction. She was discharged postoperative day 2. On postoperative day 6, she required an enema to stimulate a small bowel movement, but she continued to develop worsening abdominal pain. She proceeded to take over-the-counter magnesium citrate but vomited. She presented to the emergency department on post-op day 14. CT scan supported a diagnosis of constipation. The patient was instructed to take milk of magnesia, mineral oil, and fleet enema, as well as minimize narcotic use and anticholinergic medications. Sodium was also replaced. She was discharged on post-op day 15.

At her 4-month post-op visit, the patient's concern shifted to her fecal incontinence symptoms. Pelvic examination revealed stage 2 posterior wall prolapse, again with a positive dovetail sign. Rectal tone and contraction were both 3/5. No masses were palpated upon anorectal examination. The advanced practice nurse instructed her to modify her diet to eat a "bowel recipe" (see Sect. 11.10.3) and avoid artificial additives, such as Splenda, which the patient consumed on a daily basis. The patient also consented to try anal electrical stimulation for fecal incontinence.

At the first electrical stimulation visit, the patient reported baseline symptoms of fecal incontinence with loose or mushy stools. She complained that daily Imodium caused her constipation. She reported difficulty achieving good consistency of stool. Sometimes fecal incontinence would occur with fecal urgency, but at other times, fecal seepage would be unconscious. The advanced practice nurse performed anal electrical stimulation at 50 Hz for 30-min sessions for 6 weekly sessions 1 week apart. Amplitudes ranged from 20% to 40%, often increasing at least twice per session. Rectal tug was visualized with stimulation at each visit. At the first electrical stimulation session, the advanced practice nurse reinforced that the patient try the "bowel recipe" diet. She also instructed the patient to take 1 tablet (2 mg) of Imodium every other day or half a tablet daily or to take a probiotic daily.

The patient noticed immediate improvement the first week after the first electrical stimulation session. With subsequent sessions, the patient experienced relief for 5–6 days/week and was able to cut Imodium use down to 1–2 times/week. The patient ordered a home electrical stimulation unit, and the advanced practice nurse instructed her on use at home with recommendation to use for 30 min/day, 2–3 days/week or as tolerated for symptom relief. At her 4-month follow-up, she reported she was down to only having to use Imodium one to two times a month as needed. She reported great improvement in fecal incontinence with home electrical stimulation two to three times/ week and noticed greater improvement with three times/week. She reported that she forgot it on vacation and noticed a big difference and increase in her symptoms when she did not use her home unit at least two to three times/ week. Anorectal examination revealed rectal tone and contraction of 3/5 still. She is now using home electrical stimulation with success and is on an annual follow-up schedule.

## References

1. Bliss DZ, Mimura T, Berghmans B, Bharucha A, Chiarioni G, Emmanuel A, et al. Assessment and conservative management of faecal incontinence and quality of life in adults. In: Abrams P, Cardoso L, Wagg A, Wein A, editors. Incontinence. 6th ed. Bristol, UK: International Continence Society; 2017. p. 1993–2085.
2. Quigley EM. Impact of pregnancy and parturition on the anal sphincters and pelvic floor. Best Pract Res Clin Gastroenterol. 2007;21(5):879–91.
3. Chong AK, Hoffman B. Fecal incontinence related to pregnancy. Gastrointest Endosc Clin N Am. 2006;16(1):71–81.
4. van Brummen HJ, Bruinse HW, van de Pol G, Heintz AP, van der Vaart CH. Defecatory symptoms during and after the first pregnancy: prevalences and associated factors. Int Urogynecol J. 2006;17(3):224–30.
5. Dudding TC, Vaizey CJ, Kamm MA. Obstetric anal sphincter injury: incidence, risk factors, and management. Ann Surg. 2008;247(2):224–37.
6. Tin RY, Schulz J, Gunn B, Flood C, Rosychuk RJ. The prevalence of anal incontinence in post-partum women following obstetrical anal sphincter injury. Int Urogynecol J. 2010;21(8):927–32.

7. Pauls RN, Occhino JA, Dryfhout V, Karram MM. Effects of pregnancy on pelvic floor dysfunction and body image; a prospective study. Int Urogynecol J. 2008;19(11):1495–501.
8. Shin GH, Toto EL, Schey R. Pregnancy and postpartum bowel changes: constipation and fecal incontinence. Am J Gastroenterol. 2015;110(4):521–9.
9. Pares D, Martinez-Franco E, Lorente N, Viguer J, Lopez-Negre JL, Mendez JR. Prevalence of fecal incontinence in women during pregnancy: a large cross-sectional study. Dis Colon Rectum. 2015;58(11):1098–103.
10. Olsen IP, Wilsgaard T, Kiserud T. Development of the maternal anal canal during pregnancy and the postpartum period: a longitudinal and functional ultrasound study. Ultrasound Obstet Gynecol. 2012;39(6):690–7.
11. Walters M, Karram M. Urogynecology and reconstructive pelvic surgery. 4th ed. Philadelphia, PA: Saunders; 2015.
12. O'Boyle AL, O'Boyle JD, Magann EF, Rieg TS, Morrison JC, Davis GD. Anorectal symptoms in pregnancy and the postpartum period. J Reprod Med. 2008;53(3):151–4.
13. Svare JA, Hansen BB, Lose G. Prevalence of anal incontinence during pregnancy and 1 year after delivery in a cohort of primiparous women and a control group of nulliparous women. Acta Obstet Gynecol Scand. 2016;95(8):920–5.
14. Law H, Fiadjoe P. Urogynaecological problems in pregnancy. J Obstet Gynaecol. 2012;32(2):109–12.
15. Johannessen HH, Wibe A, Stordahl A, Sandvik L, Morkved S. Anal incontinence among first time mothers—what happens in pregnancy and the first year after delivery? Acta Obstet Gynecol Scand. 2015;94(9):1005–13.
16. Burgio KL, Borello-France D, Richter HE, Fitzgerald MP, Whitehead W, Handa VL, et al. Risk factors for fecal and urinary incontinence after childbirth: the childbirth and pelvic symptoms study. Am J Gastroenterol. 2007;102(9):1998–2004.
17. Abramowitz L, Sobhani I, Ganansia R, Vuagnat A, Benifla JL, Darai E, et al. Are sphincter defects the cause of anal incontinence after vaginal delivery? Results of a prospective study. Dis Colon Rectum. 2000;43(5):590–6.
18. Harvey MA, Pierce M, Alter JE, Chou Q, Diamond P, Epp A, et al. Obstetrical anal sphincter injuries (OASIS): prevention, recognition, and repair. J Obstet Gynaecol Can. 2015;37(12):1131–48.
19. Richter HE, Nager CW, Burgio KL, Whitworth R, Weidner AC, Schaffer J, et al. Incidence and predictors of anal incontinence after obstetric anal sphincter injury in primiparous women. Female Pelvic Med Reconstr Surg. 2015;21(4):182–9.
20. Menees SB. My approach to fecal incontinence: it's all about consistency (stool, that is). Am J Gastroenterol. 2017;112(7):977–80.
21. Heilbrun ME, Nygaard IE, Lockhart ME, Richter HE, Brown MB, Kenton KS, et al. Correlation between levator ani muscle injuries on magnetic resonance imaging and fecal incontinence, pelvic organ prolapse, and urinary incontinence in primiparous women. Am J Obstet Gynecol. 2010;202(5):488.e1–6.
22. Sultan AH, Kamm M, Hudson C, Bartram C. Third degree obstetric anal sphincter tears: risk factors and outcome of primary repair. BMJ. 1994;308(6933):887–91.
23. Kaiser AM. Cloaca-like deformity with faecal incontinence after severe obstetric injury—technique and functional outcome of ano-vaginal and perineal reconstruction with X-flaps and sphincteroplasty. Colorectal Dis. 2008;10(8):827–32.
24. MacArthur C, Glazener CM, Wilson PD, Herbison GP, Gee H, Lang GD, et al. Obstetric practice and faecal incontinence three months after delivery. BJOG. 2001;108(7):678–83.
25. Nygaard IE, Rao SS, Dawson JD. Anal incontinence after anal sphincter disruption: a 30-year retrospective cohort study. Obstet Gynecol. 1997;89(6):896–901.
26. King VG, Boyles SH, Worstell TR, Zia J, Clark AL, Gregory WT. Using the Brink score to predict postpartum anal incontinence. Am J Obstet Gynecol. 2010;203(5):486.e1–5.
27. Hoffman B, Schorge J, Shaffer J, Halvorson L, Bradshaw K, Cunningham F, et al. Gynecology. 2nd ed. New York, NY: McGraw-Hill Companies, Inc.; 2012.

28. Snooks SJ, Setchell M, Swash M, Henry MM. Injury to innervation of pelvic floor sphincter musculature in childbirth. Lancet. 1984;2(8402):546–50.
29. Wietek BM, Hinninghofen H, Jehle EC, Enck P, Franz HB. Asymmetric sphincter innervation is associated with fecal incontinence after anal sphincter trauma during childbirth. Neurourol Urodyn. 2007;26(1):134–9.
30. Guise JM, Morris C, Osterweil P, Li H, Rosenberg D, Greenlick M. Incidence of fecal incontinence after childbirth. Obstet Gynecol. 2007;109(2 Pt 1):281–8.
31. Fitzpatrick M, O'Herlihy C. Short-term and long-term effects of obstetric anal sphincter injury and their management. Curr Opin Obstet Gynecol. 2005;17(6):605–10.
32. Guise JM, Boyles SH, Osterweil P, Li H, Eden KB, Mori M. Does cesarean protect against fecal incontinence in primiparous women? Int Urogynecol J. 2009;20(1):61–7.
33. Fynes M, Donnelly V, Behan M, O'Connell PR, O'Herlihy C. Effect of second vaginal delivery on anorectal physiology and faecal continence: a prospective study. Lancet. 1999;354(9183):983–6.
34. Fitzpatrick M, Harkin R, McQuillan K, O'Brien C, O'Connell PR, O'Herlihy C. A randomised clinical trial comparing the effects of delayed versus immediate pushing with epidural analgesia on mode of delivery and faecal continence. BJOG. 2002;109(12):1359–65.
35. Frudinger A, Halligan S, Spencer JA, Bartram CI, Kamm MA, Winter R. Influence of the subpubic arch angle on anal sphincter trauma and anal incontinence following childbirth. BJOG. 2002;109(11):1207–12.
36. Sultan AH, Kamm MA, Hudson CN, Thomas JM, Bartram CI. Anal-sphincter disruption during vaginal delivery. N Engl J Med. 1993;329(26):1905–11.
37. Corton MM, McIntire DD, Twickler DM, Atnip S, Schaffer JI, Leveno KJ. Endoanal ultrasound for detection of sphincter defects following childbirth. Int Urogynecol J. 2013;24(4):627–35.
38. Harkin R, Fitzpatrick M, O'Connell PR, O'Herlihy C. Anal sphincter disruption at vaginal delivery: is recurrence predictable? Eur J Obstet Gynecol Reprod Biol. 2003;109(2):149–52.
39. Spydslaug A, Trogstad LI, Skrondal A, Eskild A. Recurrent risk of anal sphincter laceration among women with vaginal deliveries. Obstet Gynecol. 2005;105(2):307–13.
40. Elfaghi I, Johansson-Ernste B, Rydhstroem H. Rupture of the sphincter ani: the recurrence rate in second delivery. BJOG. 2004;111(12):1361–4.
41. Pollack J, Nordenstam J, Brismar S, Lopez A, Altman D, Zetterstrom J. Anal incontinence after vaginal delivery: a five-year prospective cohort study. Obstet Gynecol. 2004;104(6):1397–402.
42. Donnelly VS, O'Herlihy C, Campbell DM, O'Connell PR. Postpartum fecal incontinence is more common in women with irritable bowel syndrome. Dis Colon Rectum. 1998;41(5):586–9.
43. Dunphy L, Winland-Brown J, Porter B, Thomas D. Primary care: the art and science of advanced practice nursing. 3rd ed. Philadelphia, PA: F.A. Davis Company; 2011.
44. Hakan T. Lumbar disk herniation presented with cauda equina syndrome in a pregnant woman. J Neurosci Rural Pract. 2012;3(2):197–9.
45. Faltin DL, Boulvain M, Floris LA, Irion O. Diagnosis of anal sphincter tears to prevent fecal incontinence: a randomized controlled trial. Obstet Gynecol. 2005;106(1):6–13.
46. Faltin DL, Boulvain M, Irion O, Bretones S, Stan C, Weil A. Diagnosis of anal sphincter tears by postpartum endosonography to predict fecal incontinence. Obstet Gynecol. 2000;95(5):643–7.
47. Richter HE, Fielding JR, Bradley CS, Handa VL, Fine P, FitzGerald MP, et al. Endoanal ultrasound findings and fecal incontinence symptoms in women with and without recognized anal sphincter tears. Obstet Gynecol. 2006;108(6):1394–401.
48. Wheeler TL 2nd, Richter HE. Delivery method, anal sphincter tears and fecal incontinence: new information on a persistent problem. Curr Opin Obstet Gynecol. 2007;19(5):474–9.
49. Fitzpatrick M, Fynes M, Cassidy M, Behan M, O'Connell PR, O'Herlihy C. Prospective study of the influence of parity and operative technique on the outcome of primary anal sphincter repair following obstetrical injury. Eur J Obstet Gynecol Reprod Biol. 2000;89(2):159–63.
50. Boyle R, Hay-Smith EJ, Cody JD, Morkved S. Pelvic floor muscle training for prevention and treatment of urinary and fecal incontinence in antenatal and postnatal women: a short version Cochrane review. Neurourol Urodyn. 2014;33(3):269–76.
51. Miner PB, Donnelly TC, Read NW. Investigation of mode of action of biofeedback in treatment of fecal incontinence. Dig Dis Sci. 1990;35(10):1291–8.

52. Norton C, Cody JD. Biofeedback and/or sphincter exercises for the treatment of faecal incontinence in adults. Cochrane Database Syst Rev. 2012. https://doi.org/10.1002/14651858. CD002111.pub3.
53. Mathe M, Valancogne G, Atallah A, Sciard C, Doret M, Gaucherand P, et al. Early pelvic floor muscle training after obstetrical anal sphincter injuries for the reduction of anal incontinence. Eur J Obstet Gynecol Reprod Biol. 2016;199:201–6.
54. Vonthein R, Heimerl T, Schwandner T, Ziegler A. Electrical stimulation and biofeedback for the treatment of fecal incontinence: a systematic review. Int J Colorectal Dis. 2013;28(11):1567–77.
55. Eogan M, Daly L, O'Herlihy C. The effect of regular antenatal perineal massage on postnatal pain and anal sphincter injury: a prospective observational study. J Matern Fetal Neonatal Med. 2006;19(4):225–9.
56. Smith LA, Price N, Simonite V, Burns EE. Incidence of and risk factors for perineal trauma: a prospective observational study. BMC Pregnancy Childbirth. 2013;13:59.
57. Meyer I, Richter HE. Evidence-based update on treatments of fecal incontinence in women. Obstet Gynecol Clin North Am. 2016;43(1):93–119.
58. Doughty D. Urinary & fecal incontinence: nursing management. 2nd ed. St. Louis, MO: Mosby, Inc.; 2000.
59. Palmer KR, Corbett CL, Holdsworth CD. Double-blind cross-over study comparing loperamide, codeine and diphenoxylate in the treatment of chronic diarrhea. Gastroenterology. 1980;79(6):1272–5.
60. InfantRisk center health care mobile resource. 2017. Available from: https://www.infantrisk.com/.
61. Musial F, Enck P, Kalveram KT, Erckenbrecht JF. The effect of loperamide on anorectal function in normal healthy men. J Clin Gastroenterol. 1992;15(4):321–4.
62. Farrar D, Tuffnell DJ, Ramage C. Interventions for women in subsequent pregnancies following obstetric anal sphincter injury to reduce the risk of recurrent injury and associated harms. Cochrane Database Syst Rev. 2014. https://doi.org/10.1002/14651858.CD010374.pub2.
63. Kenton K, Brincat C, Mutone M, Brubaker L. Repeat cesarean section and primary elective cesarean section: recently trained obstetrician-gynecologist practice patterns and opinions. Am J Obstet Gynecol. 2005;192(6):1872–5.
64. Scheer I, Thakar R, Sultan AH. Mode of delivery after previous obstetric anal sphincter injuries (OASIS)—a reappraisal? Int Urogynecol J Pelvic Floor Dysfunct. 2009;20(9):1095–101.
65. Fitzpatrick M, Cassidy M, Barassaud ML, Hehir MP, Hanly AM, O'Connell PR, et al. Does anal sphincter injury preclude subsequent vaginal delivery? Eur J Obstet Gynecol Reprod Biol. 2016;198:30–4.
66. Malouf AJ, Norton CS, Engel AF, Nicholls RJ, Kamm MA. Long-term results of overlapping anterior anal-sphincter repair for obstetric trauma. Lancet. 2000;355(9200):260–5.
67. Moya P, Navarro JM, Arroyo A, Lopez A, Ruiz-Tovar J, Calpena R. Sacral nerve stimulation during pregnancy in patients with severe fecal incontinence. Tech Coloproctol. 2013;17(2):245–6.
68. Mahran A, Soriano A, Safwat AS, Hijaz A, Mahajan ST, Trabuco EC, et al. The effect of sacral neuromodulation on pregnancy: a systematic review. Int Urogynecol J. 2017;28:1357–65.
69. Vaccaro C, Clemons JL. Anal sphincter defects and anal incontinence symptoms after repair of obstetric anal sphincter lacerations in primiparous women. Int Urogynecol J Pelvic Floor Dysfunct. 2008;19(11):1503–8.
70. Halverson AL, Hull TL. Long-term outcome of overlapping anal sphincter repair. Dis Colon Rectum. 2002;45(3):345–8.
71. Lo J, Osterweil P, Li H, Mori T, Eden KB, Guise JM. Quality of life in women with postpartum anal incontinence. Obstet Gynecol. 2010;115(4):809–14.
72. Brown S, Gartland D, Perlen S, McDonald E, MacArthur C. Consultation about urinary and faecal incontinence in the year after childbirth: a cohort study. BJOG. 2015;122(7):954–62.
73. Leader-Cramer A, Kenton K, Dave B, Gossett DR, Mueller M, Lewicky-Gaupp C. Factors associated with timing of return to intercourse after obstetric anal sphincter injuries. J Sex Med. 2016;13(10):1523–9.

# Surgical Management of Fecal Incontinence and Implications for Postoperative Nursing Care

**12**

Sarah Abbott and Ronan O'Connell

**Abstract**

Surgical management of fecal incontinence is only considered following comprehensive multidisciplinary assessment and failure of conservative measures to achieve a quality of life acceptable to the client. It is important at the outset to realize that surgical intervention, except in the situation of surgical repair of an acute anal sphincter injury, can rarely restore perfect continence. Realistic expectation of outcomes is essential and requires careful explanation of the underlying causes which are often multifactorial. This chapter explains the common surgical procedures used for treating problems underlying fecal incontinence and the focused postoperative nursing care for the advanced practice continence nurse. Having a general knowledge of the repairs of the surgical procedures and of the indications for and expected outcomes of the surgeries may assist the advanced practice continence nurse in decision-making for patient referrals, postoperative management, and support of the patient. The chapter also discusses innovative and experimental procedures for fecal incontinence currently being investigated.

**Keywords**

Surgery · Postoperative care · Sphincteroplasty · Neuromodulation · Stoma

S. Abbott (✉)
Section of Surgery and Surgical Specialties, University College Dublin,
Belfield, Dublin 4, Ireland
e-mail: sarah.abbott@cdhb.health.nz

R. O'Connell
Section of Surgery and Surgical Specialties, University College Dublin,
Belfield, Dublin 4, Ireland

St. Vincent's University Hospital, Dublin 4, Ireland
e-mail: Ronan.OConnell@ucd.ie

## 12.1   Introduction

A surgical intervention should only be considered when a client understands how surgery may address the deficiencies in the continence mechanism in his/her situation. The authors always explain the results of preoperative investigations including joint viewing of radiological imaging to illustrate the abnormality, usually with the aid of a line diagram.

Surgical intervention is usually only considered in clients with incontinence that significantly interferes with quality of life. How this is determined is highly individual; however, it must be understood that minor soiling or flatal incontinence, however distressing, is not likely to improve. Indeed, there is a risk, particularly with anal sphincter repair and/or rectocele repair, that postoperative wound problems or dyspareunia could result in a worse quality of life. At the other end of the scale, some clients are best served by the recommendation to have a colostomy, an intervention that frequently in hindsight should have been considered much earlier in the client journey.

Surgical interventions can be usefully considered under five headings, sphincter repair, sphincter augmentation, sacral neuromodulation, correction of rectal intussusception, and stoma. The decision regarding which intervention to recommend is based on the nature and severity of symptoms (see Chap. 5), the presence and extent of anal sphincter disruption, the presence of pudendal neuropathy, and the presence or absence of rectal intussusception.

## 12.2   Anal Sphincter Repair and Sphincteroplasty

Anal sphincter repair describes primary repair of the anal sphincter mechanism following trauma, while anal sphincteroplasty describes secondary or delayed reconstruction. In the latter scenario, the anal sphincter injury, usually a third degree obstetric tear, was not appreciated at the time, or the initial primary repair was unsatisfactory.

### 12.2.1  Indications

The most common indication for either procedure is obstetric anal sphincter injury during vaginal delivery. In Western practice, the incidence of overt anal sphincter injury (grade 3 or 4 tear) is low, 3–5% following primiparous delivery; however, when prospectively assessed with endoanal ultrasound, the incidence is higher, perhaps up to 27% in primiparous women. Risk factors include instrumental vaginal delivery, a prolonged second stage of labor, fetal macrosomia, a persistent occiput posterior position of the fetal head, and midline episiotomy [1].

Other mechanisms of anal sphincter injury include blunt or penetrating trauma and, occasionally, anorectal surgery. Specific anorectal procedures associated with a risk of anal sphincter injury include hemorrhoidectomy, anal dilatation, fissurectomy, and fistulotomy. Particular risk factors for incontinence following fistula-in-ano surgery include high or complex fistulae and repeated procedures for recurrent disease.

## 12.2.2 Technique

Guidelines from the Royal College of Obstetricians and Gynaecologists in the UK recommend that obstetric anal sphincter injury repairs should be performed with adequate exposure, lighting, and anesthesia. This often requires transfer from the delivery suite to an operating theater [2]. The traditional repair technique involves direct opposition of the severed external anal sphincter. There is some evidence from a Cochrane review that an overlap repair of the external anal sphincter is associated with a lesser risk of fecal urgency and anal incontinence in the early period of follow-up; however, these conclusions were based on only two small trials, and as such the authors recommended further research evidence [3]. Guidelines from the American College of Obstetricians and Gynecologists state that end-to-end and overlap repairs are both acceptable [4]. There is certainly scope for cooperation and collaboration between obstetric and colorectal colleagues.

Elective anal sphincteroplasty may be undertaken following full oral mechanical bowel preparation or a preoperative enema. An indwelling urinary catheter is inserted, and broad-spectrum intravenous antibiotic prophylaxis is administered prior to skin incision. General anesthesia is preferable, and infiltration of the tissues with local anesthetic with 1:200,000 adrenaline further aids muscle relaxation and improves hemostasis. Patient position is a matter of surgeon preference; however, posterior or posterolateral sphincter defects are best approached with the patient prone with the buttocks strapped apart, while lithotomy may give better access for levatorplasty if this is to be performed in conjunction with a repair of an anterior sphincter defect.

A curvilinear incision is made parallel to the outer edge of the external anal sphincter; to provide adequate access, this usually encompasses 120°–180° of the circumference. The anoderm (and the vagina in the case of an anterior defect in a female) is mobilized from the underlying sphincter mechanism and scar, with mobilization continuing cephalad to the distal edge of the anorectal ring. It is often easiest to begin the dissection of the sphincter mechanism in an area where the planes have not been disrupted by scarring and then progress to the region of scarring. Care is taken to preserve the branches of the pudendal nerves as they enter the external anal sphincter posterolaterally. In most cases dissection of one half of the circumference of the sphincter mechanism is adequate—this wide dissection permits tension-free overlap (see Fig. 12.1).

The scar is then divided and preserved for suture placement. The divided ends are overlapped until such a point that the anal aperture fits snugly over the index finger. Four to six mattress sutures are placed, using a 2/0 synthetic absorbable suture material. There must be a minimal tendency for the divided ends to pull apart reflecting adequate mobilization. Once all sutures are placed, they are pulled tight,

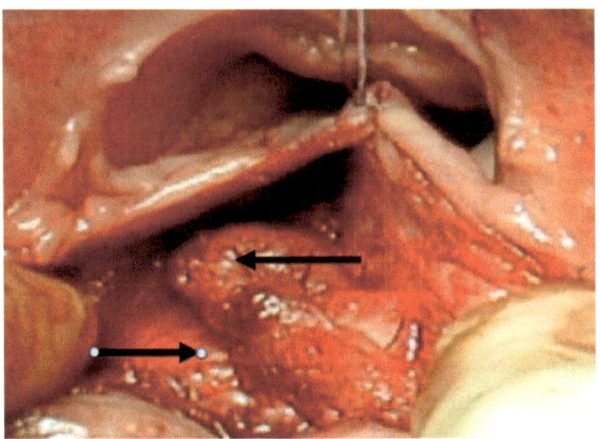

**Fig. 12.1** Overlapping anal sphincteroplasty (arrows). Repair of rectocele and posterior vaginal wall has been performed (elevated by sutures)

and there is a final check of the anal aperture and suture placement prior to tying the sutures. The knots are then covered with reconstitution of the superficial perineal muscles in order to prevent discomfort from or extrusion of the knots.

In the case of an anterior sphincter defect, a levatorplasty may be undertaken prior to the overlapping sphincteroplasty. The transverse perinei muscle and/or scar tissue is approximated to add bulk to the anovaginal area, to increase perineal length and reconstruct the perineal body.

Finally, the wound is closed with either continuous or interrupted 3/0 absorbable suture material. A small opening may be left centrally, or a drain may be placed. A vaginal pack may be inserted to reduce the incidence of vaginal vault hematoma. This is removed along with the urinary catheter on the first postoperative day.

### 12.2.3 Postoperative Nursing Care

Two randomized trials have shown benefit in the use of a laxative rather than a constipating regimen in the setting of anal sphincter repair, with a significantly earlier and less painful first bowel motion [5, 6]. There is also a reduced incidence of postoperative wound dehiscence following repair of a third or fourth degree tear and earlier hospital discharge.

There is a paucity of evidence regarding peri- and postoperative antibiotic use. Given the potential sequelae of an infectious complication, it is perhaps prudent to routinely provide broad-spectrum coverage following anal sphincter repair.

Furthermore, women should be reviewed by a specialist pelvic floor physiotherapist or nurse prior to discharge and receive ongoing follow-up after obstetric anal sphincter injury and anal sphincter repair. Following childbirth, the 6-week postpartum follow-up should include inquiry regarding wound healing, perineal pain, and ongoing continence symptoms and advice regarding resumption of sexual activity. This is often best achieved in a dedicated perineal or pelvic floor clinic [7].

There is considerable variability in postoperative regimens for patients who have undergone sphincteroplasty. Some surgeons recommend a period of oral fluids only for several days to minimize the risk disruption of the repair. Similar variability exists with regard to the use of laxatives, antibiotic use, and length of stay. It is the authors' practice to allow regular diet following surgery and to give regular laxatives to maintain soft bowel movements until the perianal wounds have healed. When possible, opioid analgesia should be avoided due to constipating effects.

Management of subsequent childbirth must consider obstetric risk factors, any ongoing symptoms of incontinence, and patient preferences. The evidence supports subsequent vaginal delivery in asymptomatic women after a previously repaired third degree tear; however, the risk of a second obstetric anal sphincter injury is increased to between 3% and 5%. Women with altered continence after first vaginal delivery are at risk of further deterioration if delivered vaginally on their second pregnancy and elective caesarian delivery should be considered [8]. There is no role for delaying sphincteroplasty until a woman has determined her family is complete.

### 12.2.4  Outcomes of Anal Sphincteroplasty

Most patients can expect a significant improvement in continence in the short-term following sphincteroplasty, with a mean of 66% reporting excellent or good results. There is no evidence that a defunctioning colostomy at the time of sphincter repair improves outcome [9].

Early failure is usually associated with a persistent defect identified using endoanal ultrasound. Unfortunately, the initial good results deteriorate in the long term with only 6% reporting excellent or good continence at 10 years as in parallel to the general population of parous women, continence deteriorates with increasing age and menopause in women with a history of a repaired third or fourth degree tear.

### 12.3    Sphincter Augmentation

### 12.3.1  Muscle Transposition Repairs

Non-stimulated and stimulated muscle transposition repairs were devised in the setting of significant tissue loss preventing anal sphincteroplasty or previous failed local repair. Unilateral and bilateral gluteoplasty (utilizing gluteus maximus) or graciloplasty were the most common non-stimulated options. Graciloplasty can be augmented by implantation of an electrical stimulator to augment contraction of the transposed muscle (dynamic graciloplasty). This may be appropriate in the context of extensive loss of sphincter (e.g., as a result of trauma) and in congenital anorectal malformation. Currently, dynamic graciloplasty is not widely used due to the high rate of morbidity and the variable success rates [10].

## 12.4    Neuromodulation

Sacral nerve stimulation, also known as sacral neuromodulation, was first used to treat fecal incontinence by Matzel et al. in 1995 [11]. Posterior tibial nerve stimulation is a more recent development in neuromodulation. The underlying principle is the enhancement of continence by electrical stimulation of the peripheral nerve supply to the anus and rectum. The precise mode of action remains uncertain, but it is likely that the observed clinical outcomes are not solely mediated by the sphincter mechanism alone, but also by central nervous system effects [12]. Objective data regarding the impact on colorectal and anal function are contradictory in part and are not entirely reproducible.

### 12.4.1 Indications

Initial trials only included those patients with an anatomically intact sphincter but functionally deficient mechanism. It has now apparent that a variety of conditions leading to fecal incontinence can be treated with sacral nerve stimulation. Patients may be selected for permanent sacral nerve stimulation based on the results of an initial percutaneous nerve evaluation.

Various studies have attempted to identify factors to predict which patients will have good symptom improvement with neuromodulation. Age, the presence of an extensive external anal sphincter defect, and an initial failure with a need for repeat procedures may correlate with a poor outcome with percutaneous nerve evaluation. Other studies have found no difference in outcome related to the extent of sphincter defect, but some have documented that stool consistency and stimulation intensity may influence outcome. A large multicenter study did not identify any determinants of success with permanent sacral nerve stimulation, other than confirming a lower failure rate in the long term in those patients with a significant reduction in incontinence scores with test stimulation [13].

There are a number of case series or case reports supporting the use of sacral nerve stimulation in fecal incontinence in a variety of other clinical scenarios including muscular dystrophy, proctocolectomy and ileal pouch-anal anastomosis, neurological dysfunction including spinal disk prolapse, rectal resection for rectal carcinoma, after neoadjuvant and adjuvant chemoradiotherapy or radiotherapy for endometrial and anorectal carcinoma, rectal prolapse repair, unilateral traumatic pudendal neuropathy, spina bifida, and external anal sphincter atrophy.

Various contraindications to sacral nerve stimulation also exist, including pathological conditions of the sacrum preventing electrode placement (e.g., spina bifida), skin disease at the area of implantation, anal sphincter damage requiring a sphincter substitute, pregnancy, bleeding diatheses, psychological instability, and inadequate cognitive capacity. Current models are not compatible with magnetic resonance imaging; however, a newer compatible model is on the horizon. The presence of an implantable defibrillator or cardiac pacemaker is a relative contraindication.

## 12.4.2 Technique

Sacral nerve stimulation is a two-stage procedure with an initial percutaneous nerve evaluation prior to implantation of the permanent device. The trial period lasts from 1 to 3 weeks. Success is commonly defined as a 50% decrease in the frequency of incontinence episodes and reversibility of this improvement upon discontinuation of stimulation. The authors' practice is to restrict permanent device implantation to those with ≥80% improvement in symptoms as this improves the long-term success rates.

There are two options for percutaneous nerve evaluation, either a temporary percutaneously placed unipolar test lead (which is subsequently removed) or a quadripolar lead (usually a "tined lead"), which, if the trial is effective, can remain in place for permanent stimulation. The lead is connected to an external pulse generator for the duration of the trial.

The second stage involves implantation of the permanent electrode (if a temporary unipolar test lead has been used) and pulse generator. This may be performed under general anesthesia without muscle relaxation or under local anesthesia with or without sedation. Intravenous antibiotic prophylaxis and strict aseptic technique are imperative. The patient is positioned prone with the buttocks strapped apart to enable visualization of the perineum. Under image intensification guidance, the permanent electrode is inserted, usually via the S3 foramina as this level seems to be the most effective (compared to S2 or S4). It is optimal to have the electrodes at the anterior table of the sacrum, ideally following the path of the nerve root on a slightly lateral course (see Fig. 12.2). Plantarflexion of the great toe and contraction of the

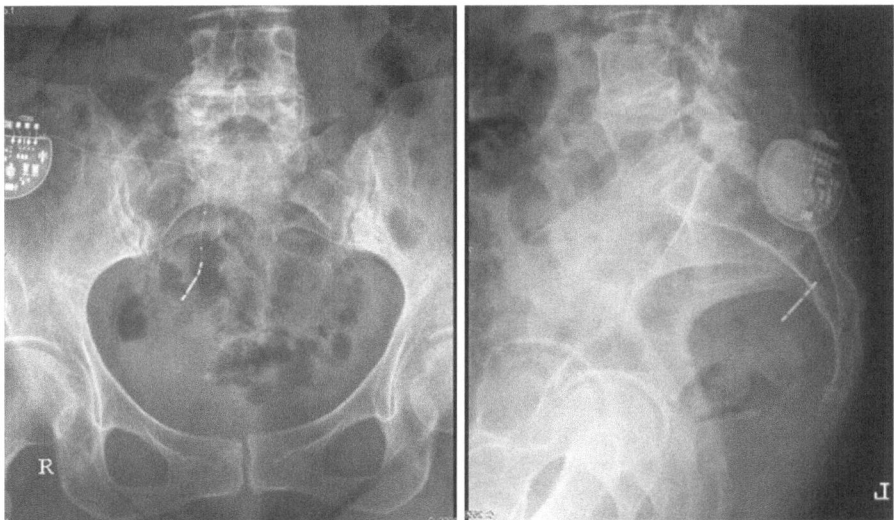

**Fig. 12.2** Anterior and lateral views of a quadripolar sacral nerve stimulation lead inserted into the left S3 foramen, following the course of the nerve (reproduced with permission, Medtronic Inc.)

pelvic floor and external anal sphincter are witnessed on stimulation of the electrode. There is no additional benefit to bilateral placement.

The pulse generator is placed in a subcutaneous pocket, usually in the gluteal region, or occasionally in the abdominal wall (see Fig. 12.2). The electrode lead is tunneled subcutaneously to the generator. A small handheld "patient programmer" contains four preset stimulation protocols, which can be adjusted. These protocols use different combinations of the four electrodes present at the tip as cathode and anode to optimize nerve root stimulation. Amplitude, pulse width, and rate can also be adjusted, although the latter two are usually constant. The patient programmer can also deactivate the device. From time to time, the pulse generator will need replacement, usually at 5–7-year intervals. This will be more frequent in patients with higher amplitude settings. In the near future, rechargeable devices will be available that use transcutaneous current induction technology.

### 12.4.3 Postoperative Nursing Care

Both stages of the procedure are day cases. Following the initial percutaneous nerve evaluation procedure, it is imperative that the patient keeps the surgical site dry. The patient must keep a diary of symptoms, which will be reviewed in the outpatient clinic and will influence the decision as to whether or not permanent sacral nerve stimulation is indicated. If a temporary unipolar test lead is used, this is simply removed in the outpatient clinic at the end of the trial period. After implantation of the permanent electrode and pulse generator, it is similarly important that the patient keeps the surgical sites clean and dry until they are healed. The responsible clinician, a clinical nurse specialist, or a representative from pulse generator company provides patient education and support regarding programming of the device.

### 12.4.4 Outcomes

A meta-analysis published by Tan et al. [14] considered studies of sacral nerve stimulation performed for fecal incontinence published between 1995 and 2008. Thirty-four studies were included, with 665 patients undergoing permanent sacral nerve stimulation after an initial 944 underwent percutaneous nerve evaluation. With permanent sacral nerve stimulation, weekly incontinence episodes and incontinence scores were significantly reduced, while the ability to defer defecation was significantly increased. Furthermore, most fecal incontinence-related quality of life domains were improved. The results were similar between the subgroups of those with an intact sphincter and an impaired sphincter. The complication rate was 15%, with 3% of patients requiring permanent explantation.

A Cochrane review was subsequently published in 2015. Four crossover trials and two parallel group trials were evaluated. The authors concluded that, in the setting of limited evidence, sacral nerve stimulation can improve continence in a proportion of patients with fecal incontinence, but that adverse events can occur. A recommendation was made for further high-quality randomized trials to more fully assess the effects of sacral nerve stimulation [15].

Multiple studies support an improvement in quality of life with sacral nerve stimulation. This is most evident when disease-specific quality of life instruments are applied. In a meta-analysis, the SF-36 was significantly increased in all categories except bodily pain across seven studies with 98–102 patients. The Fecal Incontinence Quality of Life (FIQL) score was similarly significantly increased in all categories across nine studies with 199 patients [14].

There is increasing evidence to support the use of sacral nerve stimulation in those with fecal incontinence with an anatomical defect in the sphincter mechanism, either unrepaired or after an attempted repair. However, there is no randomized trial that compares anal sphincteroplasty with sacral nerve stimulation as the primary treatment in patients with an anal external sphincter defect. Furthermore, there are relatively few data concerning the size of anal sphincter defect that should be considered for repair ahead of sacral nerve stimulation. External sphincter lesions up to 180° have been treated. A systematic review of 106 patients with a confirmed external and/or internal anal sphincter lesion on ultrasound, who subsequently received permanent sacral nerve stimulation after percutaneous nerve evaluation, demonstrated a significant reduction in incontinent episodes per week and (when evaluated) a significant increase in ability to defer defecation coupled with improvement in quality of life [16].

Sacral nerve stimulation is relatively safe. The majority of adverse events (67%) occur within the first year, with most requiring minimal or no intervention [17]. Device explantation is required in approximately 5%, due to loss of effect, symptom deterioration, pain from lead dislocation, or infection. Reimplantation may be possible at a later date.

## 12.4.5 Posterior Tibial Nerve Stimulation

Percutaneous posterior tibial nerve stimulation for the treatment of fecal incontinence was first described by Shafik et al. in 2003 [18] and was later followed by the less invasive transcutaneous approach. The former utilizes an electrode needle, while the latter involves an adhesive electrode pad placed over the posterior tibial nerve.

Thin et al. conducted a randomized pilot trial of posterior tibial nerve stimulation versus sacral nerve stimulation, with 23 patients randomized to receive sacral nerve stimulation and 17 to posterior tibial nerve stimulation. Fifteen patients progressed to permanent sacral nerve stimulation implantation, and 16 received a full course of posterior tibial nerve stimulation. Both groups experienced some clinical improvement (mean CCIS at baseline and 6 months: 16.2 and 10.4 for sacral nerve stimulation versus 15.1 and 12.1 for posterior tibial nerve stimulation) [19].

A further randomized controlled trial of posterior tibial nerve stimulation versus sham electrical stimulation (the CONFIDeNT trial) involved 227 patients with fecal incontinence who had failed conservative treatments. The authors demonstrated a similar rate of $\geq 50\%$ reduction in weekly fecal incontinence episodes across the two groups (38% in posterior tibial nerve stimulation arm versus 31% in sham arm). No significant differences were noted in the St. Mark's Incontinence Score or any quality of life measure [20]. Van der Wilt et al. have recently compared posterior tibial nerve stimulation with sham stimulation in 59 patients and found some improvement in the proportion of patients achieving 50% in the number of incontinence episodes per week [21].

These recent publications are slightly conflicting and make the role of posterior tibial nerve stimulation in the management of fecal incontinence unclear. Further high-quality studies with appropriate comparison groups and clinically meaningful outcomes measures will help to establish this treatment's utility.

### 12.4.6  Nursing Care

As part of the multidisciplinary care team, the advanced practice nurse would assess for healing of the surgical site and evaluate effectiveness of neuromodulation and change in the patient's quality of life at follow-up.

## 12.5  Correction of Intussusception

### 12.5.1  Indications

Structural causes of impaired evacuation, such as rectocele or internal rectal prolapse, may contribute to fecal incontinence. In the former, there may be trapping of fecal material with straining with subsequent leakage upon return to a resting position. In the latter, prolapse of the rectal mucosa into or beyond the anal canal may effectively compromise anal closure resulting in leakage.

It is important to consider these conditions in patients presenting with fecal incontinence as their contribution to the patient's presentation may be overlooked without appropriate clinical examination and radio-physiological studies. Similarly, patients with obstructive defecation symptoms should also be assessed for fecal incontinence.

The most commonly performed procedure for rectal intussusception is a ventral mesh rectopexy.

### 12.5.2  Technique

A detailed description of the procedure is beyond the scope of this chapter. The procedure lends itself well to a minimally invasive approach (laparoscopic or robotic). The key principles include incision of the right lateral peritoneum, dissection in the rectovaginal septum to the level of the pelvic floor, excision of the redundant peritoneum of the pouch of Douglas, fixation of the lower anterior rectum to the sacral promontory with synthetic or biologic mesh, and finally closure of the peritoneum over the prosthetic implant. It has been shown to be a safe procedure, even in the elderly.

### 12.5.3  Postoperative Nursing Care

Patients may spend one to two nights as an inpatient. It is important to avoid straining in the early postoperative period. After the initial recovery, ongoing monitoring is important for mesh-related complications (mesh erosion in particular), although these are rare and tend to occur within the first 2 years of the procedure.

### 12.5.4  Outcomes

A large multicenter observational study of 919 consecutive patients with either external rectal prolapse or high-grade internal rectal prolapse (Oxford grade III/IV) who underwent laparoscopic ventral mesh rectopexy demonstrated an improvement in fecal incontinence (37.5% vs. 11.1%, $P < 0.0001$). The mesh-related complication rate was acceptable at 4.6% [22].

Several smaller observational studies have confirmed this benefit, with objective reductions in severity scores, and some also demonstrated an improvement in the quality of life.

## 12.6    Stoma

Formation of a permanent colostomy is often viewed as the last resort and undertaken when all other interventions have failed. Despite these negative connotations, it may offer a successful management strategy for the patient with a return of independence and full social function.

### 12.6.1  Indications

The American Society of Colon and Rectal Surgeons' clinical practice guidelines for the treatment of fecal incontinence published in 2015 stated: "creation of a colostomy is an excellent surgical option for patients who have failed or do not wish to pursue other therapies for fecal incontinence" [23].

The American College of Gastroenterology clinical guideline for the management of benign anorectal disorders published in 2014 stated: "colostomy is a last resort procedure that can markedly improve the quality of life in a patient with severe or intractable fecal incontinence" [24].

## 12.6.2 Technique

In the setting of refractory fecal incontinence, the usual procedure of choice is an end sigmoid colostomy without proctectomy. This can be performed laparoscopically if safe and appropriate. The patient may be discharged from hospital once they are confident and competent in care of the stoma. A patient may occasionally require a proctectomy for symptoms such as mucous leakage, due to diversion colitis.

## 12.6.3 Postoperative Nursing Care

Stoma therapy nurses are experts in the pre- and postoperative counseling and care of the ostomate. An end sigmoid colostomy formed for refractory fecal incontinence is prone to the usual longer-term stomal complications such as a parastomal hernia, prolapse, retraction, and stenosis.

## 12.6.4 Outcomes

In view of the fact that formation of a colostomy is regarded as a failure of treatment, and therefore is not frequently performed, its effectiveness, perioperative complication rate, and its impact on patient quality of life have not been thoroughly studied.

Colquhoun et al. undertook a cross-sectional postal survey comparing quality of life in 71 patients with fecal incontinence and 39 patients with a colostomy. The indications for colostomy formation included rectal carcinoma, complicated diverticular disease, and fecal incontinence. Analysis of the SF-36 revealed higher social function score in the colostomy group, while the Fecal Incontinence Quality of Life scale demonstrated higher scores in the coping and embarrassment scales in the colostomy group, with a trend to higher scores in the lifestyle and depression scales. The authors concluded that colostomy is a viable option in patients with fecal incontinence, offering improved quality of life [25].

Finally, Norton et al. performed a questionnaire survey of patients with a colostomy which had been formed for fecal incontinence. Patients were recruited via an advertisement in the British Colostomy Association magazine and through the hospital database, with 69 patient responses obtained. Most patients felt that the stoma restricted their life "a little" or "not at all." The majority (84%) would "probably" or "definitely" choose to have a stoma again. Respondents rated their quality of life as much better overall than compared to when they suffered fecal incontinence [26].

## 12.7   Innovations

Many of the innovative strategies to be discussed in this section of the chapter are yet to gain universal approval and remain investigational or experimental as robust evidence in terms of feasibility, safety, cost-effectiveness, durability, and reproducibility is lacking.

## 12.7.1 Artificial Sphincter

At least two artificial bowel sphincter systems have been proposed over time: the artificial bowel sphincter (ABS), Acticon™ Neosphincter, and the magnetic anal sphincter reinforcement (MAS), Fenix™.

The ABS Neosphincter consists of an inflatable silicone cuff which is placed around the upper anal canal, and tubing is directed along the perineum and connected to a pump in the scrotum or labium. Further tubing connects the pump to a pressure-regulating balloon implanted in the prevesical space. The pump facilitates fluid to pass from the balloon to the cuff and vice versa. The primary concern with this device is infection, with reported rates of 20–45%. Infection and cuff perforation, reflecting the intrinsic "wear and tear," are the chief indications for explanation, with rates of up to 72%. The device is no longer commercially available.

The MAS Fenix™ is designed to augment the native anal sphincter mechanism. The dynamic circular implant is placed around the anorectal junction and consists of a series of individually linked titanium beads with magnetic cores. The magnetic beads separate temporarily with straining during defecation and magnetically self-retract afterward. The device is manufactured in different lengths based on the number of beads and is provided with a sizing tool. Most recently, Sugrue et al. have reported long-term outcomes from a multicenter cohort study. Thirty-five patients underwent magnetic anal sphincter augmentation with a median length of follow-up of 5 years. Eight patients underwent a subsequent operation secondary to device failure or complications, seven of which occurred in the first year. Therapeutic success rates were 53% at year 5. In those patients who retained their device, the number of incontinent episodes per week and Cleveland Clinic Incontinence Scale (CCIS) scores significantly decreased from baseline, with simultaneous improvement in all four scales on the Fecal Incontinence Quality of Life instrument. Adverse events were however relatively common (30 events in 20 patients), with defecatory dysfunction, pain, erosion, and infection being the most prevalent [27]. The device is currently not commercially available.

## 12.7.2 Injectable Biomaterials

Injectable agents have the advantage of being able to be implanted as an outpatient procedure, potentially without general anesthesia. The ideal agent should be biocompatible, non-allergenic, non-immunogenic, non-carcinogenic, and easy to inject and should not migrate within the tissues. There has been recent interest in solid agents such as GateKeeper™ [28] and SphinKeeper™ [29] which expand after their insertion. Injection of liquid bulk-enhancing agents has declined in popularity in recent times.

Agents include polydimethylsiloxane particles (PDMS) suspended in a bioexcretable carrier hydrogel of polyvinylpyrrolidone (Bioplastique™), cross-linked porcine dermal collagen (PDC, Permacol™), polyacrylamide hydrogel (PAH, Bulkamid®), polydimethylsiloxane elastomer silicone biomaterial (PDMS), calcium hydroxyapatite ceramic microspheres (HCM, Coaptite™), ethylene vinyl alcohol (EVOH), and pyrolytic carbon-coated zirconium oxide beads (PCZO, Durasphere®). Many have been plagued by loss of efficacy with time, and adverse effects include anal pain, infection, mucosal erosion, and material extrusion.

Two systematic reviews and a Cochrane review were not able to establish sufficient evidence to support any of these agents; the optimal bulking agent and technique of application therefore remains to be determined.

### 12.7.3 Radiofrequency Energy Treatment

This technique is thought to cause a degree of scarring or fibrosis of the anal canal, which improves the barrier function; however, recent animal studies have suggested that it induces hyperplasia and hypertrophy of smooth muscle fibers in the internal anal sphincter.

The technique was initially documented in a cohort of ten women by Takahashi et al. There was a statistically significant improvement in the Cleveland Clinic Florida Fecal Incontinence Score (CCF-FIS) in nine of the women (median 13.5–5.0, $P = 0.006$) at 12 months, with a sustained benefit at 2 and 5 years follow-up. A larger multicenter study also found a significant but less dramatic improvement in CCF-FIS 6 months following treatment ($14.5–11.1$, $P < 0.001$) [30]. Several further studies confirmed moderate benefit, with a couple questioning the longevity of the benefits induced by the technique.

### 12.7.4 Stem Cell Therapy

In the future, we may find that a biocompatible regeneration of tissue and consequent restoration of its function provides the optimal solution. Two groups have reported on the use of autologous myoblasts, and another group has engineered an internal anal sphincter using a chitosan scaffold, mature smooth muscle, and neuronal progenitor cells harvested during surgery. The possibilities are exciting; however, considerable research remains to be done.

### References

1. Donnelly V, Fynes M, Campbell D, Johnson H, O'Connell PR, O'Herlihy C. Obstetric events leading to anal sphincter damage. Obstet Gynecol. 1998;92(6):955–61.
2. Royal College of Obstetricians and Gynaecologists. The management of third and fourth degree perineal tears 2015. https://www.rcog.org.uk/globalassets/documents/guidelines/gtg-29.pdf.
3. Fernando R, Sultan AH, Kettle C, Thakar R, Radley S. Methods of repair for obstetric anal sphincter injury. Cochrane Database Syst Rev. 2006. https://doi.org/10.1002/14651858. CD002866.pub2.

4. American College of Obstetricians and Gynecologists Committee on Practice Bulletins. Practice Bulletin No. 165: prevention and management of obstetric lacerations at vaginal delivery. Obstet Gynecol. 2016;128(1):e1–e15.
5. Mahony R, Behan M, O'Herlihy C, O'Connell PR. Randomized, clinical trial of bowel confinement vs. laxative use after primary repair of a third-degree obstetric anal sphincter tear. Dis Colon Rectum. 2004;47(1):12–7.
6. Eogan M, Daly L, Behan M, O'Connell PR, O'Herlihy C. Randomised clinical trial of a laxative alone versus a laxative and a bulking agent after primary repair of obstetric anal sphincter injury. BJOG. 2007;114(6):736–40.
7. Fitzpatrick M, Cassidy M, O'Connell PR, O'Herlihy C. Experience with an obstetric perineal clinic. Eur J Obstet Gynecol Reprod Biol. 2002;100(2):199–203.
8. Fynes M, Donnelly V, Behan M, O'Connell PR, O'Herlihy C. Effect of second vaginal delivery on anorectal physiology and faecal continence: a prospective study. Lancet. 1999;354(9183):983–6.
9. Bravo Gutierrez A, Madoff RD, Lowry AC, Parker SC, Buie WD, Baxter NN. Long-term results of anterior sphincteroplasty. Dis Colon Rectum. 2004;47(5):727–31.
10. Chapman AE, Geerdes B, Hewett P, Young J, Eyers T, Kiroff G, et al. Systematic review of dynamic graciloplasty in the treatment of faecal incontinence. Br J Surg. 2002;89(2):138–53.
11. Matzel KE, Stadelmaier U, Hohenfellner M, Gall FP. Electrical stimulation of sacral spinal nerves for treatment of faecal incontinence. Lancet. 1995;346(8983):1124–7.
12. Carrington EV, Evers J, Grossi U, Dinning PG, Scott SM, O'Connell PR, et al. A systematic review of sacral nerve stimulation mechanisms in the treatment of fecal incontinence and constipation. Neurogastroenterol Motil. 2014;26(9):1222–37.
13. Maeda Y, Norton C, Lundby L, Buntzen S, Laurberg S. Predictors of the outcome of percutaneous nerve evaluation for faecal incontinence. Br J Surg. 2010;97(7):1096–102.
14. Tan E, Ngo N-T, Darzi A, Shenouda M, Tekkis PP. Meta-analysis: sacral nerve stimulation versus conservative therapy in the treatment of faecal incontinence. Int J Colorectal Dis. 2011;26(3):275–94.
15. Thaha MA, Abukar AA, Thin NN, Ramsanahie A, Knowles CH. Sacral nerve stimulation for faecal incontinence and constipation in adults. Cochrane Database Syst Rev. 2015. https://doi.org/10.1002/14651858.CD004464.pub3.
16. Ratto C, Litta F, Parello A, Donisi L, De Simone V, Zaccone G. Sacral nerve stimulation in faecal incontinence associated with an anal sphincter lesion: a systematic review. Colorectal Dis. 2012;14(6):e297–304.
17. Mellgren A, Wexner SD, Coller JA, Devroede G, Lerew DR, Madoff RD, et al. Long-term efficacy and safety of sacral nerve stimulation for fecal incontinence. Dis Colon Rectum. 2011;54(9):1065–75.
18. Shafik A, Ahmed I, El-Sibai O, Mostafa RM. Percutaneous peripheral neuromodulation in the treatment of fecal incontinence. Eur Surg Res. 2003;35(2):103–7.
19. Thin NN, Taylor SJ, Bremner SA, Emmanuel AV, Hounsome N, Williams NS, et al. Randomized clinical trial of sacral versus percutaneous tibial nerve stimulation in patients with faecal incontinence. Br J Surg. 2015;102(4):349–58.
20. Horrocks EJ, Bremner SA, Stevens N, Norton C, Gilbert D, O'Connell PR, et al. Double-blind randomised controlled trial of percutaneous tibial nerve stimulation versus sham electrical stimulation in the treatment of faecal incontinence: CONtrol of Faecal Incontinence using Distal NeuromodulaTion (the CONFIDeNT trial). Health Technol Assess. 2015;19(77):1–164.
21. van der Wilt AA, Giuliani G, Kubis C, van Wunnik BPW, Ferreira I, Breukink SO, et al. Randomized clinical trial of percutaneous tibial nerve stimulation versus sham electrical stimulation in patients with faecal incontinence. Br J Surg. 2017;104(9):1167–76.
22. Consten ECJ, van Iersel JJ, Verheijen PM, Broeders IAMJ, Wolthuis AM, D'Hoore A. Long-term outcome after laparoscopic ventral mesh rectopexy: an observational study of 919 consecutive patients. Ann Surg. 2015;262(5):742–7.

23. Paquette IM, Varma MG, Kaiser AM, Steele SR, Rafferty JF. The American Society of Colon and Rectal Surgeons' clinical practice guideline for the treatment of fecal incontinence. Dis Colon Rectum. 2015;58(7):623–36.
24. Wald A, Bharucha AE, Cosman BC, Whitehead WE. ACG clinical guideline: management of benign anorectal disorders. Am J Gastroenterol. 2014;109(8):1141–57.
25. Colquhoun P, Kaiser R Jr, Efron J, Weiss EG, Nogueras JJ, Vernava AM 3rd, et al. Is the quality of life better in patients with colostomy than patients with fecal incontience? World J Surg. 2006;30(10):1925–8.
26. Norton C, Burch J, Kamm MA. Patients' views of a colostomy for fecal incontinence. Dis Colon Rectum. 2005;48(5):1062–9.
27. Sugrue J, Lehur P, Madoff RD, McNevin S, Buntzen S, Laurberg S, Mellgren A. Long-term experience of magnetic anal sphincter augmentation in patients with fecal incontinence. Dis Colon Rectum. 2017;60(1):87–95.
28. Ratto C, Buntzen S, Aigner F, Altomare DF, Heydari A, Donisi L, et al. Multicentre observational study of the Gatekeeper for faecal incontinence. Br J Surg. 2016;103(3):290–9.
29. Ratto C, Donisi L, Litta F, Campennì P, Parello A. Implantation of SphinKeeper(TM): a new artificial anal sphincter. Tech Coloproctol. 2016;20(1):59–66.
30. Takahashi T, Garcia-Osogobio S, Valdovinos MA, Belmonte C, Barreto C, Velasco L. Extended two-year results of radio-frequency energy delivery for the treatment of fecal incontinence (the Secca procedure). Dis Colon Rectum. 2003;46(6):711–5.

# Management of Skin Damage Associated with Fecal and Dual Incontinence

13

Mikel Gray, Donna Z. Bliss, and Sheila Howes Trammel

**Abstract**

The skin problems of dermatitis and pressure injury are common sequelae of fecal incontinence. The advanced practice nurse prevents and treats these problems while managing fecal incontinence. This chapter describes the manifestations of incontinence-associated dermatitis and pressure injury and how to make a differential diagnosis and assess their severity. It explains the association of incontinence to pressure injury along with other risk factors. The chapter summarizes the interventions used for prevention and treatment of both skin problems highlighting the expected outcomes for the advanced practice nurse to evaluate.

M. Gray
Department of Urology,
University of Virginia School of Medicine,
Charlottesville, VA, USA

Department of Acute and Specialty Care,
University of Virginia School of Nursing,
Charlottesville, VA, USA
e-mail: mg5k@virginia.edu

D. Z. Bliss (✉)
University of Minnesota School of Nursing,
Minneapolis, MN, USA
e-mail: bliss@umn.edu

S. H. Trammel
Hennepin County Medical Center,
Minneapolis, MN, USA

WEBWOC Nursing Education Program,
Minneapolis, MN, USA

© Springer International Publishing AG, part of Springer Nature 2018
D. Z. Bliss (ed.), *Management of Fecal Incontinence for the Advanced Practice Nurse*,
https://doi.org/10.1007/978-3-319-90704-8_13

## 13.1    Incontinence and Skin Damage

A holistic approach to management of fecal incontinence by the advanced practice nurse encompasses prevention and treatment of associated skin damage. Fecal incontinence is a major risk factor for incontinence-associated dermatitis and pressure injury, including full-thickness injuries [1–3]. This risk is highest in patients with dual fecal and urinary incontinence [4–6]. Inflammation of the skin in the presence of fecal or urinary incontinence is referred to as diaper or nappy dermatitis in infants. In adults it is commonly referred to as incontinence-associated dermatitis; other terms for this condition over time have included perineal dermatitis, moisture lesions, or incontinence-associated skin damage. Incontinence-associated dermatitis is a form of moisture-associated skin damage; this umbrella term is defined as inflammation and erosion of the skin caused by prolonged exposure to various sources of moisture, including urine or stool, perspiration, wound exudate, mucus, or saliva [7]. A pressure injury, historically referred to as a pressure ulcer, pressure sore, or decubitus ulcer, is defined as a localized area of damage to the skin or underlying tissue that occurs in the presence of pressure or pressure in combination with shearing forces [8, 9]. In this chapter, the terms pressure injury and incontinence-associated dermatitis (IAD) will be used. Advanced practice nurses in some countries can chart in health records and bill for clinical services using the ICD-10 code L24.89 (irritant dermatitis due to other agents) for patients with incontinence-associated dermatitis and the ICD-10 code L89.XX (pressure ulcer) when diagnosing a patient with a pressure injury.

## 13.2    Incontinence-Associated Dermatitis

Incontinence-associated dermatitis (IAD) has been reported in patients in a variety of clinical settings, including 20–35% of hospitalized patients [10, 11], 50% or more of critically ill patients [11, 12], and 3–8% of residents in nursing homes and long-term acute care facilities [4, 6, 13, 14]. Approximately 40% of individuals living in the community who have fecal incontinence experience episodes of IAD [1, 15]. Risk or associated factors for IAD in addition to incontinence include limitations in mobility, toileting, or communication abilities, deficits in cognitive functioning (due to sedation or dementia), poor nutritional status, severity of illness and comorbidities, alkaline skin pH, lack of prevention for IAD, and presence of pressure injury [10, 13, 16–20].

Knowledge of diagnosing, assessing, and treating IAD will assist the advanced practice nurse in managing this problem in patients in their own practice or consulting to nursing staff in other settings. The most common signs of IAD are erythema and erosion of superficial skin layers, i.e., the epidermis and sometimes the subepidermis. Erythema manifests as pink, purple, or red coloring of the skin (see Figs. 13.1 and 13.3); it can also appear as a lighter or darker tone of affected areas of a darker skin (see Fig. 13.2). There may be some local swelling. Loss of skin can result in serous drainage and a shiny, glistening appearance of the area (see Fig. 13.3).

**Fig. 13.1** Pink on upper buttocks and in the crease

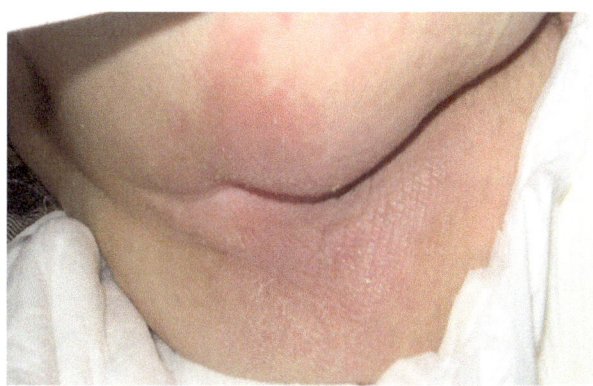

**Fig. 13.2** IAD on buttocks and thighs of medium-toned skin

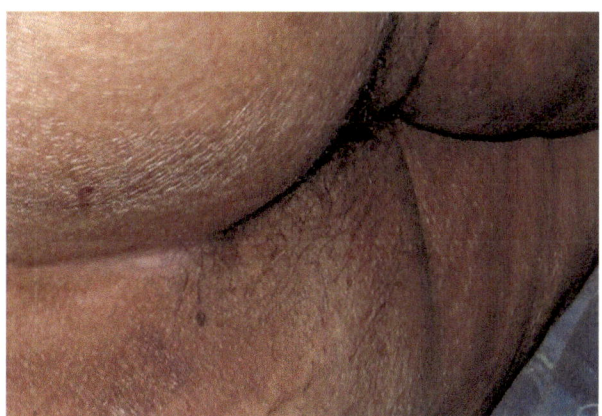

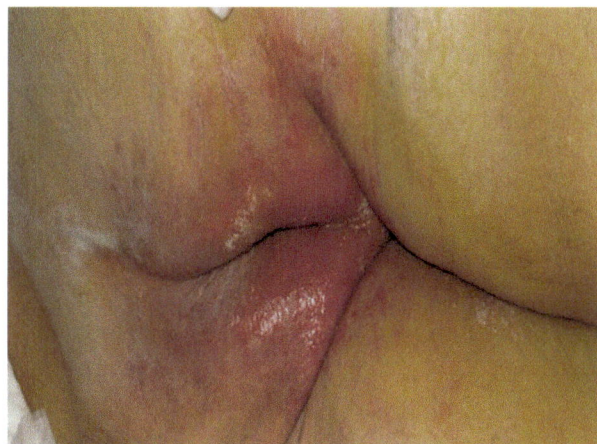

**Fig. 13.3** Redness and skin loss in the perianal area and lower buttocks

**Fig. 13.4** Rash on the left
lower buttocks

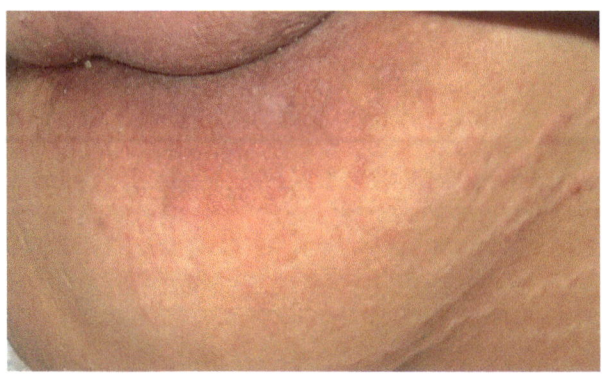

A rash may develop from fungal or bacterial infection as the protective function of the skin barrier is impaired. The rash is typically raised and papular, red in color, and on the periphery of IAD damage; hence it is often described as "satellite lesions" (see Fig. 13.4). The edges of skin loss and rash are irregular. Patients with IAD may feel a variety of symptoms including degrees of soreness, discomfort, or pain, itching, or a burning sensation that has been described as feeling similar to a sunburn [1, 12, 13, 21].

## 13.3 Differential Diagnosis of IAD

Despite improved understanding of cutaneous sequelae of fecal incontinence, patients and clinicians are often reluctant to discuss and assess the genital and perineal skin because of the psychosocial and cultural implications of lesions in this area [22]. Nevertheless, assessment of the genital, perineal, and perianal skin is essential in patients with fecal incontinence because of the risk for IAD and pressure injury, along with other dermatoses that may be producing local symptoms. Assessment includes a history focused on identification of contributing factors, inspection of the skin including determination of the location, size, depth, and character of damaged skin and immediately adjacent skin, and referral for additional evaluation in selected cases. This chapter focuses on differential diagnosis of IAD versus pressure injury, two of the more prevalent forms of genital skin damage seen in patients with fecal incontinence.

Incontinence-associated dermatitis, as its name implies, occurs only in patients experiencing fecal, urinary, or dual fecal and urinary incontinence [6, 10, 23]. Inflammation occurs in areas where the skin is exposed to fecal matter, urine, or a combination of stool and urine, resulting in indistinct borders. In patients with fecal incontinence, IAD has been most commonly reported in the perianal fold of the buttocks [1, 15, 21], suggesting it originates here and spreads to adjacent areas based on the contours of body-worn absorptive products used to contain stool or urine or severity of IAD and skin exposure. In critically ill and community-living patients with fecal incontinence, however, Bliss et al. [1, 20] reported that the initial presentation of IAD varied in severity and spread and was not contained to one body area; additional surveillance is needed to fully describe the course of IAD. Incontinence-associated dermatitis also may extend to the crease between the genitalia and the thighs and the inner folds of the thighs. Affected areas in persons with lighter skin tones will be bright red, and erythema will be more subtle in persons with darker skin tones. Affected skin may appear to glow because of serous exudate associated with damage to the skin's moisture barrier. The skin may develop areas of erosion or denudation that may appear as isolated areas of skin loss or may affect large portions of the exposed skin in severe cases. Denuded skin is typically bright red regardless of underlying skin tone. Damaged skin in patients with large areas of erosion also may contain yellow debris; this finding should not be confused with necrotic fat (slough) seen in full-thickness wounds (stage 3, stage 4, and unstageable pressure injuries) that extend well below the dermis. Rather, IAD creates partial-thickness skin loss, and the yellow material in the wound bed is an inflammatory discharge rather than a necrotic tissue.

A proportion of patients with IAD will have a secondary fungal rash; reported prevalence rates vary from 15% to 18% in the hospital setting and 17% in the critical care setting [2, 20, 24]. These rashes are characterized by darker red area in the middle with satellite lesions superimposed on the inflammation with or without the erosion characteristic of IAD. Although their location varies, they are particularly common in skin folds such as the inner thighs, beneath the abdominal pannus of obese individuals, or beneath the scrotum in males.

Several characteristics aid the advanced practice nurse to differentiate IAD from a pressure injury. While both pressure injuries and IAD share a common risk factor (fecal or urinary incontinence), pressure injuries typically are attributable to a combination of a set of reasonably well-defined risk factors including immobility, impaired sensory perceptions, poor nutrition, and exposure to shearing forces [25]. Unlike IAD that occurs in the skin exposed to fecal matter, pressure injuries are found over bony prominences or underneath a medical device that lies in contact with the skin [9]. Stage 1 pressure injuries may cause redness that does not turn to a lighter tone when gently pressed with the fingers (non-blanchable erythema) similar to that seen with IAD, but it will be located over a bony prominence or underneath a medical device. Similar to IAD, stage 2 pressure injuries are partial-thickness wounds, but their location will also be over a bony prominence or underneath a medical device. In addition, a stage 2 pressure injury will have distinct border unlike the diffuse borders caused by IAD with secondary denudation of affected skin. Stage 3 and 4 pressure injuries differ from IAD because they are full thickness, extending into the subcutaneous tissues or exposing underlying bone. Unstageable pressure injuries are also full-thickness wounds characterized by true slough (necrotic fatty tissue) or black eschar not seen in IAD. A deep tissue pressure injury is characterized by a deep red, maroon, or purple lesion with a dark wound bed or blood-filled blister. These injuries can be differentiated from IAD both by their color and location.

## 13.4    Assessment of IAD Severity

The severity of IAD (or IASD) is assessed by inspection. An instrument to guide nursing staff in assessing IAD and in monitoring its worsening or improvement is the incontinence-associated skin damage severity instrument (IASD.D.2) [26–28]. Version IASD.D.2 of the instrument has been tested for use with skin tones ranging from light to dark [27, 29]. The instrument provides a single score of IAD severity ranging from 0 to 56. The score of the IASD.D.2 instrument is based on the main observable signs of IAD (redness, skin loss, and rash) weighted for severity and 14 body areas that it has identified as locations of IAD occurrence (see Fig. 13.5). The score also considers the spread of IAD. The instrument's components and scoring were developed using evidence from research with experts and current literature [26–28].

The IASD.D.2 instrument has numerous guidance or educational features. The 14 body areas of IAD are numbered on figures with different body shapes (see Fig. 13.5). There is a chart showing a range of colors of the signs of IAD on light, medium, and dark skin tones, which was created using pixels from digital photos of patients' skin. There is good validity and reliability of the IASD.D.2 instrument reported from testing using photograph cases and different types of nurses, for example, wound ostomy and continence nurse specialists and general staff nurses [26, 27, 29]. The advanced practice nurse can use the IASD.D.2 instrument without any fees to educate clinical staff about IAD and in research and quality improvement studies [28]. The instrument can also be licensed for use in practice.

### IASD.D.2 Instrument

**THE INCONTINENCE ASSOCIATED SKIN DAMAGE AND ITS SEVERITY INSTRUMENT (I.A.SD.D.2)**

**LOCATION**
The 14 body locations of IASD
(IASD = Incontinence Associated Skin Damage)

1.   Perianal skin
2.   Crease between buttocks
3.   Left upper buttock
4.   Right upper buttock
5.   Left lower buttock
6.   Right lower buttock
7.   Left Posterior thigh
8.   Right posterior thigh
9.   Genitalia (labia/scrotum)
10.  Lower abdomen/suprapubic
11.  Left Crease between genitalia and thigh
12.  Right Crease between genitalia thigh
13.  Left inner thigh
14.  Right inner thigh

Note: "Left" and "Right" refer to
the patient's left and right as shown.

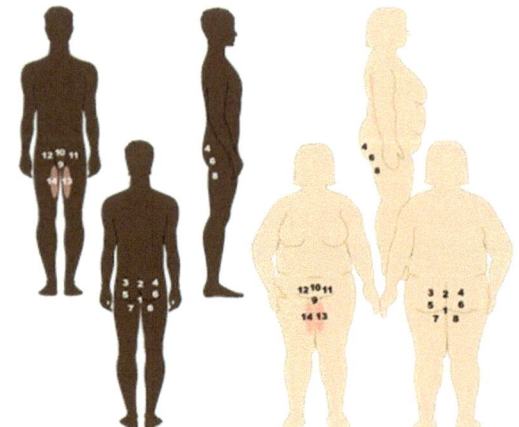

**Fig. 13.5** Part of the incontinence-associated skin damage severity instrument (IASD.D.2). Copyright University of Minnesota. All rights reserved 2015. Reprinted with permission

## 13.5     Prevention and Management of IAD

Because IAD is associated with fecal or urinary incontinence, its prevention and management focus on the treatment of incontinence, preventing stool from coming into contact with the skin, and a structured skin care program [23, 30]. Treatment of fecal incontinence is discussed in detail in other chapters of this book. In addition to interventions to treat or prevent fecal incontinence, research indicates that more severe IAD is associated with more severe fecal incontinence, especially when the individual experiences uncontrolled discharge of liquid stool [15]. Therefore, steps to prevent diarrhea or change stool consistency from liquid to soft and formed are also recommended for prevention and management of IAD. This chapter will focus on strategies to contain fecal incontinence and interventions to alleviate or prevent damage to the skin via a structured skin care program.

### 13.5.1  Containment Strategies

Several strategies may be used to prevent or alleviate IAD by diverting or preventing stool from coming into contact with the skin. Several indwelling devices have been developed that are placed in the rectal vault and drain liquid stool into a collection bag. These devices are designed for short-term use, typically 29 days or less, in persons experiencing high-volume liquid stool multiple times daily [31, 32]. They are mainly employed in patients in the acute or critical care setting (see Chap. 10). These devices have been shown to prevent IAD and pressure injuries in patients with fecal incontinence [33, 34]. Nevertheless, clinical experience demonstrates that these devices move within the rectal vault, often resulting in seepage of stool from the anus, requiring application of an ointment-based occlusive moisturizer (skin protectant) or terpolymer acrylate film to the perianal skin [35]. Nevertheless, insertion of an indwelling stool containment device creates clinically relevant interface pressures between the retention balloon and rectal vault [36], and cases of rectal bleeding from these devices have been reported that may contribute to mucosal injuries to the rectal vault [37]. In addition, several cases of bleeding requiring urgent intervention have been reported [38–41].

An anal pouch incorporates components of a one-piece ostomy pouching system; a wafer is adhered to the perianal skin that is attached to a pouch that stores fecal materials. These pouches have been found to delay time to onset of IAD or occurrence rates of IAD when compared to usual care (absorptive products and routine skin cleansing) [42, 43]. Limitations to their use include challenges in safe application of the adhesive wafer to denuded skin in patients with more severe IAD, the need for frequent changes as the fecal pouch is filled, and difficult emptying of solid fecal material from the pouch. A more recent study of a drainable pouch that can be irrigated with saline and is attached to wall suction shows initial promise in overcoming several limitations of current designs [44].

Absorptive products, also referred to as incontinence pads, were historically designed to limit exposure of the skin to urinary or fecal materials and to protect clothing and bedding. They are widely used for containing incontinence in the acute- and long-term care settings and in the community [45, 46]. Absorbent products can be used as an adjunct to ongoing continence care, as containment when more aggressive interventions are not feasible, and as a means to preserve dignity in persons with incontinence. These products may be categorized based on application (body worn versus bed or chair) or their intended function (products intended for light or moderate to heavy incontinence) [47]. Current best evidence indicates that no single product is superior for containing fecal or dual fecal and urinary incontinence. Selection of the best absorptive product is based on several factors including gender, type and severity of incontinence, and time of day (i.e., use during waking hours versus use while sleeping) [48, 49]. Few products are available that are specifically designed to contain fecal incontinence. An anorectal dressing originally designed to absorb postoperative discharge was preferred to a traditional body-worn absorptive pad by a group of community-dwelling men [50]. Findings from a systematic review and meta-analysis suggest that women tend to prefer pull-up absorptive briefs (similar to underpants) for moderate to heavy fecal or dual incontinence, while men prefer more traditional style absorptive briefs (diapers) especially at night [49]. Nevertheless, the authors acknowledged insufficient research exists to draw firm conclusions concerning the performance of various products or classes of products for management of fecal incontinence, and research in this area should be a priority for continence clinicians and researchers.

Advances in the design of absorbent products aim to maintain skin integrity and health. These include high absorbency of liquids with minimal bulking, a soft smooth layer against the skin, breathable materials, and a range of sizes and styles to ensure a good fit with less leaking and to satisfy personal preferences. Individuals with fecal incontinence identified desired features to improve the performance of absorbent briefs for fecal incontinence [11]. These features include better odor control, higher absorption in the rear near the perianal area, allowing easier, discrete change or removal, and the ability to shield the skin from irritation from solid and particulate matter. A recent advancement in absorbent products is the inclusion of a spiral-shaped cellulosic fiber that maintains an acidic pH of the product as well as the skin when wet with an alkaline solution mimicking urine or feces [18]. Acidifying the skin may have a potential to prevent IAD or promote its healing, but further clinical studies are needed.

Evidence concerning the simultaneous use of leave-on skin products and absorptive products is mixed. For example, a laboratory study using healthy volunteers evaluated the effects of a petrolatum-based ointment on the pores of an absorbent product and found that it reduced their absorptive ability [51]. In contrast, a second study of two cream and ointment-based products found minimal product transfer onto the absorptive product [52]. Additional research is needed to provide evidence that advanced practice nurses can synthesize into clinical decision-making in patients with fecal incontinence who regularly use body-worn or other absorptive products.

Due to the variety of styles and types of absorbent products, community-living individuals with fecal incontinence and their caregivers may need assistance with selection [53]. A web-based, interactive product advisor website is available as a reference for the advanced practice nurses and as a resource for advising nurses and individual patients [54]. The website guides an individual toward options in style, absorbency, and fit depending on their incontinence needs.

## 13.5.2 Structured Skin Care Regimen

Current best evidence indicates that use of a structured skin care protocol for preventing and managing IAD is superior to soap and water alone [11, 18, 30, 55, 56]. Research further indicates that interventions designed for prevention cannot be readily distinguished from those aimed at management [30, 55]. Two principle-based approaches to a structured skin care program have been proposed to aid in designing such a program; they are "cleanse, moisturize, and protect" [6] and "cleanse, protect, and restore" [23]. Each is based on regular cleansing at least daily and following fecal incontinence episodes, followed by the application of a leave-on product that protects the skin against further exposure to irritants, and the selection of a skin product or products that enhance the skin's moisture barrier.

Cleansing should remove fecal matter, urine, microorganisms, and additional soiling from the surface of the skin. In persons with fecal incontinence, the skin should be cleansed daily and after episodes of fecal incontinence. The optimal cleanser should closely reflect the acidic nature (acid mantle) of the surface of healthy skin, whose pH normally ranges from 5.4 to 5.9 [6]. An acidic pH contributes to numerous protective functions of the skin; it promotes growth of certain species of bacteria while exerting antimicrobial activity against coliform and other bacterial, fungal, and viral pathogens. The skin's acid mantle activates enzyme function and promotes cohesion and layering of lipid cells necessary to maintain optimal moisture of levels within the stratum corneum of the skin and regulate transepidermal water loss levels [57]. Bar soaps consist of alkalis and fatty acids; they effectively remove irritants and dirt from the skin by releasing free alkali and insoluble acid salts when mixed with water; soaps are alkaline with a pH varying from 8.0 to 11.0 [58]. Bathing with bar soap and water transiently raises the pH of the skin, increasing its vulnerability to colonization with pathogenic bacterial or fungal species found in the gastrointestinal tract, reducing adhesion of the lipid and protein barrier of the stratum corneum, and altering enzymatic activity in the skin that negatively influences cell adhesion [59]. This transient effect is not harmful in persons who bathe daily, but it is more pronounced when fecal or urinary incontinence create the need for more frequent bathing. A variety of personal and incontinence cleansers are available whose pH ranges are similar to that of normal skin, and their use is recommended for cleansing the perineal and perianal areas, over bar soap and water, in persons with fecal incontinence. Many of these products are designed as no rinse products that do not require rinsing with water and drying with a towel as does cleansing with soap and water. Research in healthy subjects suggests that these products are equally effective in removing pathogenic microorganisms when compared to soap and water [60]. Research also suggests that cleansing persons with moderate to heavy incontinence or IAD should minimize the friction associated with the use of bar soap, a reusable wash cloth, and towel drying because they impair the skin's protective barrier in patients who require frequent cleansing [61].

Protection of the skin typically involves the use of leave-on products containing one or multiple ingredients creating a cream, ointment, or liquid polymer acrylate [55]. Cream-based products are emulsions with a water base, and ointment-based products are oil-based emulsions. Liquid polymer acrylates, including the terpolymer acrylates, are synthetic products that may be combined with other ingredients in various leave-on skin products or applied as a liquid that dries to form a thin, flexible, and transparent protective layer over the skin.

Three common ingredients are commonly used in ointments and cream formulations for prevention and treatment of IAD: petrolatum, dimethicone, and zinc oxide (see Table 13.1). Petrolatum is a semisolid mixture of hydrocarbons obtained from petroleum; it was discovered in 1859 and initially marketed for its healing properties when applied to the skin [62]. It is hydrophobic and reduces transepidermal water loss from the skin by 99%. Petrolatum exerts multiple actions that restore the skin's moisture barrier and enhance repair of skin damaged by exposure to fecal matter or urine [63]. Dimethicone is one of the family of silicones (silicas) that are derived from quartz, granite, or sand. Similar to petrolatum, dimethicone is impermeable to water in its liquid formulation but permeable to water vapor which is important in simultaneously protecting the skin from additional exposure to irritants while maintaining adequate transepidermal water loss needed to manage the hyperhydration of the perineal and perianal skin especially when covered with an absorptive product. Zinc oxide is a white powder that can be processed to form variably sized granules; it is mixed with other products to create an ointment or cream-based paste that is frequently used to treat diaper or nappy dermatitis in infants and IAD in adults. Zinc is particularly effective as a barrier to irritants, but it may create an opaque white layer blocking visual assessment of damaged skin and is resistant to removal using soap and water or no rinse perineal or incontinence cleansers. Application of topical zinc oxide is considered to have wound healing properties, and it is incorporated into a variety of tropical products varying from 1% to 25% [57]. However, evidence concerning its wound healing properties is sparse and inconclusive [64]. A study in healthy volunteers examined each of these three common ingredients and found that zinc oxide exerted the most protective effects against exposure to a standardized irritant, followed by petrolatum and dimethicone [65]. However, dimethicone maintained skin hydration better than zinc oxide or petrolatum. While it is tempting to use this study as a basis for judging the efficacy of various leave-on products used to prevent or treat IAD, it must be remembered that skin care product performance must be evaluated based on the entire formulation rather than the performance of a single ingredient in a laboratory-based study.

Additional ingredients used to restore the skin's moisture barrier included emollients and humectants [66] (see Table 13.1). Emollients form a lipid or oil barrier on the skin to protect against loss of water (i.e., water repellent) and irritants and to supply/restore lipids of the skin barrier. Humectants enhance the skin moisture barrier by attracting moisture to the skin.

**Table 13.1** Ingredients of skin moisturizers and barriers/protectants

| Humectants | Hydrophilic (attract water) into the epidermis and from the dermis and a humid external environment<br>Oil repellent | Glycerine (glycerol), propylene glycol, or 70% sorbitol solution, and trihydroxylated glycerine |
|---|---|---|
| Hydrating agents | Oil repellent<br>Protect against oils, varnishes, and organic solvents | |
| | Oil repellent | Sodiumbischlorophenyl sulfamine and aluminum chlorohydrate |
| | Act as a physical protective layer<br>Oil repellent | Inorganic substances such as talc, zinc oxide, kaolin, and the organoclay quaternium-18 bentonite |
| | Oil repellent<br>Prevent absorption of nickel, chromium, and copper | EDTA (disodium ethylenediaminetetraacetic acid) and pentetic acid (diethylenetriamine pentaacetic acid) |
| | Antioxidant | Botanicals such as Vitis vinifera extract and Rosa canina |
| | Moisturizes skin | Urea and allantoin |
| | Moisturizes skin | Natural moisturizing factor |
| | Attracts and holds water maintaining skin hydration | Hyaluronic acid |
| | Wet skin<br>Protect against irritants | Film-forming polymers soluble or dispersible in water, e.g., VP/eicosene copolymer and ammonium acryloyldimethyltaurate/VP copolymer |
| | Water and oil repellent;<br>Form a thin film that does not clog pores to protect the skin | Synthetic polymers such as FOMBLIN HC(R) |
| Emollients | Highly occlusive<br>Water repellent<br>Protect against acids, alkalies, soaps, water-soluble irritants, and detergents | Petrolatum (paraffinum liquidum, mineral oil)<br>Paraffin waxes (petrolatum jelly, white petrolatum)<br>Lanolin<br>Dimethicone |
| | Naturally synthesized for inclusion in the skin barrier for healing | Ceramides |
| Anti-inflammatory ingredients | | Plant derivatives or botanical extracts: Glycyrrhetinic acid (a root licorice extract), bisabolol (derived from chamomile), and *Butyrospermum parkii* butter (shea butter) |

There are a variety of commercially available skin care product formulations/applications that are used to treat and prevent IAD [55]. Each product must be judged based on the specific formulation rather than extrapolation of the actions of a single ingredient, and none has proved superior for management of IAD. For example, a study of 981 nursing home residents compared ointment and cream-based formulations to a terpolymer acrylate and found that all improved IAD while none emerged as superior based on clinical outcomes alone [11]. Innovations in skin care products for IAD aim to increase cost-effectiveness by decreasing nursing work. For example, some cleansers no longer need to be rinsed off with water, and a disposable wipe combining a cleanser, a skin protectant, and ingredients to restore the skin's moisture barrier was found more effective than pH neutral soap and water for prevention of IAD in nursing home residents [67]. Other important features of skin care products for treating IAD relate to whether they contain fragrance or alcohol, are hypoallergenic, or have ingredients that are left on the skin [66]. Important nursing and patient self-care actions that are components of a skin care protocol are timely cleansing of soiled skin, gentle cleansing, and complete, gentle drying. Usual care that relies on nurse preferences can be inadequate and inconsistent as general nursing staff often lack knowledge about the types and use of skin care products available in their clinical facilities [19, 68].

## 13.6    Educating Nursing Staff

In addition to increasing their own knowledge and expertise about identifying and assessing IAD to support their own practice and consultations, the advance practice continence nurse may participate in educating nursing staff about IAD. Education topics for nursing staff are understanding risks for IAD, assessing signs and symptoms and severity, treatment and prevention approaches, and benefit of a structured skin care protocol as needed. In clinical facilities utilizing nursing assistants, nursing assistants should be prepared to recognize the presence of skin damage and empowered to communicate the information to the nurse who can perform an assessment. The advance practice continence nurse may be called upon to manage severe or non-healing cases. Given turnover rates of approximately 50% of nursing staff in US nursing homes [69, 70], staff education is a continuous need. Web-based educational modules about risk factors and assessment of IAD using video gaming aspects are available [71]. Educational strategies such as this allow for an individual and interactive approach for IAD education in a way that may be time efficient.

## 13.7    Expected Clinical Outcomes

Time to healing of IAD can vary among individuals and patient groups. Mild IAD manifested by pink or red skin is most common across all patient groups from community-living residents to critical care patients [1, 17, 20, 72]. Approximately half of residents in long-term care and acute long-term care healed IAD within 2 weeks of observation [12, 20, 21]. Median time to healing IAD was about 1 week in community-living individuals [17] and nearly 2 weeks in critically ill patients [20]. Lack of progress in healing suggests the need for a change in approach, which may range from achieving less exposure of the skin to leaked urine and/or feces or using different skin care or absorbent products. Observations of community-living individuals with fecal incontinence show IAD reoccurs after healing [1–4] and supports the need for prevention after healing. Prevention IAD in nursing home residents with incontinence significantly reduced the odds of developing IAD by about half [17].

## 13.8    Recommendations for Management of IAD for the Advanced Practice Nurse

- The advanced practice nurse has a role in managing IAD in patients in their own practice and when consulting to nursing staff in a variety of clinical settings.
- The advanced practice nurse should develop expertise in diagnosing IAD, assessing its severity, and treating and preventing it.
- The IASD.D.2 instrument can be useful in assessing IAD severity, monitoring IAD worsening and improvement, and educating nursing staff about IAD.
- Consultation about IAD includes evaluating the use and components of a structured skin care protocol and, as needed, recommending modifications based on the needs of patients, staff, and the care model/setting.
- The advanced practice nurse should be knowledgeable about the options of skin care and absorbent products available to patients and a clinical facility and the actions/features of these.
- Skin care protocols for managing IAD typically include products for cleansing and softening skin, replacing water and lipids in the epidermal skin barrier, and protecting skin from losing moisture and irritants. Maintaining an acidic pH of skin while using skin care and/or absorbent products is recommended.
- Educating nursing staff about IAD and the role for the advanced practice nurse may facilitate better patient outcomes.
- Prevention of IAD is critical to maintain skin integrity and to reduce recurrence of skin damage. Protocols are similar as those for treating IAD.

## 13.9    Pressure Injury and Fecal Incontinence

Incontinence is a risk factor in the development of pressure injury in any healthcare setting due to the increase in moisture and temperature to the perineal skin, making it a higher risk for damage from pressure. Therefore, understanding how pressure injuries develop, how to identify each patient's individual risk factors, and the proper management to prevent and treat pressure injuries is part of the comprehensive management of fecal incontinence.

### 13.9.1   Background about Pressure Injury

The development of a pressure injury has significant impact on the quality and duration of a patient's life as well as the economic burden for the patient and the healthcare system. Approximately 60,000 patients die each year from pressure injury complications [73]. Pressure injury complications are the cause of death in 80% of people over 75 years of age [73, 74]. Septicemia occurs in 39.7% of pressure injury-associated deaths. The pressure injury mortality rates are higher in African Americans than in other racial groups [74]. Each year, more than 2.5 million people in the United States develop pressure injuries. These skin injuries cause pain, associated risk for serious infection, and increased healthcare utilization.

The annual cost of a pressure injury management in the United States (US) in 2011 was estimated to be as much as $11 billion [73]. For an individual patient, the cost of care per pressure injury was $20,900–$151,700, depending on its stage. Medicare (US third party payor for healthcare of older adults) data reports $43,180 per pressure ulcer [73]. Hospital stay was longer for patients with pressure injuries, and more than half of these patients were discharged from a hospital to a long-term care facility/nursing home, which is three times the rate as that from hospitalizations for all other diagnoses [75]. More than 20% of residents who have been in long-term care facilities for 2 or more years will develop at least one pressure ulcer [76]. The cost of treating pressure injury is 2.5 times the cost of preventing them [77].

## 13.10  Pressure Injury Risk Assessment and Prevention

An important role for nurses, especially for continence nurse specialists and advanced practice nurses, has been to identify the patients at risk for pressure injury and order or implement a prevention plan targeting the identified risk factors. Patients should be assessed on admission to any healthcare setting: hospital, acute long-term care, nursing home, rehabilitation, and home care. At specific intervals per healthcare setting, the risk assessment should be repeated as an ongoing evaluation. The risk assessment scale provides a score that assists the nurse in identifying areas of risk in order to implement a prevention plan. There are three validated pressure injury risk assessment tools with scales that are most commonly used: Waterlow, Norton, and Braden scales.

- The Waterlow scale consists of seven items to evaluate risk for pressure injury development. Those seven areas are height, weight, skin assessment, sex/age, continence, mobility, and appetite. There are also special risk areas including tissue malnutrition, neurological deficit, medications, and surgery/trauma [78].
- The Norton scale evaluates five areas of risk: physical condition, mental condition, activity, mobility, and incontinence [79].
- The Braden scale has six subscales identified as key risk factors to predict overall level of risk for developing pressure injury. The six subscales are sensory, moisture, activity, mobility, nutrition, and friction and shear. It lists the presence of moisture versus urinary and fecal incontinence per se as other scales do as a contributing factor [3]. The skin has increased moisture with incontinence which weakens the epidermis and with the addition of pressure and/or shear can cause a pressure injury to develop.

The Braden scale is most widely used in the United States to identify patients risk for developing pressure injury in various settings. Therefore, it may be readily available for the advanced practice nurse to review during an assessment of fecal incontinence. Based on the overall score [1–23] of a particular patient and each subscale score (1–4 or 1–3 for friction/shear), an individualized care plan for prevention can be developed to address the risk factors with appropriate targeted interventions. A prevention plan can be implemented as a team approach. A higher score on the Braden scale means a lower risk of developing a pressure injury.

The advanced practice nurse should be cognizant of the strategies needed to prevent the development of a pressure injury in patients that are high risk. A generalist nurse usually will evaluate the patient on admission to the healthcare setting via a risk assessment scale such as those noted above and implement prevention measures based on the results. Nurses are responsible for providing a daily skin care protocol and assessment, continence care, turning, and repositioning. Because risks for skin damage can be dynamic, the ongoing assessment and updating of a care plan are done regularly by the nursing staff.

Incontinence care with skin care products (i.e., cleansers, moisturizers, protectants/moisture barrier) that are gentle and maintain the natural acidic pH of skin is recommended after every incontinence episode. Interventions that preserve the protective functions of the skin are crucial for prevention of skin injury in incontinent patients. Turning and repositioning are currently recommended and should be done based on patients' individual needs and at a minimum of every 2 h. The turning and repositioning do not eliminate the pressure but do reduce the duration of the pressure. The amount of time the pressure is present on the skin is a critical element in the development of the pressure injury.

Prevention involves a multidisciplinary team, and if one is not in place, the advanced practice nurse can order appropriate consults. For example, a dietician conducts a nutritional assessment making recommendations to ensure adequate nutrition and hydration. Physical and occupational therapists implement a plan to improve the patient's mobility status and, if needed, recommend a seating surface and proper equipment for turning and repositioning. The advanced practice nurse ensures that all areas have been adequately addressed and a treatment plan is in place for each area assessed as being a risk.

### 13.10.1   Nutrition

Nutrition plays an important role in the prevention and healing of pressure injury. The dietitian or nutritional support nurse's thorough nutritional assessment and ongoing review is an important part of the team approach. They assist in screening for malnutrition risk on admission and for significant changes in condition afterward using a valid and reliable nutritional screening tool. They address nutritional deficits with adequate protein, vitamins, and minerals and adequate hydration through a comprehensive nutritional plan (see Box 13.1). Assessing fluid and caloric intake may require a 48-h calorie count for accuracy [8]. As many as 56% of residents in nursing facilities require assistance to eat [80]. Dental problems, ill-fitting dentures, swallowing problems, dementia, depression, and Parkinson's disease are all potential reasons for poor nutritional intake.

> **Box 13.1: Nutrition Plan**
> - Screen patients with pressure injury or at high risk for pressure injury for malnutrition risk.
> - Assess nutritional status and intake of these patients.
> - Develop and implement a nutrition support plan.
>   - Provide and encourage intake of sufficient calories.
>   - Provide and encourage intake of adequate protein to achieve positive nitrogen balance.
>   - Provide and encourage adequate fluid intake for hydration.
>   - Provide adequate vitamins and minerals, especially vitamins C and A and zinc.
> - Reassess nutritional status for pressure injuries that are not progressing in healing and modify plan according to findings.

## 13.10.2 Sensory and Mobility

Limitations in mobility and sensory impairments are addressed by an individualized turning and repositioning schedule and by using a support surface that redistributes pressure in a chair, wheelchair, and/or bed. There are numerous products that claim to provide this redistribution of pressure and prevent shearing. Consulting physical and/or occupational therapy to evaluate the patient's functional level and make recommendations is helpful in selecting an appropriate product.

## 13.10.3 Shear and Friction

An example of how a shearing injury can occur is as follows: If the head of the patient's bed is elevated greater than 30 degrees, and the patient slides down in bed due to gravity forces, then mechanical damage to the skin and pressure injury can develop. Shear presents as linear extensions or undermining in a pressure injury. To eliminate shearing forces, keep the head of the bed elevated less than 30° with the knee area notched or elevated to prevent sliding down in bed. Lifting or moving a patient with turning sheets, not dragging, and/or the use of a trapeze or lift equipment will decrease both friction and shearing.

Friction is the surface damage caused by skin layers rubbing against another surface. Friction can occur from frequent and aggressive cleansing of the skin after incontinent episodes. Friction damages the epidermis and top dermal layers of the skin. It presents in the fleshy part of the buttocks as superficial red patchy areas. Gentle cleansing after incontinent episodes using an appropriate skin cleanser decreases the risk of friction [81].

## 13.10.4 Moisture

Moisture has a role in the formation of pressure injury. Skin become waterlogged (or overhydrated) from frequent exposure to moisture, which results in skin maceration (or thinning). With friction, erosion of macerated skin occurs very easily. Moist skin is five times more likely to form a pressure injury than dry skin [82]. Most commonly, the moisture in an incontinent patient is from fecal or urinary incontinence or both. Additionally, when wearing an incontinent brief, skin pH can increase (can become alkaline) from the increased heat, occlusion, and exposure to urine and feces (which have an alkaline pH) [18]. An alkaline skin pH promotes the action of fecal enzymes in "digesting" the protective lipoprotein matrix of the skin [83].

A management plan for urinary and fecal incontinence is critical for long-term elimination or reduction of this risk factor. However, in the short term, it is important to use a structured skin care program for patients with incontinence, which includes cleansing, moisturizing, and protecting the skin barrier against moisture loss. It is also crucial to use high-quality incontinence pads or briefs with moisture wicking, super absorbency, and air permeability properties and that maintain an acidic skin pH and offer a good fit. Additional risk factors for the development of pressure injury that need to be managed include extrinsic factors such as limitations in mobility, movement, transferring, toileting abilities, and cognitive functioning, decreased circulation, tissue perfusion and oxygenation, and diminished sensation [84].

## 13.11 Description and Manifestations of Pressure Injury

Pressure injury is defined by the National Pressure Ulcer Advisory Panel as a localized damage to the skin and underlying soft tissue, usually over a bony prominence caused by pressure or pressure with shear [85]. Signs of pressure injury can range from intact non-blanchable erythema of the skin to full-thickness skin loss. The tolerance of the skin for pressure and shear injury can be affected by nutrition, perfusion, comorbidities, microclimate, and condition of the skin at the baseline.

The staging of pressure injury (from 1 to 4) is differentiated by the degree of tissue damage at the wound base [83] (see Box 13.2). Pressure injuries are the only wounds that are staged. Other types of wounds are described as partial-thickness or full-thickness wounds. Since the correct staging of pressure injury requires an evaluation at the base of the wound, if the wound base is covered with necrotic tissue (either slough or eschar), the wound is considered an unstageable pressure injury. A deep tissue injury is also not staged because it is a persistent non-blanchable deep red, maroon, or purple intact skin discoloration. This area may resolve or evolve into a stageable pressure injury.

**Box 13.2: Stages of Pressure Injury** [85]
- Stage 1 pressure injury is intact skin with non-blanchable erythema. The damaged skin may have changes in temperature and firmness compared to adjacent tissue. Stage 1 may difficult to determine on darker skin tones.
- Stage 2 pressure injury is partial-thickness skin loss (see Fig. 13.6a). Partial thickness is damage to the epidermal skin which can extend *into* the dermal layer but not *through* the dermis. Stage 2 pressure injury heals through epithelialization, which means the tensile strength is not affected. Stage 2 pressure injury may easily be confused with incontinence-associated dermatitis if relying on appearance only, so knowing the etiology (i.e., if pressure was a factor) is important.
- Stages 3 and 4 are full-thickness tissue injuries. Stage 3 pressure injury extends *through* the dermis into the subcutaneous tissue. Stage 4 involves the muscle, fascia, tendon, and possibly bone (see Fig. 13.6b). Full-thickness wounds leave a healed area weakened because they heal with scar formation. The healed area never reaches more than 70% tensile strength and therefore is at risk to recur.

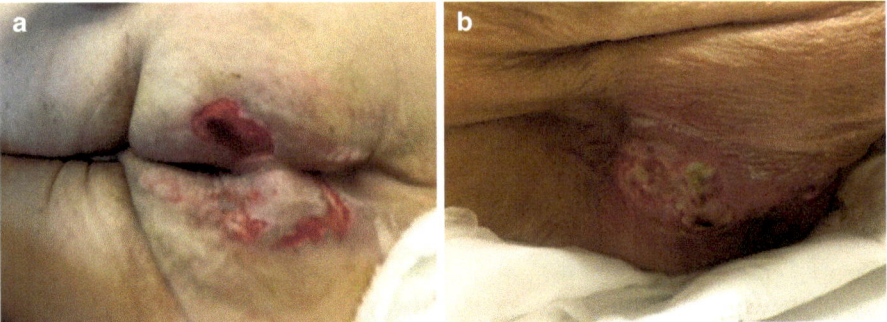

**Fig. 13.6** (**a**) Stage 2 pressure injury on the right buttock with slough and granulation tissue (Permission for reprinting images obtained from patient). (**b**) Stage 4 pressure injury on the right ischial area with eschar, slough, and granulation and periwound erythema present (Permission for reprinting images obtained from patient)

In 2014, an analysis of a survey of incontinence and hospital-acquired pressure injury concluded that facility-acquired pressure injuries were more likely to be full thickness in incontinent patients than in those who were continent [3].

## 13.12  Differential Diagnosis

### 13.12.1  Differentiating Pressure Injuries from Incontinence-Associated Dermatitis

The differentiation of pressure ulcers from incontinence-associated dermatitis can be simplified if you consider the etiology and the characteristics of these two types of skin damage. Moisture, friction, shear, and pressure are mechanical factors that cause skin damage. Moisture and friction cause damage top down. In other words, when the damage occurs on the surface (epidermis) with moisture (from incontinence) and/or friction, the result is incontinence-associated dermatitis. In contrast, shear and pressure occur from the inside out. The forces on the blood vessels and muscles become ischemic when the damage is done inside, extending to the surface which occurs from the pressure and/or shear.

The location of the ulcer is another characteristic that differentiates the two types of skin damage. Incontinence-associated dermatitis is considered a top-down skin injury which is typically in the perineal area as the cause is from incontinence (moisture). In contrast, pressure injury occurs over a bony prominence and is a localized skin damage occurring bottom-up. Pressure injuries are lesions that have well-defined borders and are present over a bony prominence, for example, the sacral or ischial area. Incontinence-associated dermatitis should not be classified or staged as a pressure injury (see Table 13.2).

**Table 13.2** Characteristics and treatment of incontinence-associated dermatitis and pressure injury associated with incontinence

| | Incontinence-associated dermatitis | Pressure injury |
|---|---|---|
| | 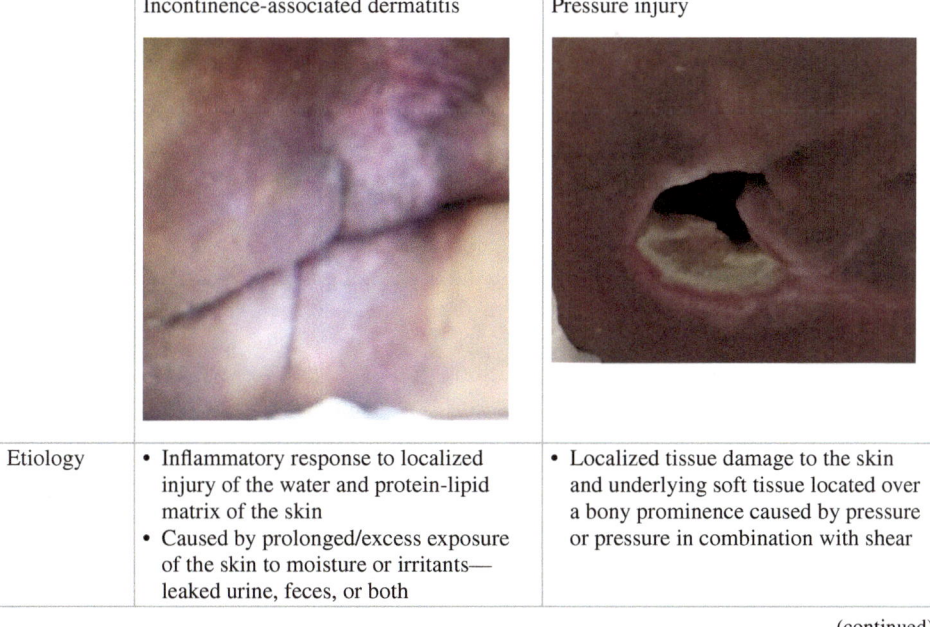 | |
| Etiology | • Inflammatory response to localized injury of the water and protein-lipid matrix of the skin<br>• Caused by prolonged/excess exposure of the skin to moisture or irritants—leaked urine, feces, or both | • Localized tissue damage to the skin and underlying soft tissue located over a bony prominence caused by pressure or pressure in combination with shear |

(continued)

**Table 13.2** (continued)

|  | Incontinence-associated dermatitis | Pressure injury |
|---|---|---|
| Location | Fourteen areas (see assessment tool in Sec. 13.4): perianal, buttocks, groin, perineum, inner thighs | Over a bony prominence, mainly sacrum, ischium, trochanters |
| Skin damage signs | Color change (erythema: pink, red, or darker or lighter shades of underlying skin tone of medium or darker skin), irregular shape/edges, superficial, partial-thickness erosion: local swelling, oozing, vesiculation, crusting, and scaling | Distinct borders, round ulcer/wound, partial or full thickness, necrotic tissue |
| Periwound | Inflammation: bright red or hyperpigmented skin; secondary infection: fungal or bacterial | Intact, induration, erythema, maceration, denuded (i.e., skin loss) |
| Symptoms | Discomfort, soreness, pain, burning, tingling, and/or itching | Discomfort and/or pain |
| Treatment | Structured skin care regimen (e.g., cleansers, moisturizers as needed, protectants/moisture loss barriers), use of quality containment products, promotion of acidic pH, interventions to reduce/eliminate incontinence | Reduce/eliminate contributing factors with appropriate interventions, pressure relief system (e.g., repositioning, special beds/mattresses), topical wound treatment plan |

## 13.13   Assessment of Pressure Injury

The wound assessment and documentation of a pressure injury should be very detailed. The documentation elements must include location; stage of the wound; wound measurement (length, width, and depth) including measurements of undermining or tunneling; wound base tissue; amount and type of exudate; and the periwound skin. Detailed documentation provides objectivity to the efficacy of the interventions and evaluates the wound healing progress. Documentation must be the exact anatomical location of the pressure injury measuring the length (head to toe), width (side to side), and depth including the measurements of undermining or tunneling.

Describe the location of the tunneling and undermining by using the location on the face of a clock with 12 o'clock being the head of the patient. Tunneling is tissue destruction occurring in any direction from the wound surface, which results in dead space. Tunneling must be lightly packed with a dressing to prevent abscess formation. Undermining is the area of tissue destruction extending under the intact skin along the periphery of a wound edge. The cause of undermining is shear forces.

The tissue in the wound base is described as granulation, slough, or eschar with the percentage of each (e.g., 25% slough and 75% granulation tissue). Granulation tissue is the beefy red tissue. There are two types of necrotic or nonviable tissue: slough and eschar. Slough is the white (or yellowish) stringy necrotic tissue, and eschar is the leathery black necrotic tissue. Document the amount of drainage from the wound (small, moderate, large) and the type of drainage (serous, serosanguinous, and sanguinous). Adequate documentation will not only record effectiveness of the treatments but is often the basis for reimbursement of products and services by health insurance companies. Figure 13.7 shows characteristics of a pressure injury.

## 13.14  Management of Pressure Injury

An advanced practice nurse who is developing a management plan for pressure injuries must realize that wound healing occurs best when all of the patient's systemic risk factors have been adequately addressed (see Box 13.3). There are many wound care products on the market, and the features they have for wound healing vary. However, the most expensive dressing will not heal a wound if the patient has poor nutrition, unstable glucose levels, or poor oxygenation and continues to experience pressure and shear or if the skin continues to be exposed to moisture from drainage or incontinence.

If the wound is not healing or it is getting worse, like any other chronic disease, it is important to reevaluate all the factors that affect the wound healing process.

---

**Box 13.3: Local and Systemic Factors Impeding Wound Healing**

| Local factors | Systemic factors |
|---|---|
| • Hypothermia | • Decreased tissue oxygenation and perfusion |
| • Moisture | • Malnutrition |
| • Bacterial load | • Infection |
| • Foreign bodies in wound | • Diabetes mellitus |
| • Rolled wound edges | • Obesity |
| • Necrotic tissue or hypergranulation tissue | • Medications |
| | • Older age |
| | • Immunosuppression |
| | • Pain or emotional or psychosocial stress |
| | • Lack of pressure redistribution |

---

There are three wound healing principles that can guide the advanced practice nurse in managing pressure injury wounds:

1. Control or eliminate causative factors.
   (a) Offload the lying or sitting surface, decrease friction and shear, and protect from moisture.
2. Provide systemic support to reduce the existing and potential cofactors.
   (a) Optimize nutrition and hydration, control blood sugar, and promote blood flow, i.e., eliminate nicotine, caffeine, pain.
3. Maintain a physiological moist wound environment.
   (a) Prevent/manage infection, cleanse wound, remove nonviable tissue, eliminate dead space, control odor, protect periwound skin, and address pain.

Whether the wound is dry or moist also influences the treatment goals and selection of dressings (see Table 13.3).

**Table 13.3** Types of dressings by wound characteristics

| Wound characteristic | Dry wound | Wet wound | Increased critical bacterial colonization | Wound with necrotic tissue |
|---|---|---|---|---|
| • Type of treatment recommended and reason | • Keep wound moist<br>– prevents cell death<br>– promotes cell migration<br>– protects, add moisture<br>– promotes closure without necrosis | • Absorb excess drainage<br>– protects surrounding skin | • Provide sustained antimicrobial activity<br>– bacteria interfere with healing | • Use autolytic or enzymatic debridement<br>– removes necrotic tissue so healing can occur |
| *Primary dressing* | | | | |
| Transparent film | X | | | X |
| Hydrocolloid | X | X | | X |
| Foam | X | X | | X |
| Gel | X | | | X |
| Calcium alginate | | X | | |
| Honey-based dressing | X | X | X | |
| Silver dressing | | | X | |
| Enzymatic debrider | | | | X |
| Gauze | X | X | | X |
| *Secondary dressing* | | | | |
| Transparent film | X | | | X |
| Hydrocolloid | X | X | | X |
| Foam | X | X | | X |
| Gauze | X | X | | X |

## 13.14.1 Topical Wound Management: TIME

The TIME framework [86, 87] can be used to guide the topical management of pressure injury wounds. The T refers to tissue management, which is the removal (or debridement) of nonviable tissue, slough, and eschar, from the wound bed. Necrotic tissue is a culture medium for bacterial growth and it impedes the healing process by prolonging the inflammatory phase. The debridement of the necrotic tissue can be performed surgically or conservatively using sharp, mechanical, autolytic or enzymatic procedures.

Surgical debridement occurs in the operating room with a surgeon debriding the wound. This converts a wound to an acute wound again and therefore initiates the clotting cascade. Certainly this is not an available option to all patients due to comorbidities which preclude them from being a surgical candidate.

Conservative sharp debridement occurs at the bedside with sterile equipment by a registered nurse, advanced practice nurse, or physical therapist. The necrotic tissue is removed with minimal invasion into the healthy tissue. This option is not as aggressive as a surgical debridement but can be very successful in situations where surgical debridement is not an option.

Mechanical debridement is accomplished with wet-to-dry gauze, monofilament fiber pads, wound irrigation, low-frequency ultrasound, or ultrasonic mist. Wet to dry debridement is rarely used as it is painful and has not shown to enhance the wound healing process. The use of monofilament fiber pads is effective with the removal of slough tissue but has low evidence on increased wound healing. The use of ultrasound provides mechanical and hydrodynamic effects to the wound bed, which have shown to increase the wound healing process but is not reimbursed in all healthcare settings [81].

Autolytic debridement uses an occlusive dressing such as transparent film or hydrocolloid to collect fluid under the dressing that allows the body to use its own enzymes and WBC to debride the necrotic tissue. This is a noninvasive but slower process of debridement.

Enzymatic debridement uses a prescription enzymatic debrider that is applied with every dressing change to debride the necrotic tissue. This product can be slow and expensive. This type of product is only effective for 12 h and cannot be used with silver and iodine products.

The goal of debriding a wound is to rid the wound bed of necrotic tissue that slows down the healing process. Necrotic tissue in the wound slows down the healing process by increasing the risk of infection, prolonging the inflammatory process, increasing metabolic load, and losing nutrients through the exudate from the wound.

The I of the TIME framework refers to inflammation and infection control. All chronic wounds are contaminated, but when the colonization rises to a high level, it interferes with wound healing. Maintaining a bacterial balance in chronic wounds through debridement of necrotic tissue, proper wound cleansing, and perhaps an intervention such as an antimicrobial dressing may be needed. An antimicrobial dressing could include but is not limited to silver, honey or cadexomer iodine dressings. The wound can also have a local infection or a systemic infection. Local infection signs and symptoms include a period of 2 weeks with no healing and an increase in the amount of exudate, odor, granulation tissue that is friable, and necrotic tissue. The increase in bacterial load in a wound will impede the progression of wound healing. The use of an antimicrobial cleanser and/or an antimicrobial dressing would be an option to decrease the bacterial load in the wound bed.

Systemic infection would have the following signs and symptoms: increased drainage or wound size, odor, induration or erythema >2 cm periwound, increased odor, elevated WBC, and fever. This would require the wound culture and the treatment with an oral antibiotic based on the culture and sensitivities.

The M of the TIME framework refers to moisture balance, which is required for a wound to heal. A moist wound healing environment is achieved by creating a moisture balance in the wound. To create that moisture balance, a dressing may need to absorb, donate, or maintain moisture at the wound surface according to the amount of drainage occurring. The guiding principle of providing a moist wound healing environment means that initially it is important to determine if the wound is wet or dry. A wound that has excess drainage will require a dressing choice that will be able to absorb the exudate between the dressing changes (see Table 13.3).

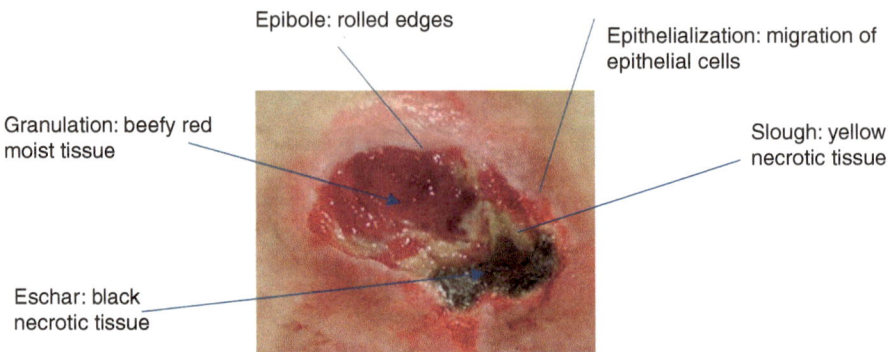

Epibole: rolled edges

Epithelialization: migration of epithelial cells

Granulation: beefy red moist tissue

Slough: yellow necrotic tissue

Eschar: black necrotic tissue

**Fig. 13.7** Characteristics of a pressure injury

A wound that is dry must have a dressing applied that will donate moisture to the wound bed and keep it moist between dressing changes.

The E refers to wound edges. The wound edge must be open to facilitate epithelial migration. If the wound edges are rolled (called epibole) (see Fig. 13.7), the body interprets the wound as being healed and no epithelial migration occurs. To restart the healing process, the rolled edges of the wound would need to be removed in order for healing to occur. Removal of the epibole or healed edges can be accomplished with silver nitrate or surgical removal.

Determining the appropriate topical dressing management for a pressure injury can be a very daunting task. Table 13.3 lists common types of dressings used for pressure injury wounds and the reason for their use. The limitations will start with the availability of the products in a specific setting. Healthcare reimbursement and cost-efficiency play a very important role in wound dressing choices. Using products within guidelines can improve cost-effective treatment for wound care.

## 13.14.2 Dressings

The first step of managing a pressure injury wound is to cleanse the wound. The use of normal saline or a noncytotoxic wound cleanser is ideal. Avoid irrigating a wound if the entire wound base cannot be visualized. Antimicrobial wound cleanser can also be used to decrease bacterial burden in the wound. Acetic acid solution 0.5–1.0% or Dakin's solution can decrease the odor and control bacterial burden but should be used for a very short period of time such as 72 h to 1 week as they can impede healing if used in the long term.

Wound dressings are classified as either primary or secondary (see Table 13.3). A primary dressing is applied directly to the wound bed (hydrocolloid, foam, transparent film, gauze, manuka honey products). Some primary dressings will require a secondary dressing (hydrogels, calcium alginate, manuka honey products). A secondary dressing is placed over a primary dressing to secure its place or provide a

**Table 13.4**  Treatment goals and types of dressings for moist and wet wounds

|  | Partial thickness | Full thickness |
|---|---|---|
| Dry wound | *Goal*: hydrate wound<br>*Dressings*: transparent film, hydrocolloid, foams, hydrogel, honey-based dressing | *Goal*: hydrate wound<br>*Dressings*: hydrogel, transparent film, foam, hydrocolloid, honey-based dressing |
| Moist wound | *Goal*: control drainage to prevent further skin damage, absorb excess drainage for moist balance<br>*Dressings*: calcium alginate, foam, hydrocolloid, gauze, honey-based dressing | *Goals*: control drainage, prevent periwound skin damage, absorb excess drainage for moist balance<br>*Dressings*: calcium alginate, foam, gauze, honey-based dressing |

barrier for the wound (hydrocolloid, foam or transparent films, gauze). Dressings for wounds in sacral or ischial area are available in oval versus square to better accommodate the difficulty of applying dressings in this area of the body. Antimicrobials are dressing that have silver impregnated or manuka honey in the properties.

When choosing a dressing for basic wound management, the first step would be to determine the level of moisture (drainage) in the wound bed (see Table 13.4). Is the wound dry or wet? For a wound that is dry, the options include foams, transparent film, hydrocolloid, and hydrogel. The goal of these dressings is to add moisture to create a moist wound healing environment that prevents cell death and promotes cell migration. For a wound that is wet, dressing options include hydrocolloid, calcium alginate, foam, gauze or negative pressure wound therapy. The primary goals would be to absorb excess drainage while providing a moist wound environment and protecting the periwound skin.

## 13.15   Expected Outcomes

### 13.15.1   Acute Wounds

Acute wounds heal at a predictable rate as they move through the four stages of wound healing: hemostasis, inflammation, proliferation, and remodeling. The wound healing process is best understood as a cascade of events. Injury of the skin immediately triggers clot formation which stops the bleeding in the hemostasis phase. The clot formation then releases growth factors activating the neutrophils and macrophages to move to the wounded site in the inflammatory phase. In this phase, edema, warmth, and exudate develop, and phagocytosis of bacteria occurs. The proliferative phase continues the production and recruitment of growth factors. In this phase, granulation tissue and contraction of the wound occur. The last phase is the remodeling phase when the maturation of the wound occurs.

Acute wounds heal in a timely way in about four weeks. Chronic wounds are considered wounds that have not healed in that time frame. Often the chronic wound "gets stuck" in the inflammation process for various reasons. These reasons can include the patient's lifestyle, for example, smoking, poor nutrition, comorbidities such as diabetes and COPD, and an increased number of bacteria in the wound (i.e., bioburden).

## 13.15.2  Chronic Wounds

Chronic wounds have a prolonged inflammatory phase, no initial bleeding events to trigger fibrin and growth factors, cellular senescence, deficiency of growth factor receptor sites, and high level of proteases. Chronic wounds fail to progress through an orderly and timely process of wound healing. The various characteristics of the individual and their environment can facilitate or impede the wound healing process. One of the activities of the advanced practice nurse is to identify and modify any roadblocks to chronic wounds from healing.

Boxes 13.4 and 13.5 describe case studies about skin damage in patients with fecal incontinence and the care provided by an advanced practice nurse.

---

**Box 13.4: Case Study 1**

Mr. Geer is a 72-year-old widower who had a stroke at his home. He is an obese man that has right-sided hemiplegia, aphasia, and dysphagia. He requires maximum assistance with bed positioning and a mechanical lift for transfers. He frequently slides down in bed. He is out of bed in the wheelchair once a day. Mr. Geer has a gastrostomy tube for tube feeding which runs 20 h a day for nutritional support due to dysphagia. The head of his bed is elevated at 45° because of the tube feeding. His last prealbumin was 11 mg/dL. His weight is 265 pounds (120.5 kg). His blood glucose ranges from 200 to 360 mg/dL. He is currently incontinent of urine and feces with loose stools at least three times per day. His vital signs are stable and he is afebrile. The advanced practice continence specialist nurse performs the assessment and interventions, and evaluation below.

*Past health history*: Diabetes, hypertension, obesity

*Skin assessment reveals*

- A non-blanchable erythematous area on his sacrum.
- An open area of length = 0.5 cm by width = 1.0 cm by depth = 0.25 cm on his right ischial area, with a red wound base and minimal drainage. The periwound skin has maceration and erythema.
- There are erythema and circular open areas (less than 0.25 cm) scattered on scrotum and bilateral inner thigh.

*Braden scale score: 9 = very high risk*
Sensory = 2 Constantly moist = 1 Activity = 1 Mobility = 1 Nutrition = 3 Friction and Shear = 1

*Interventions:*

1. Address risk factors for skin damage.
   (a) Order use of a skin care cleanser and topical protectant/barrier cream every 2 h and with a pad change and evaluate the incontinent pad for proper fit and quality.

(b) Evaluate the cause of diarrhea and treat. For example, assess if tube feeding contains dietary fiber or if a medication administered by feeding tube contains sorbitol, which can result in diarrhea. Assess changes in frequency of stooling and in stool consistency using a standardized scale in response to treatment. Start a bowel program aimed at achieving a regular stool pattern.

(c) Order use of a pressure redistribution device on the bed and a specialty wheelchair cushion to reduce pressure. Protect heels and elbows from pressure, friction, and shear. Order maximum time in chair to be 45 min at a time.

(d) Order a position change every 2 h. Keep the head of his bed at 30°. Use a mechanical lift moving or transferring the patient.

2. Adjust medications to keep blood glucose below 180 mg/dL.

3. Topical skin treatments:

(a) Sacrum stage 1 pressure injury: assess and cleanse area and apply a topical protectant/moisture barrier every shift.

(b) Right ischial stage 2 pressure injury: cleanse with wound cleanser or normal saline, apply a hydrocolloid or foam dressing with border tape, and change dressing every 3 days.

(c) Incontinence-associated dermatitis around wound and on scrotum and thigh: cleanse with every incontinent episode (or every 2–4 h) and apply a topical protectant barrier product.

*Outcomes*

The evaluation of Mr. Geer in 72 h after the implementation of the above plan shows:

- Sacral area damage is resolved.
- On the right ischial area, the maceration and erythema have resolved. Open area measures length = 0.75 cm by width = 1.0 cm by depth = 0.5 cm. This is larger than the previous assessment. This could be from the decreased erythema in the area. Continue with the same treatment.
- Assessment shows no erythema on the scrotum or inner thigh; skin loss areas on the scrotum are resolved, and bilateral inner thigh skin loss areas are healing. Continue with current plan.

*Follow-up*

- Review the turning schedule with the nursing staff; check that the head of his bed is 30° and his time up in the wheelchair is not more than 45 min at a time.
- Assess the pressure redistribution products.
- Assess progress on his bowel program, diarrhea, and stool frequency and consistency.
- Order blood glucose to be drawn.

**Box 13.5: Case Study 2**

Mrs. Somner is a 70-year-old woman with a hip fracture. She has been admitted to the hospital for surgical repair. She has been sitting in the wheelchair 4 h, twice per day. She ambulates with a front wheel walker up to 25 ft. She has difficulty transferring to the commode or toilet and requires assistance of one person. She slides down in bed regularly. She requires assistance with bed mobility of 2–4 people due to pain. She is alert and oriented, but incontinent of urine twice each night and occasionally during the day. She has had constipation but complains of itching of her "bottom." She has a poor appetite, eating only a few bites of each meal and drinks a small amount of a liquid feeding supplement each day. She is underweight at 105 pounds and her prealbumin = 2 mg/dL. Her vital signs are stable and she is afebrile. Her hemoglobin = 10 g/dL. The advanced practice continence specialist nurse performs the assessment and interventions, and evaluation below.

*Past health history*: smoking, malnutrition, COPD, osteoporosis
*Skin assessment*:

- Full-thickness skin loss on her sacral area (length = 3 cm, width = 2 cm, depth = 2 cm). The ulcer presents as a deep crater with no undermining. Gauze dressings are saturated twice a day with serosanguinous drainage, no odor, and the wound base is yellow slough with a small amount of granulation tissue. Periwound skin is erythematous and macerated with a rash present.
- Perianal and crease between the buttocks are red and erythematous with a rash present around her perianal area.

*Braden scale score: 15 = preventable risk*
Sensory = 4 Moist = 2 Activity = 3 Mobility = 2 Nutrition = 2 Friction and Shear = 2

*Interventions*

1. Address risk factors for skin damage:
   (a) Order use of a skin care cleanser with topical protectant barrier cream at night and with a pad change and evaluate the incontinent pad for proper fit and quality.
   (b) Protect heels from pressure, shear, and friction. Evaluate the need for a trapeze to assist with moving in bed.
   (c) Consult dietician for poor nutrition and anemia.
2. Topical Skin Care:
   (a) Sacral area stage 3 pressure injury with fungal infection: apply light dusting of topical antifungal powder to the periwound skin, apply calcium alginate gauze into the wound, and cover with foam border dressing. Change every day.

(b) Incontinence-associated dermatitis with fungal infection: order use of a skin cleanser and a topical antifungal powder twice during the day and at night covered with a protectant/barrier cream.

*Outcomes*
On evaluation 72 h later

- Sacral area stage 3 pressure injury with fungal infection; maceration, erythema, and rash have been resolved. The wound measures length = 3 cm, width = 2 cm, and depth = 2.5 cm, and slough is present in 25% of the wound base with 75% granulation tissue. When the calcium alginate was removed, it was 50% dry. This indicates that the dressing can be changed less frequently. Discontinue the antifungal powder, apply calcium alginate gauze into the wound, and cover with foam border dressing. Change every other day.
- Incontinence-associated dermatitis with fungal infection: the perianal rash has decreased but is still present perianally, but there is no more itching. Incontinence-associated dermatitis in the buttocks crease has resolved. Continue to apply antifungal powder twice during the day perianally and at night apply antifungal powder covered with a topical protectant/moisture barrier.

# References

1. Bliss DZ, Funk T, Jacobson M, Savik K. Incidence and characteristics of incontinence associated dermatitis in community-living individuals with fecal incontinence. J Wound Ostomy Cont Nurs. 2015;42:525–30.
2. Gray M, Giuliano KK. Incontinence associated dermatitis and immobility as pressure injury risk factors: a multisite epidemiologic analysis. J Wound Ostomy Cont Nurs. 2017;45(1):63–7.
3. Lachenbruch C, Ribble D, Emmons K, VanGilder C. Pressure ulcer risk in the incontinent patient: analysis of incontinence and hospital-acquired pressure ulcers from the International Pressure Ulcer Prevalence™ Survey. J Wound Ostomy Cont Nurs. 2016;43(3):235–41.
4. Beeckman D, Van Lancker A, Van Hecke A, Verhaeghe S. A systematic review and meta-analysis of incontinence-associated dermatitis, incontinence, and moisture as risk factors for pressure ulcer development. Res Nurs Health. 2014;37(3):204–18.
5. Bliss DZ, Savik K, Harms S, Fan Q, Wyman JF. Prevalence and correlates of perineal dermatitis in nursing home residents. Nurs Res. 2006;55(4):243–51.
6. Gray M, Beeckman D, Bliss DZ, Fader M, Logan S, Junkin J, et al. Incontinence-associated dermatitis: a comprehensive review and update. J Wound Ostomy Cont Nurs. 2012;39(1):61–74.
7. Gray M, Black JM, Baharestani MM, Bliss DZ, Colwell JC, Goldberg M, et al. Moisture-associated skin damage: overview and pathophysiology. J Wound Ostomy Cont Nurs. 2011;38(3):233–41.
8. National Pressure Ulcer Advisory Panel, European Pressure Ulcer Advisory Panel, Pan Pacific Pressure Injury Alliance. Prevention and treatment of pressure ulcers: Quick reference guide. Emily Haesler, editor. Cambridge Media, Perth, Australia; 2014. https://www.npuap.org/.../2014/...Updated-10-16-14-Quick-Reference-Guide-DIGITAL-NPUP-EPUAP-PPPIA-16Oct2014.pdf.

9. Edsberg LE, Black JM, Goldberg M, McNichol L, Moore L, Sieggreen M. Revised national pressure ulcer advisory panel pressure injury staging system: revised pressure injury staging system. J Wound Ostomy Cont Nurs. 2016;43(6):585–97.

10. Black JM, Gray M, Bliss DZ, Kennedy-Evans KL, Logan S, Baharestani MM, et al. MASD part 2: incontinence-associated dermatitis and intertriginous dermatitis: a consensus. J Wound Ostomy Cont Nurs. 2011;38(4):359–70.

11. Bliss DZ, Zehrer C, Savik K, Smith G, Hedblom E. An economic evaluation of four skin damage prevention regimens in nursing home residents with incontinence: economics of skin damage prevention. J Wound Ostomy Cont Nurs. 2007;34(2):143–52.

12. Bliss DZ, Zehrer C, Savik K, Thayer D, Smith G. Incontinence-associated skin damage in nursing home residents: a secondary analysis of a prospective, multicenter study. Ostomy Wound Manage. 2006;52(12):46–55.

13. Brown DS, Sears M. Perineal dermatitis: a conceptual framework. Ostomy Wound Manage. 1993;39(7):20–2. 4-5

14. Gray M, Bliss DZ, Doughty DB, Ermer-Seltun J, Kennedy-Evans KL, Palmer MH. Incontinence-associated dermatitis: a consensus. J Wound Ostomy Cont Nurs. 2007;34(1):45–54.

15. Rohwer K, Bliss DZ, Savik K. Incontinence-associated dermatitis in community-dwelling individuals with fecal incontinence. J Wound Ostomy Cont Nurs. 2013;40(2):181–4.

16. Brown DS. Perineal dermatitis risk factors: clinical validation of a conceptual framework. Ostomy Wound Manage. 1995;41(10):46. -8, 50, 2-3

17. Bliss DZ, Mathiason MA, Gurvich O, Savik K, Eberly LE, Fisher J, et al. Incidence and predictors of incontinence-associated skin damage in nursing home residents with new-onset incontinence. J Wound Ostomy Cont Nurs. 2017;44(2):165–71.

18. Bliss DZ, Bland P, Wiltzen K, Gannon A, Wilhelms A, Mathiason MA, et al. Incontinence briefs containing curly fiber lower (acidify) skin pH of older nursing home residents reducing risk for incontinence associated skin damage. J Wound Ostomy Cont Nurs. 2017;44(5):475–80.

19. Kottner J, Surber C. Skin care in nursing: a critical discussion of nursing practice and research. Int J Nurs Stud. 2016;61:20–8.

20. Bliss DZ. Incontinence-associated dermatitis in critically ill adults: time to development, severity, and risk factors. J Wound Ostomy Cont Nurs. 2011;38(4):433–45.

21. Arnold-Long M, Reed LA, Dunning K, Ying J. Incontinence-associated dermatitis in a long-term acute care facility. J Wound Ostomy Cont Nurs. 2012;39(3):318–27.

22. Edwards L, Lynch PJ. Genital dermatology atlas. Philadelphia, PA: Lippincott Williams & Wilkins; 2010.

23. Beeckman D, Campbell J, Campbell K, Chimentao D, Coyer F, Domansky R, et al. Proceedings of the Global IAD Expert Panel-Incontinence associated dermatitis: Moving prevention forward. London: Wounds International; 2015. www. woundsinternational.com.

24. Junkin J, Selekof JL. Prevalence of incontinence and associated skin injury in the acute care inpatient. J Wound Ostomy Cont Nurs. 2007;34(3):260–9.

25. Kelechi TJ, Arndt JV, Dove A. Review of pressure ulcer risk assessment scales. J Wound Ostomy Cont Nurs. 2013;40(3):232–6.

26. Borchert K, Bliss DZ, Savik K, Radosevich DM. The incontinence-associated dermatitis and its severity instrument: development and validation. J Wound Ostomy Cont Nurs. 2010;37(5):527–35.

27. Bliss DZ, Hurlow J, Cefalu J, Mahlum L, Borchert K, Savik K. Refinement of an instrument for assessing incontinent-associated dermatitis and its severity for use with darker-toned skin. J Wound Ostomy Cont Nurs. 2014;41(4):365–70.

28. Rockwood TH, Church JM, Fleshman JW, Kane RL, Mavrantonis C, Thorson AG, et al. Patient and surgeon ranking of the severity of symptoms associated with fecal incontinence: the fecal incontinence severity index. Dis Colon Rectum. 1999;42(12):1525–32.

29. Bliss DZ, Hurlow J, Cefalu JE, Gurvich OV, Wiltzen KR, Gannon A, et al. Validity and reliability of the Incontinence Associated Skin Damage Severity Instrument.D.2. when used by hospital and nursing home nursing staff. Abstract accepted for presenation at Wound Ostomy and Continence Nurses Society conference; 2018.

30. Doughty D, Junkin J, Kurz P, Selekof J, Gray M, Fader M, et al. Incontinence-associated dermatitis: consensus statements, evidence-based guidelines for prevention and treatment, and current challenges. J Wound Ostomy Cont Nurs. 2012;39(3):244–7.
31. Whiteley I, Sinclair G, Lyons AM, Riccardi R. A retrospective review of outcomes using a fecal management system in acute care patients. Ostomy Wound Manage. 2014;60(12):37–43.
32. Powers J, Bliss DZ. Product options for faecal incontinence management in acute care. J World Council Enterostomal Ther. 2012;32(1):20–3.
33. Pittman J, Beeson T, Terry C, Kessler W, Kirk L. Methods of bowel management in critical care: a randomized controlled trial. J Wound Ostomy Cont Nurs. 2012;39(6):633–9.
34. Benoit RA Jr, Watts C. The effect of a pressure ulcer prevention program and the bowel management system in reducing pressure ulcer prevalence in an ICU setting. J Wound Ostomy Cont Nurs. 2007;34(2):163–75.
35. Sammon MA, Montague M, Frame F, Guzman D, Bena JF, Palascak A, et al. Randomized controlled study of the effects of 2 fecal management systems on incidence of anal erosion. J Wound Ostomy Cont Nurs. 2015;42(3):279–86.
36. Marchetti F, Corallo JP Jr, Ritter J, Sands LR. Retention cuff pressure study of 3 indwelling stool management systems: randomized study of 10 healthy subjects. J Wound Ostomy Cont Nurs. 2011;38(5):569–73.
37. Monge FJC, Angorrilla IÁ, Aguado ES, Ruiz FR. Rectal ulceration due to using the Fexi-Seal fecal management system: a case report. Rev Esc Enferm USP. 2011;45(5):1256–9.
38. Sparks D, Chase D, Heaton B, Coughlin L, Metha J. Rectal trauma and associated hemorrhage with the use of the ConvaTec Flexi-Seal fecal management system: report of 3 cases. Dis Colon Rectum. 2010;53(3):346–9.
39. Bright E, Fishwick G, Berry D, Thomas M. Indwelling bowel management system as a cause of life-threatening rectal bleeding. Case Rep Gastroenterol. 2008;2(3):351–5.
40. Mulhall AM, Jindal SK. Massive gastrointestinal hemorrhage as a complication of the Flexi-Seal fecal management system. Am J Crit Care. 2013;22(6):537–43.
41. Page BP, Boyce SA, Deans C, Camilleri-Brennan J. Significant rectal bleeding as a complication of a fecal collecting device: report of a case. Dis Colon Rectum. 2008;51(9):1427–9.
42. Denat Y, Khorshid L. The effect of 2 different care products on incontinence-associated dermatitis in patients with fecal incontinence. J Wound Ostomy Cont Nurs. 2011;38(2):171–6.
43. Palmieri B, Benuzzi G, Bellini N. The anal bag: a modern approach to fecal incontinence management. Ostomy Wound Manage. 2005;51(12):44–52.
44. Zhou X-L, He Z, Chen Y-H, Zuo L-E. Effect of a 1-piece drainable pouch on incontinence-associated dermatitis in intensive care unit patients with fecal incontinence: a comparison cohort study. J Wound Ostomy Cont Nurs. 2017;44(6):568–71.
45. Bliss DZ, Lewis J, Hasselman K, Savik K, Lowry A, Whitebird R. Use and evaluation of disposable absorbent products for managing fecal incontinence by community-living people. J Wound Ostomy Cont Nurs. 2011;38(3):289–97.
46. Palese A, Regattin L, Venuti F, Innocenti A, Benaglio C, Cunico L, et al. Incontinence pad use in patients admitted to medical wards: an Italian multicenter prospective cohort study. J Wound Ostomy Cont Nurs. 2007;34(6):649–54.
47. Fader M, Cottenden A, Brooks R. The CPE network: creating an evidence base for continence product selection. J Wound Ostomy Cont Nurs. 2001;28(2):106–12.
48. Fader M, Bliss DZ, Cottenden A, Moore K, Norton C. Continence products: research priorities to improve the lives of people with urinary and/or fecal leakage. NeurourolUrodyn. 2010;29(4):640–4.
49. Fader M, Cottenden AM, Getliffe K. Absorbent products for moderate-heavy urinary and/or faecal incontinence in women and men. Cochrane Database Syst Rev. 2008. https://doi.org/10.1002/14651858.CD007408.
50. Bliss DZ, Savik K. Use of an absorbent dressing specifically for fecal incontinence. J Wound Ostomy Cont Nurs. 2008;35(2):221–8.
51. Zehrer CL, Newman DK, Grove GL, Lutz JB. Assessment of diaper-clogging potential of petrolatum moisture barriers. Ostomy Wound Manage. 2005;51(12):54–8.

52. Dykes P, Bradbury S. Incontinence pad absorption and skin barrier creams: a non-patient study. Br J Nurs. 2016;25(22):1244–8.
53. Rolnick SJ, Bliss DZ, Jackson JM. Healthcare providers' perspectives for promoting communication with family caregivers and patients with dementia about incontinence and skin damage. Ostomy Wound Manage. 2013;59(4):62–7.
54. Continence Product Advisor. International Continence Society, International Consultation on Incontinence, University College London, University of Southampton; https://www.continenceproductadvisor.org/
55. Beeckman D, Van Damme N, Schoonhoven L, Van Lancker A, Kottner J, Beele H, et al. Interventions for preventing and treating incontinence-associated dermatitis in adults. Cochrane Database Syst Rev. 2016;11:CD011627.
56. Park KH, Kim KS. Effect of a structured skin care regimen on patients with fecal incontinence: a comparison cohort study. J Wound Ostomy Cont Nurs. 2014;41(2):161–7.
57. Gray M. Optimal management of incontinence-associated dermatitis in the elderly. Am J Clin Dermatol. 2010;11(3):201–10.
58. Abbas S, Goldberg JW, Massaro M. Personal cleanser technology and clinical performance. Dermatol Ther. 2004;17(s1):35–42.
59. Ali SM, Yosipovitch G. Skin pH: from basic science to basic skin care. Acta Derm Venereol. 2013;93(3):261–9.
60. Rönner A-C, Berland CR, Runeman B, Kaijser B. The hygienic effectiveness of 2 different skin cleansing procedures. J Wound Ostomy Cont Nurs. 2010;37(3):260.
61. Voegeli D. The effect of washing and drying practices on skin barrier function. J Wound Ostomy Cont Nurs. 2008;35(1):84–90.
62. Aboud A, Khachemoune A. Vaseline: a historical perspective. Dermatol Nurs. 2009;21(3):143–4.
63. Draelos ZD. Active agents in common skin care products. Plast Reconstr Surg. 2010;125(2):719–24.
64. O'Connor S, Murphy S. Chronic venous leg ulcers: is topical zinc the answer? A review of the literature. Adv Skin Wound Care. 2014;27(1):35–44.
65. Hoggarth A, Waring M, Alexander J, Greenwood A, Callaghan T. A controlled, three-part trial to investigate the barrier function and skin hydration properties of six skin protectants. Ostomy Wound Manage. 2005;51(12):30–42.
66. Corazza M, Minghetti S, Bianchi A, Virgili A, Borghi A. Barrier creams: facts and controversies. Dermatitis. 2014;25(6):327–33.
67. Beeckman D, Verhaeghe S, Defloor T, Schoonhoven L, Vanderwee K. A 3-in-1 perineal care washcloth impregnated with dimethicone 3% versus water and pH neutral soap to prevent and treat incontinence-associated dermatitis: a randomized, controlled clinical trial. J Wound Ostomy Cont Nurs. 2011;38(6):627–34.
68. Peterson KJ, Bliss DZ, Nelson C, Savik K. Practices of nurses and nursing assistants in preventing incontinence dermatitis in acutely/critically-ill patients. Am J Crit Care. 2006;15(3):333.
69. American Health Care Association. American Health Care Association 2012 staffing report. 2012. https://www.ahcancal.org/research_data/staffing/.../2012_Staffing_Report.pdf.
70. Nursing Solutions Inc. National healthcare retention and RN staffing report. East Petersburg, PA; 2016. www.nsinursingsolutions.com/.../retention.../NationalHealthcareRNRetentionReport2016.pdf.
71. VitalSims. Incontinence associated skin damage. http://www.vitalsims.com/product/incontinence-associated-skin-damage/
72. Boronat-Garrido X, Kottner J, Schmitz G, Lahmann N. Incontinence-associated dermatitis in nursing homes: prevalence, severity, and risk factors in residents with urinary and/or fecal incontinence. J Wound Ostomy Cont Nurs. 2016;43(6):630–5.
73. Berlowitz D, Lukas VC, Parker V, Niederhauser A, Silver J, Logan C, et al. Preventing pressure ulcers in hospitals: a toolkit for improving quality of care. Rockville, MD: Agency for Healthcare Research and Quality; 2012. https://www.ahrq.gov/sites/default/files/publications/files/putoolkit.pdf

74. Redelings MD, Lee NE, Sorvillo F. Pressure ulcers: more lethal than we thought? Adv Skin Wound Care. 2005;18(7):367–72.
75. Russo CA, Steiner C, Spector W. Hospitalizations related to pressure ulcers among adults 18 years and older, 2006: Statistical brief #64. 2008 Dec. In: Healthcare Cost and Utilization Project (HCUP) statistical briefs. Rockville, MD: Agency for Healthcare Research and Quality; 2006. https://www.ncbi.nlm.nih.gov/books/NBK54557/
76. Voss AC, Bender SA, Ferguson ML, Sauer AC, Bennett RG, Hahn PW. Long-term care liability for pressure ulcers. J Am Geriatr Soc. 2005;53(9):1587–92.
77. Lyder CH, Ayello EA. Pressure ulcers: A patient safety issue. In: Hughes R, editor. Patient safety and quality: an evidenced-based handbook for nurses. Rockville, MD: Agency for Healthcare Research and Quality; 2008. https://archive.ahrq.gov/professionals/clinicians-providers/resources/nursing/resources/nurseshdbk/nurseshdbk.pdf.
78. Waterlow Scale. http://www.health.vic.gov.au/__data/assets/file/0009/233667/Waterlow-scale.pdf.
79. Norton Pressure Sore Risk Assessment Scale Scoring System. www.health.vic.gov.au/__data/assets/file/0010/233668/Norton-scale.pdf.
80. Posthauer ME. Nutrition: fuel for pressure ulcer prevention and healing. Nursing. 2014;44(12):67–9.
81. Wound Ostomy & Continence Nurses Society. Guidelines for prevention and management of pressure ulcers (injuries). Mount Laurel, NJ: Wound Ostomy & Continence Nurses Society; 2016.
82. Allman RM. Pressure ulcers among the elderly. N Engl J Med. 1989;320(13):850–3.
83. Andersen PH, Bucher AP, Saeed I, Lee PC, Davis JA, Maibach HI. Faecal enzymes: In vivo human skin irritation. Contact Dermatitis. 1994;30(3):152–8.
84. Braden B, Bergstrom N. A conceptual schema for the study of the etiology of pressure sores. Rehabil Nurs. 1987;12(1):8–12.
85. National Pressure Ulcer Advisory Panel (NPUAP). NPUAP position statement on staging -2017 Clarifications. 2017 [1–6]. http://www.npuap.org/wp-content/uploads/2012/01/NPUAP-Position-Statement-on-Staging-Jan-2017.pdf.
86. Leaper DJ, Schultz G, Carville K, Fletcher J, Swanson T, Drake R. Extending the TIME concept: What have we learned in the past 10 years? Int Wound J. 2012;9(s2):1–19.
87. Dowsett C, Newton H. Wound bed preparation: TIME in practice. Wounds UK. 2005;1(3):58.

# Management of Urinary Incontinence in the Presence of Fecal Incontinence

## 14

Sandra Engberg

**Abstract**

Fecal and urinary incontinence share a number of risk factors, and there is a high prevalence of concurrent urinary incontinence among individuals with fecal incontinence. Coexisting urinary incontinence should be considered when assessing patients with fecal incontinence and, if present, needs to be considered in the treatment plan. This chapter addresses the assessment and management of urinary incontinence in patients with fecal (i.e., dual incontinence). Interventions with some research to suggest that they may be beneficial for both conditions are highlighted.

**Keywords**

Dual incontinence · Double incontinence · Urinary incontinence
Fecal incontinence

## 14.1 Introduction

The bowel and bladder both develop from the embryologic hindgut, and studies of bowel and bladder physiology support a functional relationship between these two organs [1]. Botlero, Bell, Urquhart, and Davis [2] examined the relationship between fecal incontinence and urinary incontinence in community-dwelling women aged 26–82 years and reported that 68% of women with fecal incontinence reported also having urinary incontinence. Bliss et al. [3] showed that 51% of a sample of 189 community-living men and women with fecal incontinence also had urinary

S. Engberg
University of Pittsburgh School of Nursing, Pittsburgh, PA, USA
e-mail: sje1@pitt.edu

© Springer International Publishing AG, part of Springer Nature 2018
D. Z. Bliss (ed.), *Management of Fecal Incontinence for the Advanced Practice Nurse*,
https://doi.org/10.1007/978-3-319-90704-8_14

incontinence. This knowledge is useful for the advanced practice nurse in assessing and managing the patient with fecal incontinence, as urinary incontinence will also need to be addressed.

## 14.2   Prevalence of Dual Incontinence

In studies examining the prevalence of dual incontinence in community-dwelling adult populations, estimated rates vary from 3% to 8.8% [4–10]. Across studies, a variety of characteristics have been examined for their association with dual incontinence in community dwelling adults, mostly older adults. Characteristics associated with an increased odds of dual incontinence in two or more studies were older age [4, 5, 7–9], female sex (in studies including both men and women) [4, 6, 10], depressive symptoms [6, 7, 9, 10], presence or number of comorbidities [4, 6], diabetes [5, 9], and functional impairment [4, 6, 7, 9]. In a study examining the prevalence of dual incontinence during pregnancy and postpartum [11], the prevalence rate of dual incontinence was 8.6% during pregnancy and decreased to 3.5% postpartum (women ($n = 1128$) were nulliparous and followed for an average of 7 weeks postpartum).

The prevalence of dual incontinence in noncommunity settings is more limited. In a study of 9,861 hospitalized patients, the prevalence of dual incontinence was 5.2%. While the overall prevalence was similar to that reported in community-dwelling adults, the prevalence was much higher in patients in intensive care units where it was 18.9% [12].

The prevalence of dual incontinence in nursing home residents is much higher than in the community. In one of the largest studies of nursing home residents, Bliss et al. [13] reported a prevalence of 39.7% in a sample of 59,588 residents in 555 nursing homes in the United States (US) while investigating dermatitis associated with incontinence. Chiang et al. reported a prevalence of 54% among 413 residents in 20 US nursing homes [14]. Saga et al. observed that 40.2% of their sample of 930 residents from 27 nursing homes in Norway had dual incontinence [15]. Characteristics associated with dual incontinence in both studies were length of stay in the nursing home, cognitive impairment, and functional impairment.

In one of the few studies of incidence of dual incontinence, Bliss et al. [16] investigated data on 39,181 nursing home admissions without dual incontinence on admission. The incidence of dual incontinence at 6 months after admission was 28%, and, at 1 year, 42% of residents developed dual incontinence. Predictors of time to develop dual incontinence were having urinary incontinence on admission, age, more comorbidities, greater functional impairment, and more severe cognitive impairment [16].

While the prevalence of dual incontinence varies across settings, it is relatively common in adults and probably even more common in those with fecal incontinence. The possibility of coexisting urinary incontinence needs to be considered when evaluating patients with fecal incontinence and, if present, should be considered in the treatment plan.

## 14.3 Urinary Incontinence Types

Urinary incontinence, defined as "the complaint of any involuntary loss of urine" [17] (p. 500), is a symptom of a bladder storage problem. Urinary incontinence is classified according to patient descriptions about when involuntary urine loss occurs. The most common types of urinary incontinence are stress urinary incontinence, involuntary urine loss with effort or exertion or when sneezing or coughing; urge urinary incontinence, involuntary urine loss accompanied or immediately preceded by urgency; and mixed urinary incontinence, involuntary urine loss associated with urgency and also during effort, exertion, coughing, or sneezing. Table 14.1 presents the definitions of urinary incontinence by type and subtype according to the 6th International Consultation on Incontinence and the International Continence Society [17]. While there is wide variation in the reported prevalence rates of urinary incontinence in community-dwelling women, in most studies, it is between 25% and 45%, and, stress urinary incontinence is the most common subtype of urinary incontinence, followed by mixed incontinence and isolated urge urinary incontinence. Studies examining age-related differences in the prevalence of urinary incontinence consistently report that the prevalence increases

**Table 14.1** Classification of urinary incontinence[a]

| Type or subtype of urinary incontinence | Definition |
|---|---|
| Urgency | Complaints of involuntary urine loss associated with urgency |
| Stress | Complaints of involuntary urine loss with effort or physical exertion or upon sneezing or coughing |
| Mixed | Complaints of involuntary urine loss with urgency and also with effort or physical exertion or upon coughing or sneezing |
| Postural | Complaints of involuntary urine loss occurring with changes in body position such as rising from a seated or lying position |
| Incontinence associated with chronic retention of urine | Complaints of involuntary loss of urine that occurs in conditions where the bladder does not empty completely as indicated by a significantly high residual urine volume and/or a non-painful bladder which remains palpable after the individual has passed urine |
| Nocturnal enuresis | Complaints of involuntary urine loss during sleep |
| Continuous | Complaints of continuous involuntary urine loss |
| Insensible | Complaints of involuntary urine loss without the individual being aware of how it occurred |
| Coital | Complaints of involuntary urine loss during coitus |
| Functional | Complaints of involuntary urine loss from inability to reach the toilet due to cognitive, functional, or mobility impairment in the presence of an intact lower urinary tract system |
| Multifactorial | Complaints of involuntary urine loss related to multiple interacting risk factors, including factors within and outside the lower urinary tract such as comorbidities, medications, age-related physiologic changes, and environmental factors |

[a]According to the 6th International Consultation on Incontinence and the International Continence Society [17] (pp. 500–501)

with age, and most studies report that mixed urinary incontinence becomes the predominate subtype. Body mass index (BMI) and mode of delivery (vaginal) are the two risk factors other than aging that have the most research supporting their association with urinary incontinence in women [18].

Less is known about the rate of urinary incontinence in men than in women, but the prevalence appears to be much lower (urinary incontinence is probably at least twice as common in women than men). Similarly, regarding dual incontinence in men, Bliss et al. [19] surveyed 1,352 community-living older adults and found that 55% of women versus 28% of men had dual incontinence [19]. As with fecal incontinence, there is a steady increase in the prevalence of urinary incontinence as men age [20]. The most common type of urinary incontinence in men is urge urinary incontinence, followed by mixed urinary incontinence and stress urinary incontinence.

## 14.4    Risk Factors for Urinary Incontinence

In addition to increasing age, other lower urinary tract symptoms, urinary tract infections, cognitive and functional impairment, diabetes, alcohol intake, neurologic disorders, and prostatectomy have been shown to increase the risk for urinary incontinence in men [18]. Some of the risk factors for urinary incontinence in men and/or women are also risk factors for fecal incontinence although research supporting this is not as strong as it is for urinary incontinence. The risk factor with the most support for both urinary incontinence and fecal incontinence is aging. Diabetes and neurological diseases such as Parkinson's disease and stroke have also been associated with an increased risk for both urinary incontinence and fecal incontinence as have cognitive and ADL impairments. While studies show a consistent association between obesity and urinary incontinence, those examining the association with fecal incontinence are inconsistent [18].

## 14.5    Assessment of Urinary Incontinence

Given that many patients with fecal incontinence are also likely to have urinary incontinence, it is important for the advanced practice nurse to include questions about bladder function when assessing patients with fecal incontinence. Many patients with urinary incontinence do not report this problem to a health-care provider unless directly asked about bladder function. Questions that may be helpful in eliciting the presence of urinary incontinence include asking about problems with bladder control, involuntary urine loss, and the use of pads and why they are being used. In patients experiencing urinary incontinence, a careful history should be the first step in assessing the problem (see Table 14.2). Questions should be asked to determine the type (factors that precipitate involuntary urine loss), frequency, and amount (indicators of severity) of urinary incontinence; day- and nighttime voiding frequency as well as nocturia; fluid intake (amount and type); measures used to

**Table 14.2** History taking for urinary incontinence

| *Continence history* | |
| --- | --- |
| Duration | Duration and progression of symptoms |
| Frequency | How often involuntary urine loss occurs; self-reported number of incontinent episodes per day, week, or month |
| Severity | How much typically leaks with urinary incontinence episodes—a few drops, enough to make clothing or pad damp, or soaks pad or clothing |
| Precipitating factors | When does involuntary urine loss occur—coughing, sneezing, laughing, lifting, exercise, urgency, sight or thought of the toilet, "key in the door," running water, changing position, during sexual activity, continuous leaking, leaking without awareness of precipitating factor identifiable, involuntary urine loss while sleeping (enuresis) |
| Voiding frequency | How frequently voids typically occur during the day<br>How many times a patient gets up from sleep to void (nocturia), does urgency wake up patient, impact of loss of sleep |
| Fluid intake | Fluid intake during the day and the evening<br>Type of fluid intake; ask specially about caffeine and alcohol intake and amount |
| Urine containment measures | Measures used to contain involuntary urine loss—specific products used (with frequency changed/used) |
| Associated symptoms | Pain or burning on urination (dysuria), blood in urine (hematuria), lower abdominal pain, difficulty emptying bladder, pelvic organ prolapse symptoms |
| Previous treatment | Previous/current treatments for urinary incontinence and effectiveness |
| Impact on quality of life | Impact on personal and social life |
| *General medical history* | |
| Functional limitations | Mobility and cognition |
| Comorbidities | Diabetes, heart failure, neurologic disorders |
| Medications | Medications currently taking |
| *Past medical history* | |
| Obstetric history (women) | Number of pregnancies, type of delivery, complications |
| Previous surgery/radiation | Abdominal, pelvic, prostate (men) |
| *Treatment expectations* | |
| Desire for treatment | Including acceptable treatment options |
| Treatment expectations | Consider in relation to reductions in urinary incontinence and other lower urinary tract symptoms |

contain leakage; impact of urinary incontinence on quality of life; previous treatment for urinary incontinence and its effects; as well as comorbid conditions, medications being taken, functional impairments, the desire and goals for treatment, and treatment expectations.

**Table 14.3** Focused physical examination for urinary incontinence

| Physical examination | |
| --- | --- |
| Abdominal exam | Suprapubic dullness, tenderness, or palpable bladder |
| Neurologic exam | |
| Pelvic exam in women | Pelvic floor muscle tone and strength<br>Pelvic organ prolapse |
| Rectal exam in men | Prostate enlargement or nodules |
| Bladder diary (2–3 days) | |
| Additional tests as indicated, e.g., post-void residual urine, urinalysis, urodynamic testing | |

The advanced practice nurse should perform a focused physical examination when evaluating urinary incontinence, which includes an abdominal exam, neurologic exam, a pelvic exam in women, and a rectal exam in men. A bladder diary is very useful in establishing the type, frequency, and severity of urinary incontinence as well as voiding frequency, volume, and fluid intake. If feasible, patients should complete a 2- to 3-day diary. In addition to its usefulness in the diagnostic process, the bladder diary is very helpful in monitoring the effectiveness of treatment [17] (see Table 14.3).

## 14.6 Interventions for Urinary Incontinence

While some interventions may have beneficial effects on both fecal incontinence and urinary incontinence, the advanced practice continence nurse needs to consider the patient's and, if relevant, caregivers' preferences when developing an intervention plan for dual incontinence. Which symptoms are most bothersome to the patient? What do they want to focus on during the initial treatment? Which treatments are acceptable? What are their outcome expectations relative to treatment? In a systematic review, Riemsma et al. [21] examined cure rates following various treatments for urinary incontinence and fecal incontinence. "Cure was defined as no leakage (urinary incontinence) and/or no episodes of fecal incontinence at trial specified time points, of at least 3 months" [21] (p. 2). Based on their findings that cure rates were relatively low for most interventions examined for both urinary incontinence and fecal incontinence, improvement is a more realistic goal than cure for many patients with both types of incontinence.

There are many treatment options for urinary incontinence with the choice of interventions based on the type and severity of urinary incontinence as well as patient preferences. This chapter will focus on conservative management of urinary incontinence, interventions not involving surgical or pharmacological approaches [22], and some management approaches that are similar to those for fecal incontinence addressed in other chapters of this book. These interventions are summarized in Table 14.4. They include lifestyle modifications, pelvic floor muscle training, electric stimulation, posterior tibial nerve stimulation, and toileting programs. Conservative interventions are generally recommended as the initial treatment approach for urinary incontinence and for those for whom other treatments are inappropriate.

**Table 14.4** Conservative treatment options for urinary incontinence

| Intervention | Evidence supporting for urinary incontinence | Evidence supporting for fecal incontinence |
|---|---|---|
| Lifestyle modifications | | |
|   Weight reduction | Strong evidence for overweight and obese women; some evidence for men | Inconsistent |
|   Fluid intake | Some evidence to support minor reductions as long as intake is not <30 mL/kg/day | Has not been examined |
|   Reduce caffeine intake | Some evidence to support | Has not been examined |
| Behavioral therapies | | |
|   Pelvic floor muscle training | Strong evidence to support in individuals able and willing to actively participate | Limited evidence |
|   Bladder training | Some evidence to support effectiveness in women able and willing to actively participate | Not applicable |
|   Toileting programs (for individuals unable to actively participate in self-management activities) | Strong evidence of short-term benefit of prompted voiding when caregivers adhere to treatment protocol; limited research examining scheduled toileting and habit training | Limited evidence |
| Electrical stimulation | Limited evidence to suggest may be better than no treatment | Very limited evidence; low-frequency estim does not appear to be helpful Medium frequency may be beneficial but additional research is needed to confirm |
| Posterior tibial nerve stimulation | Limited evidence to suggest may be effective for urge urinary incontinence | No evidence to support use in clinical practice |

## 14.6.1 Lifestyle Interventions for Urinary Incontinence

Lifestyle interventions such as weight loss, dietary and fluid modifications, smoking cessation, and the avoidance of constipation are low-cost and noninvasive options for treating urinary incontinence. While these interventions are often recommended as part of the treatment program for urinary incontinence, many lack adequate research to draw conclusions about their effectiveness. The lifestyle intervention that has sufficient current research evidence to support its effectiveness in reducing urinary incontinence is weight loss in overweight and obese women. The 6th International Consultation on Incontinence gave recommending weight loss in overweight and obese women a grade A recommendation based on level 1 evidence (evidence from the meta-analysis of randomized controlled trials (RCTs) or well-designed RTCs). There is also some evidence to support recommending weight loss for overweight or obese men with urinary incontinence, but it is much more limited than research examining this intervention in women. While it is possible that, in addition to improving urinary incontinence in overweight or obese women and men with dual incontinence, weight loss may also improve the coexisting fecal incontinence, research findings supporting this beneficial effect are inconsistent [22]. Although not as strong as the evidence related to weight loss, there is some evidence to support that reducing caffeine intake may reduce urinary incontinence. There is also some evidence to support recommending minor reductions in fluid intake (by 25%) as long as baseline fluid intake is not less than 30 mL/kg per day [22]. The effects of restricting caffeine intake and reducing fluid intake have not been examined in relation to fecal incontinence [23].

While there are many good health reasons to recommend that patients stop smoking, there is a lack of research examining the impact of smoking cessation on urinary incontinence. Constipation has been associated with fecal incontinence, and there is limited evidence from small observational studies to suggest that it may be a risk factor for urinary incontinence. Some notions are that a bowel filled with feces presses on the bladder reducing its capacity or creating a sense of urgency and straining during constipation weakens pelvic floor muscles. While clinicians often recommend measures to treat or prevent constipation in individuals with urinary incontinence, there is a lack of research examining the effect of this recommendation [22]. One of the first-line nonconservative treatments for urge urinary incontinence and overactive bladder is antimuscarinic drugs. One of the bothersome side effects of these medications is constipation [24]. When treating patients with dual incontinence, clinicians need to carefully review the medications that patients are taking and weigh their risk-benefit ratio in relation to both urinary incontinence and fecal incontinence.

### 14.6.2 Behavioral Therapies for Urinary Incontinence

Behavioral therapies, pelvic floor muscle training, bladder (re)training, and toileting programs are widely recommended conservative approaches to managing urinary incontinence that the advanced practice continence nurse can perform. The pelvic floor muscles provide structural support for the pelvic organs including the bladder and lower bowel and their openings. Improving the strength of these muscles is hypothesized to improve this support [22]. Pelvic floor muscle training includes assessing the ability to contract these muscles, education about how to perform pelvic floor muscle exercises, and instructions on the active use of the muscles to prevent involuntary urine loss. Across research studies, pelvic floor muscle training programs vary in terms of clinician supervision, the intensity of the training, instructional method, type of training, and inclusion of other treatment modalities. Based on a recent review of these studies, pelvic floor muscle training with regular clinician supervision is considered better than training with little or no supervision [22]. There is no clear benefit from using biofeedback to teach pelvic floor muscle exercises, and while research is more limited, adding other modalities to the pelvic floor muscle training regimen does not appear to enhance its beneficial effects [22].

Once patients learn to contract and relax their pelvic floor muscles, if they have stress urinary incontinence, they should be taught to contract their muscles during activities that produce involuntary urine loss such as coughing and sneezing. If they have urge urinary incontinence, they can be taught to contract their pelvic floor muscles to suppress urgency and then walk to the toilet at a normal pace, which decreases the likelihood of involuntary urine loss. Pelvic floor muscle training techniques for urinary incontinence and fecal incontinence are similar and may reduce fecal incontinence as well as urinary incontinence although there is less research evidence to support efficacy for fecal incontinence than there is for urinary incontinence [23].

In contrast to urinary incontinence, where the evidence does not support the use of biofeedback, the 6th International Consultation on Incontinence recommends biofeedback, usually in combination with pelvic floor muscle training, as a second-line therapy for fecal incontinence when pelvic floor muscle training alone and other conservative therapies have not provided adequate symptom relief [23].

Bladder training, also called bladder retraining, can be another effective intervention for urinary incontinence, particularly urge urinary incontinence and mixed urinary incontinence with concurrent urgency and urinary frequency (i.e., overactive bladder). The goal of this intervention is to improve bladder capacity and reduce urinary frequency. The patient is instructed to void at fixed intervals ("by the clock") based on their average baseline voiding interval. Alternately, some clinicians have the patient begin by voiding every hour. The voiding interval is gradually increased by 15–30 min with the goal of achieving a more normal voiding interval, usually every 3–4 h. Individuals are instructed to void at the scheduled times even if there is no urge to urinate, and if urgency occurs prior to the scheduled voiding time, they are instructed to try to suppress the urgency using distraction techniques or by contracting their pelvic floor muscles. There is limited evidence from randomized clinical trials to suggest that bladder training may be an effective intervention for urinary incontinence in women, and it received a recommendation (grade A) as a first-line conservative treatment by the 6th International Consultation on Incontinence [22]. Like pelvic floor muscle training, bladder training is more likely to be effective when there is direct clinician supervision [22].

### 14.6.3 Neuromodulation for Urinary Incontinence

Electrical stimulation, generally a clinic-based intervention, increases proprioception and/or muscle strength when used to treat stress urinary incontinence, while the goal when used to treat urge urinary incontinence is often to inhibit detrusor overactivity. Based on studies comparing electrical stimulation to no active treatment, electrical stimulation might be better than no treatment for stress urinary incontinence and urge urinary incontinence (grade B recommendation, evidence from consistent low-quality randomized clinical trials, meta-analysis of good quality cohort, retrospective case-control or case series studies) [22]. There is a need for more well-designed clinical trials to establish whether or not electrical stimulation is effective in treating urinary incontinence. There is very limited research examining the effectiveness of electrical stimulation for fecal incontinence, but low level (100 Hz) electrical stimulation does not appear to be helpful [23]. The findings from two randomized controlled trials suggest that triple therapy combining medium-frequency electrical stimulation and biofeedback is superior to EMG biofeedback alone and to low-frequency electrical stimulation [25, 26]. Additional research is needed to confirm this.

Posterior tibial nerve stimulation is a form of neuromodulation that provides indirect access to the sacral plexus through intermittent, electrical stimulation of the posterior tibial nerve through insertion of fine needles close to the nerve, or through surface electrodes applied to the area of the medial malleolus. Treatments are usually administered weekly for a period of 2–3 months. Studies examining posterior tibial nerve stimulation have small sample sizes, and were assessed by the 6th International Consultation on Incontinence as having a high risk of bias [22]. Based on this, they concluded that posterior tibial nerve stimulation may be more effective than no treatment for symptom control in women with urge urinary incontinence and overactive bladder [22]. Due to a lack of evidence supporting the use of posterior tibial nerve stimulation for fecal incontinence, it cannot be recommended for clinical practice [23].

Most urinary incontinence intervention research studies have been conducted in community-dwelling women. There is much less research in men and what has been done has primarily focused on post-prostatectomy urinary incontinence. According to the 6th International Consultation on Incontinence, treatment recommendations for men with urinary incontinence include weight loss for those who are obese or overweight, smoking cessation for those who smoke, reducing caffeine intake, and pelvic floor muscle training [22]. Adding electrical stimulation to pelvic floor muscle training does not appear to improve outcomes. Posterior tibial nerve stimulation is a potential treatment option for men with urge urinary incontinence and overactive bladder who do not achieve satisfactory outcomes with lifestyle changes and pelvic floor muscle training. For all of these recommendations, evidence is limited [22].

## 14.7    Managing Urinary Incontinence in the Frail Older Adult

Frail older adults constitute a group where the prevalence of both urinary incontinence and dual incontinence are higher than among healthy adults. Many frail older individuals have coexisting disabilities and comorbidities. These can both contribute to urinary incontinence and to response to urinary incontinence-specific interventions. Management of urinary incontinence in this population needs to start by identifying and treating comorbid conditions and impairments that may be contributing to the incontinence [27]. While there is no research examining the effects of lifestyle interventions in treating urinary incontinence in this population, these interventions may be appropriate in select frail older adults with some caveats [28]. For example, weight loss may be inappropriate, and caution should be exercised in

> **Box 14.1: Toileting Programs for Urinary Incontinence**
> - *Prompted voiding*—which combines regular prompts to void with positive feedback for appropriate toileting. The goals are to increase awareness of the need to urinate and self-initiated toileting.
> - *Scheduled toileting*—which is regular toileting without prompts or reinforcement for appropriate voiding.
> - *Habit training*—which matches the toileting schedule to the individual's voiding pattern established during a baseline assessment (bladder diary/ wet checks) to determine the frequency of continent and incontinent voids. The goal is to preempt incontinent episodes.

recommending fluid restriction as many frail elders are at risk for inadequate fluid intake and dehydration, particularly long-term care residents.

Because of their minor side effects, behavioral interventions are generally considered a first-line treatment for urinary incontinence in this population. Toileting programs are recommended for frail older adults with cognitive or physical impairments that limit their ability to actively participate in self-care activities, but may be used in other frail elders as well. Toileting programs for urinary incontinence include prompted voiding, scheduled toileting, and habit training (see Box 14.1).

Toileting interventions for urinary incontinence all depend on active caregiver involvement. The intervention that has been examined most often in research studies is prompted voiding. Research on habit training and scheduled toileting is very limited. Based on current evidence, it is uncertain if these interventions reduce urinary incontinence in frail older individuals. There is evidence, primarily from studies conducted in long-term care settings, that prompted voiding is effective as a short-term treatment for daytime incontinence when caregivers adhere to the treatment protocol (level 1 evidence) [28]. There is a lack of research examining the long-term effect of this intervention. Given that prompting voiding increases caregiver burden, it is important to target it to those most likely to benefit. It is not recommended for individuals who need the assistance of more than one person during toileting, those who cannot follow one-step commands, and those who have less than a 20% reduction in wet checks or toilet appropriately less than 66% of the time during a 3-day trial of the intervention [28]. There is also good evidence to support combining toileting and functional training when treating urinary incontinence in nursing home residents. There is limited research examining the effect of toileting interventions on concurrent fecal incontinence. Multicomponent interventions in nursing home settings that included a toileting program did not reduce fecal incontinence, although bowel frequency and the number of continent bowel movements improved [28].

For frail individuals who are cognitively intact and able to actively participate in bladder-related self-care, bladder training and pelvic floor muscle training may be effective treatment options. There is, however, limited research examining these interventions in this population. Talley et al. [29] conducted a systematic review of conservative treatments for urinary incontinence in frail community-dwelling older adults. They identified three studies, with only one randomized controlled clinical trial, that examined multicomponent behavioral interventions that included pelvic floor muscle training and bladder training. All three studies reported significant reductions in urinary incontinence episodes at the end of the interventions (75–80% reductions). Engberg and Sereika [30] compared the effectiveness of biofeedback-taught pelvic floor muscle training in reducing urinary incontinence in frail (homebound) and non-frail community-dwelling older adults and reported that there was no significant difference in the median percent reduction in urinary incontinence episodes in the two groups (64.5% in the frail and 70.4% in the non-frail subjects).

## 14.8 Environmental Factors

Environmental factors, specifically lack of easy access to the toilet and timely toileting assistance, are risk factors for urinary incontinence particularly in caregiver-dependent individuals. Improving access to the toilet (e.g., use of bedside commodes) and providing toileting aids such as grab bars and raised toilet seats may improve continence (both urinary and fecal) in individuals with mobility and functional impairments. Increasing toilet visibility or adding signage or images to show where the toilet is may be effective in increasing appropriate toileting in individuals with cognitive and visual-perceptual impairments [28]. In caregiver-dependent individuals, the need for timely toileting assistance is a critical but often neglected risk factor for urinary incontinence. For individuals who cannot toilet independently, the availability of timely toileting assistance is critical to the success of all other interventions for both urinary incontinence and fecal incontinence.

## 14.9 Products for Containing or Collecting Incontinent Urine

As previously noted, complete cure of dual incontinence may not be a realistic goal for many individuals, and even when effective, interventions often take time to work. Consequently, continence products that contain or collect leaked urine have a role in incontinence management for many adults. They should not, however, be a substitute for active assessment and treatment of urinary incontinence or dual incontinence. Available products vary by country and include toileting products (commodes, bedpans, handheld urinals), absorbent products, external urine collection devices, mechanical devices, and catheters (intermittent and indwelling). The choice of products will vary with availability, the severity and type of incontinence, functional ability, and personal preferences (patient and caregiver). A combination of products is often the best option for managing incontinence [31]. There is an interactive web site available to provide current product-related evidence to help users and health-care providers in the selection of products and how to best use them [32].

Body-worn absorbent pads are the most commonly used products to manage urinary incontinence. Clinicians need to remember that pad use is not without risks including increased risk for new onset and worsening incontinence, urinary tract infections, and incontinence-associated dermatitis (see Chap. 13). There are a wide variety of absorbent products available, and the best product for any given individual varies with a variety of characteristics including the frequency and severity of incontinence, whether it occurs during the day or night, sex (men or women), pad changing position, personal priorities and preferences, lifestyle, and caregiver needs and preferences [31]. While there are pads made specifically for fecal incontinence, the individual with dual incontinence will often elect to wear a pad that is also effective in containing urine leakage [3].

## 14.10 Summary

Many patients with fecal incontinence will also have urinary incontinence. Thus, it is important for the advanced practice nurse to ask patients with fecal incontinence about coexisting urinary incontinence. If urinary incontinence is also present, it needs to be considered when planning and initiating a plan of management/treatment for fecal incontinence. While there are unique interventions for each type of incontinence, there are some interventions that may helpful in reducing both urinary and fecal incontinence.

## References

1. Kaplan S, Dmochowski R, Cash B, Kopp Z, Berriman S, Khullar V. Systematic review of the relationship between bladder and bowel function: implications for patient management. Int J Clin Pract. 2013;67(3):205–16.
2. Botlero R, Bell RJ, Urquhart DM, Davis SR. Prevalence of fecal incontinence and its relationship with urinary incontinence in women living in the community. Menopause. 2011;18(6):685–9.
3. Bliss DZ, Lewis J, Hasselman K, Savik K, Lowry A, Whitebird R. Use and evaluation of disposable absorbent products for managing fecal incontinence by community-living people. J Wound Ostomy Cont Nurs. 2011;38(3):289–97.
4. Wu JM, Matthews CA, Vaughan CP, Markland AD. Urinary, fecal, and dual incontinence in older U.S. adults. J Am Geriatr Soc. 2015;63(5):947–53.
5. Chang TC, Chang SR, Hsiao SM, Hsiao CF, Chen CH, Lin HH. Factors associated with fecal incontinence in women with lower urinary tract symptoms. J Obstet Gynaecol Res. 2013;39(1):250–5.
6. Markland AD, Goode PS, Burgio KL, Redden DT, Richter HE, Sawyer P, et al. Correlates of urinary, fecal, and dual incontinence in older African-American and White men and women. J Am Geriatr Soc. 2008;56(2):285–90.
7. Matthews CA, Whitehead WE, Townsend MK, Grodstein F. Risk factors for urinary, fecal, or dual incontinence in the Nurses' Health Study. Obstet Gynecol. 2013;122(3):539–45.
8. Teunissen TA, van den Bosch WJ, van den Hoogen HJ, Lagro-Janssen AL. Prevalence of urinary, fecal and double incontinence in the elderly living at home. Int Urogynecol J Pelvic Floor Dysfunct. 2004;15(1):10–3.

9. Yuaso DR, Santos JL, Castro RA, Duarte YA, Girão MJ, Berghmans B, et al. Female double incontinence: prevalence, incidence, and risk factors from the SABE (health, wellbeing and aging) study. Int Urogynecol J. 2017;29:1–8.

10. Santos CR, Santos VL. Prevalence of self-reported double incontinence in the urban population of a Brazilian city. Neurourol Urodyn. 2011;30(8):1473–9.

11. Espuña-Pons M, Solans-Domènech M, Sánchez E. Double incontinence in a cohort of nulliparous pregnant women. Neurourol Urodyn. 2012;31(8):1236–41.

12. Shahin ES, Lohrmann C. Prevalence of fecal and double fecal and urinary incontinence in hospitalized patients. J Wound Ostomy Cont Nurs. 2015;42(1):89–93.

13. Bliss DZ, Savik K, Harms S, Fan Q, Wyman JF. Prevalence and correlates of perineal dermatitis in nursing home residents. Nurs Res. 2006;55(4):243–51.

14. Chiang L, Ouslander J, Schnelle J, Reuben DB. Dually incontinent nursing home residents: clinical characteristics and treatment differences. J Am Geriatr Soc. 2000;48(6):673–6.

15. Saga S, Vinsnes AG, Morkved S, Norton C, Seim A. What characteristics predispose to continence in nursing home residents? A population-based cross-sectional study. Neurourol Urodyn. 2015;34(4):362–7.

16. Bliss DZ, Gurvich OV, Eberly LE, Harms S. Time to and predictors of dual incontinence in older nursing home admissions. Neurourol Urodyn. 2017;37(1):229–36.

17. Diaz DC, Robinson D, Bosch R, Costantini E, Cotterill N, Espuna-Pons M, et al. Initial assessment of urinary incontinence in adult male and female patients. In: Abrams P, Cardozo L, Wagg A, Wein A, editors. Incontinence. 6th ed. Bristol: International Continence Society; 2017. p. 497–540.

18. Milsom A, Altman D, Cartwright R, Lapitan MC, Nelson R, Sjostrom S, et al. Epidemiology of urinary incontinence (UI) and other lower urinary tract symptoms (LUTS), pelvic organ prolapse (POP) and anal (AI) incontinence. In: Abrams P, Cardozo L, Wagg A, Wein A, editors. Incontinence. 6th ed. Bristol: International Continence Society; 2017. p. 1–142.

19. Bliss DZ, Fischer LR, Savik K. Managing fecal incontinence: self-care practices of older adults. J Gerontol Nurs. 2005;31(7):35–44.

20. Shamliyan T, Wyman J, Bliss DZ, Kane RL, Wilt TJ. Prevention of urinary and fecal incontinence in adults. Evid Rep Technol Assess. 2007;161:1–379.

21. Riemsma R, Hagen S, Kirschner-Hermanns R, Norton C, Wijk H, Andersson K-E, et al. Can incontinence be cured? A systematic review of cure rates. BMC Med. 2017;15(1):63.

22. Dumoulin C, Adewuyi T, Booth J, Bradley C, Burgio K, Hagen S, et al. Adult conservative management. In: Abrams P, Cardozo L, Wagg A, Wein A, editors. Incontinence. 6th ed. Bristol: International Continence Society; 2017.

23. Bliss DZ, Mimura T, Berghmans B, Bharucha A, Chiarioni G, Emmanuel A, et al. Assessment and conservative management of faecal incontinence and quality of life in adults. In: Abrams P, Cardozo L, Wagg A, Wein A, editors. Incontinence. 6th ed. Bristol: International Continence Society; 2017. p. 1993–2085.

24. Andersson KE, Cardozo L, Cruz F, Lee KS, Sahai A, Wein AJ. Pharmacological treatment of urinary incontinence. In: Abrams P, Cardozo L, Wagg A, Wein A, editors. Incontinence. 6th ed. Bristol: International Continence Society; 2017. p. 805–957.

25. Schwandner T, Konig IR, Heimerl T, Kierer W, Roblick M, Bouchard R, et al. Triple target treatment (3T) is more effective than biofeedback alone for anal incontinence: the 3T-AI study. Dis Colon Rectum. 2010;53(7):1007–16.

26. Schwandner T, Hemmelmann C, Heimerl T, Kierer W, Kolbert G, Vonthein R, et al. Triple-target treatment versus low-frequency electrostimulation for anal incontinence: a randomized, controlled trial. Dtsch Arztebl Int. 2011;108(39):653–60.

27. Engberg S, Li H. Urinary incontinence in frail older adults. Urol Nurs. 2017;37(3):119–26.

28. Wagg A, Chen LK, Johnson IIT, Kirschner-Hermanns R, Kuchel G, Markland A, et al. Incontinence in frail older persons. In: Abrams P, Cardozo L, Wagg A, Wein A, editors. Incontinence. 6th ed. Bristol: International Continence Society; 2017. p. 1309–441.

29. Talley KM, Wyman JF, Shamliyan TA. State of the science: conservative interventions for urinary incontinence in frail community-dwelling older adults. Nurs Outlook. 2011;59(4):215–20.
30. Engberg S, Sereika SM. Effectiveness of pelvic floor muscle training for urinary incontinence: comparison within and between nonhomebound and homebound older adults. J Wound Ostomy Cont Nurs. 2016;43(3):291–300.
31. Cottenden A, Fader M, Beeckman D, Buckley B, Kitson-Reynolds E, Moore K, et al. Management using continence products. In: Abrams P, Cardozo L, Wagg A, Wein A, editors. Incontinence. 6th ed. Bristol: International Continence Society; 2017. p. 2303–426.
32. Continence Product Advisor. 2018. https://www.continenceproductadvisor.org/.

# Epilogue

As Dr. Norton noted in the foreword, bowel dysfunction and fecal incontinence have long been neglected conditions in the world of medical research and technological advancement. We have lacked clear terminology and definitions of the various conditions that are included in the broad categories of "fecal incontinence" and "bowel dysfunction." We have had relatively few diagnostic tools and sometimes conflicting guidelines as to their use and interpretation. Treatment options have been limited, lacking adequate research evidence, and often ineffective. Add to this the intense embarrassment and shame associated with loss of bowel control, and it is not surprising that many individuals have sought to cover up and deny having this problem rather than to seek treatment. Similarly, many practitioners have adopted a "don't ask, don't tell" approach to problems of bowel elimination because why ask about a problem if you have relatively little to offer in the way of solutions?

The good news is we have come a long way, and that progress is both reflected and enhanced by this much-needed text! The ICS and ICI have developed clear definitions and terminology to classify and describe the types of fecal incontinence, the first step in managing any problem effectively. This updated terminology is used in this book and will serve to educate healthcare providers and patients.

A second major challenge is "consciousness-raising" about fecal incontinence, and this text is a major step forward in increasing awareness about this problem to advanced practice nurses and other primary care providers. However, there needs to be more progress in public awareness. While many health conditions (including erectile dysfunction) are openly discussed on television and in print media, disorders of elimination remain largely taboo. This is beginning to change, as evidenced by increased openness in discussion of overactive bladder symptoms and advertisements for absorptive pads and medications for inflammatory bowel disease and constipation. Nevertheless, urinary leakage seems a much more acceptable condition and topic than bowel leakage, as evidenced by the media silence on this topic (at least in the USA) and by many patients' reluctance to seek treatment. Nurses can help bridge the gap by routinely asking their patients about bowel problems, pursuing research into the pathology, presentation, impact, and management of fecal incontinence, and delivering podium presentations and contributing to the professional and lay literature with their findings.

© Springer International Publishing AG, part of Springer Nature 2018    307
D. Z. Bliss (ed.), *Management of Fecal Incontinence for the Advanced Practice Nurse*,
https://doi.org/10.1007/978-3-319-90704-8

A third major challenge is accurate diagnosis and management of the various types of fecal incontinence. Until recently, assessment and management strategies have been heavily focused on sphincter dysfunction. Continued research into behavioral, pharmacologic, and surgical therapies is needed. However, we also need research into other factors potentially affecting bowel function and fecal continence including the impact of motility disorders, the role of various neurotransmitters, the gastrointestinal microbiome, and genetics. Increased knowledge regarding the pathology of fecal incontinence can stimulate the development of medications, biological agents, and procedures to correct the underlying pathology, and will offer clinicians and patients an increasing array of treatment options.

Finally, we need to develop more effective strategies for symptom and self-management of "uncorrectable" fecal incontinence. There have been major advancements in containment and absorptive products for urinary incontinence; as a result, we now have an increasing variety of containment products for both men and women with features designed to maximize skin protection, minimize leakage, and control odor. In contrast, we have are fewer products to offer the individual or caregiver specifically for fecal incontinence, which poses unique problems compared to urinary leakage. The anal plug, anal insert, and the vaginal bowel device are innovative steps forward. Collaboration between researchers, clinicians, and manufacturers is encouraged to design needed products.

In summary, this text represents significant progress in our knowledge about assessment and management of fecal incontinence as well as the evolution of nursing practice at an advanced level into this area—all of which is very exciting! It is my hope that nurses will continue to be leaders in continence care and research to "push the envelope" forward. Hopefully, there will be future editions of this book reflecting increasing scientific evidence about fecal incontinence and management options benefitting our patients!